Innovations in Urologic Surgery

Second Edition

Edited by

Rudolf Hohenfellner
Department of Urology,
University of Mainz, Mainz, Germany

Andrew Novick
Professor and Chairman,
Department of Urology,
Cleveland Clinic Foundation,
Cleveland, Ohio, USA

Jan Fichtner
Department of Urology,
University of Mainz, Mainz, Germany

I S I S
MEDICAL
MEDIA
—
Oxford

British Library Cataloguing in Publication Data
A catalogue record for this title is available from the British Library

ISBN 1 899066 47 0

Hohenfellner R (Rudolf)
Innovations in Urologic Surgery/
Rudolf Hohenfellner, Andrew Novick and Jan Fichtner

Always refer to the manufacturer's Prescribing Information before prescribing drugs cited in this book

Typeset by
Marksbury Multimedia Ltd., Midsomer Norton, UK

Printed by
Dah Hua Printing Press Co. Ltd., Hong Kong

Distributed by
Oxford University Press
Saxon Way West
Corby, Northants, NN18 9ES, UK

Preface

Surgical atlases and operative textbooks which are often produced with a great deal of effort seldom elude an all too rapid ageing process. The more dilatory the co-authors participating, the longer the period of time it takes from planning and production to the finished product. From this sorrowful realization was born the concept of *Innovations in Urologic Surgery*. The aim was to produce a stimulating operative textbook with an animated interpretation of technical advancements and innovations or supplements, modifications and improvement proposals for standardized and new procedures.

The first edition, published in 1994, was limited and published only in the German language. The huge national and international interest which followed, led to two further German reprints in the same year and translations into Italian, Japanese, Portuguese, Spanish and now English.

For the purpose of limiting and systematizing the text, we completely revised the first German publication into categories according to indication, contraindication, instruments, approach, step by step technique, operative tricks, post-operative care and special features.

Reviews from surgeons familiar with the specific problems of each procedure provide an objective approach and at the same time contributed towards the evaluation of each respective technique. Three stars (***) represent standardized, proven over many years, recommended procedures; two stars: technically largely standardized, details could be improved upon, proven regarding reproducibility and long-term results with guaranteed data; 1 star: a new procedure, possibly useful and reproducible although without conclusive results.

In accordance with the concept described in the introduction, we reevaluated the already published procedures. Analysis of information from congresses and operation seminars proved particularly helpful in this respect. The interest and demand for a particular technique can be calculated from the number of lectures, poster and video contributions. Additionally, the published complications demonstrated the reproducibility as well as possible technical shortcomings. For example, an analysis of 'neuralgic ureter implantation sites' in continent urinary reservoirs showed the occurrence of a predominantly short-term postoperative obstruction rate of up to 8%. Accordingly there was considerable interest in the antirefluxive 'Hassan implantation' with a minimal complication rate including also dilated, thick-walled ureters. Despite the comparative short follow-up of only two years, this alternative procedure was included.

The reader will undoubtedly search in vain for some of the more traditionally employed 'gold standard' techniques, which have proved their worth and from which there is no reason to deviate. Consequently, the reader will most probably not miss these all too familiar techniques. Nevertheless the editors are particularly grateful for comments and correspondence on these subjects. It is only through continuous dialogue with operating surgeons that these animated operative techniques can fulfil the original intentions.

Many authors who participated in the first German edition will miss their contributions in this English language version. The prevailing reasons were either high published complication rates or technical improvements developed in alternative procedures. The emphasis lies deliberately on a 'selection' of operative techniques; an undoubtedly problematic undertaking. On the other hand the reader may feel spoiled for choice in view of, for example, the 300 surgical procedures for hypospadias correction published up until 1995. If only 20 from this number were reproduced, as is the case in the average surgical atlas, the situation would not be any better. Should the reader not systematically follow for example, "hypospadiology", he or she may not realise, that a procedure perhaps favoured by an institution for over 10 years and published in various national and international surgical textbooks has been abandoned due to a high late complication rate. *Innovations in Urologic Surgery* seeks to do justice to such a situation.

At this point we would like to express our gratitude to Mr Brammer who, apart from his artistic skills, possesses the necessary capacity and composure to produce high quality illustrations under the exacting demands of deadline pressure. Furthermore, we thank the reviewer for their critical and time consuming work. Last but not least, our thanks go to Mrs Hug who ran the entire scientific secretariat superbly.

R. Hohenfellner
A. Novick
J. Fichtner

Contents

II Ureter

III Bladder

VI Special Techniques

Kidney

I

Supracostal Approach and Pyeloplasty

F. Steinbach[a], R. Stein, H. Riedmiller[b],
R. Hohenfellner
Department of Urology,
University of Mainz School of Medicine,
Mainz, Germany
[a]*University of Magdeburg, Magdeburg, Germany*
[b]*University of Marburg, Marburg, Germany*

Supracostal Approach

Introduction

The supracostal incision (Figures 1–11) provides good exposure of the kidney, adrenal gland and proximal ureter depending on the height of the incision. In benign disease of the kidney the 11th intercostal space is used, and in malignant disease the 10th intercostal space. For unilateral adrenalectomy a supracostal incision above the 11th, 10th or 9th rib is used; in those with an exceptionally large tumor, a thoracoabdominal approach may be advantageous.

Advantages

- Preservation of the intercostal vessels and nerves as well as the ilioinguinal and iliohypogastric nerves
- Minimal incision of the external oblique, internal oblique and transverse muscles
- Extraperitoneal approach
- No resection of the rib
- Excellent exposure of the kidney and proximal ureter
- Simple closure of the wound, with high strength through preservation of the rib

Disadvantages

- Risk of pleural laceration
- Risk of rib fracture

Diagnostics

- Electrocardiography and radiography of the chest
- Pulmonary function test in patients with suspected lung disease

Special instruments and materials

- Wickham retractor, Balfour retractor or Finochetto rib retractor
- Absorbable monofilament suture material: 5/0 for small pleural lacerations and 4/0 for larger defects, e.g. polyglyconate (Maxon, Davis and Geck, Gosport, UK)
- Absorbable twisted suture material: 1/0 for suture of the fascia in adults and 2/0 for children, e.g. polyglycolic acid (Dexon, Davis and Geck)
- Soft silastic tube drain (12–20 Fr)

Repair of pleural lacerations

- At the end of the operation the tension is released and the retractor removed
- Small laceration: Closure with 5/0 polyglyconate interrupted sutures
- Larger laceration: a part of the diaphragm muscle is included in the suture
- Before the last suture is knotted, the lung is fully distended by positive high-pressure ventilation until it becomes visible. Then the last suture is tied
- The wound is filled with fluid and inspected for air bubbles to check for leakage
- Where the pleural laceration is very lateral (and therefore difficult to close) a chest tube is inserted during the operation
- Postoperative chest radiography: pneumothorax of 1–2 cm is treated conservatively; if there is a larger pneumothorax a chest tube is inserted

Postoperative care

- Extreme traumatic pain: infiltration of the intercostal nerves with local anesthetic (during or after the operation)
- Division of sensitive skin nerves: reversible paresthesia and hyperreflexia (sensation often disappears after 3–6 months)
- Injury of motor nerves: temporary paralysis of the muscle mimicking a scar hernia

Pyeloplasty

Introduction

Ureteropelvic obstruction may be congenital or secondary. Congenital causes include aberrant ureter crossing vessels and intrinsic stenosis (e.g. fibrous adhesion between the ureter and the renal pelvis as well as segmental dysfunction of the ureter). Secondary causes include distal obstruction of the ureter resulting in dilatation of the ureter, development of loops of the ureter and, in the long term, fixation of these loops resulting in stenosis. In children, obstruction is mostly associated with vesicorenal reflux (which should always be excluded by voiding cystourethrography before operation).

Indications

- Objective stenosis (on radiography, ultrasonography and isotopic studies)
- Symptomatic stenosis (recurrent flank pain after fluid load)
- Complicated stenosis (infection, stone, bleeding)
- Increasing dilatation and reduction of renal function after initial conservative treatment
- Bilateral stenosis (the kidney with the better function is operated on first)

Diagnosis

- Ultrasonography documentation and follow-up of the dilatation of the renal pelvis and calyces
- Intravenous pyelography (not necessary in children): documentation of the morphology of the kidney, ureter and opposite kidney, with radiography after 12–24 hours if there is poor opacification of the kidney
- Voiding cystourethrography: exclusion of vesicorenal reflux (secondary stenosis)
- Renography, e.g. with mercaptoacetyltriglycerin (MAG 3): split renal function, outwash of the isotopic agents after administration of furosemide
- Retrograde pyelography (only on the day of operation under anesthesia): in adults with insufficient documentation of the ureter and unknown reason and/or extent of the stenosis; contraindicated in small children, especially boys, because of the risk of urethral injury

Special instruments and materials

- Pott's scissors
- Atraumatic suture material: 6/0 or 7/0 chromic catgut
- 6 Fr silastic ureter splint
- 8 Fr silastic pyelostomy
- Magnifying glasses

Operative technique step by step

The dismembered pyeloplasty of Anderson and Hynes as modified by Sigel (Figures 12–16) is a useful and simple technique.

- Gerota's fascia and the perirenal fat are opened, a retractor inserted, and the ureter prepared up to the renal pelvis
- Adhesions, scars and ureter loops are carefully divided with preservation of the adventitia of the ureter. Aberrant pole vessels of the kidney are surrounded by vessel loops
- The anterior and posterior renal pelvis are separated from the surrounding fibrous tissue
- Stay sutures are placed at the medial insertion of the ureter, the cranial angle of the renal pelvis and in the region of the lateral adventitia of the ureter below the ureteropelvic stenosis. A longitudinal incision is made in the renal pelvis, and the stenosis is resected (circularly around the ureter)
- The renal pelvis is inspected (e.g. for stones), with irrigation of the renal pelvis if necessary
- Sigel's modification: 12–15 mm cranially to the lower pelvic margin an incision is made on either side measuring 12–18 mm. The ureter is spatulated laterally
- To prevent injury to the extrarenal opening of the calyces, resection of the redundant renal pelvis should be minimal
- The ureter is spatulated at the medial margin down to the poststenotic dilatation (up to 3 cm)
- An anchor suture is placed at the deepest point of the opened renal pelvis and the spatulated ureter
- The pyelostomy tube (8–10 Fr) is inserted, with the end in the upper calyces and the ureter splint (6 Fr) passing out through the dorsal part of the renal pelvis, and fixed with catgut sutures (4/0)
- The posterior wall of the renal pelvis and the ureter are anastomosed with interrupted suture. The posterior wall of the renal pelvis is closed with interrupted sutures or, if the wound is large, with running sutures
- The tightness and free drainage of the pyelostomy and the splint are checked
- The renal pelvis with the anastomosis is embedded in the surrounding fat. In patients with nearly no fat tissue, a pedicle omentum flap can be used after opening the peritoneum if necessary
- A Silastic drainage tube (Dow Corning, Reading, UK) is inserted and the wound closed

Advantages

Temporary urinary diversion by minimal pyelostomy and ureter splint
- Prevents blockage of the ureter leading to extravasation, urinoma, and the formation of scar tissue with the risk of secondary stenosis
- Allows pressure measurements within the renal pelvis after removal of the ureter splint

Aberrant pole vessels
- Avoids division, with the risk of segmental renal ischemia
- Good performance of the anastomosis anterior to the vessel with insertion of fat tissue or of a pedicle omentum flap between the vessel and the anastomosis

Tandem kidney
- Folding of a tandem kidney with a thin but well functioning parenchyma by atraumatic capsule sutures
- Reduction of the dead space volume of the collecting system and a move of the ureteropelvic anastomoses down to the deepest point of the renal pelvis

Complications

- Bleeding: mostly caused by nephrostomy. Larger hematomas in the region of the renal pelvis require revision
- Acute pyelonephritis: mostly caused by a combination of obstruction and infection. Guarantee free drainage by pyelostomy and ureter splint and antibiotic treatment
- Urinary extravasation for more than 1 week: mostly caused by insufficiency of the anastomosis. Insert a ureter splint

Postoperative care

- Antibiotic treatment in patients with infection or stone disease, with prophylactic trimethoprim or nitrofurantoin for some months
- Removal of the perirenal drainage step by step (in children in one step) on days 3 and 4, depending on the drainage fluid
- Removal of the ureter splint on day 8
- Pressure measurement of the renal pelvis on the next day. If the pressure is below 12–15 cmH$_2$O and ultrasonography indicates no increase in renal dilatation compared with preoperative results or if in adults there is documentation of free drainage in the intravenous urogram, the pyelostomy is removed. If the pressure is elevated the pyelostomy is left for one additional week (with occasional treatment with diclofenac) and the measurements are then repeated.

Control examinations

- Ultrasonography at 3–4 weeks and then at 3–6 month intervals
- Isotopic renography for documentation of free drainage on an individual basis. If there is no or only minimal dilatation on ultrasonography this is not necessary.

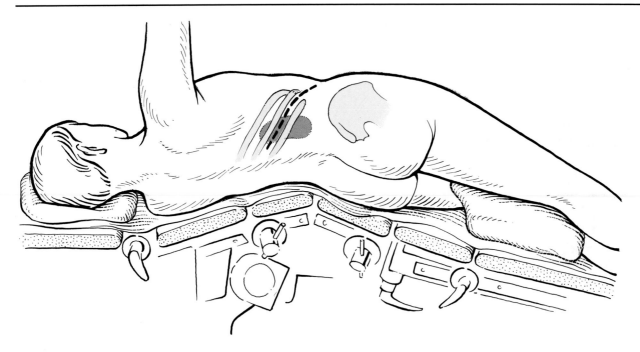

Figure 1. *The patient is in an overstretched lateral position.*

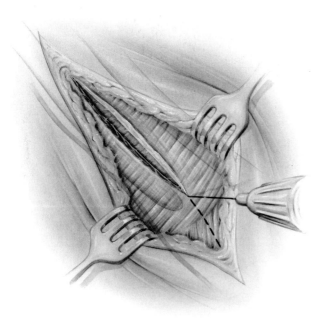

Figure 2. *Skin incision along the 12th rib, from the margin of the erector spinae muscle down to about 7 cm (in children about 3 cm) ventral to the tip of the 12th rib. Incision of the latissimus dorsi and the underlying inferior posterior serratus muscle, closely following the easy palpable upper rim of the 12th rib.*

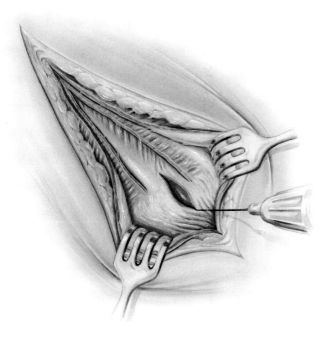

Figure 3. *Incision of the deep layer of the lumbodorsal fascia.*

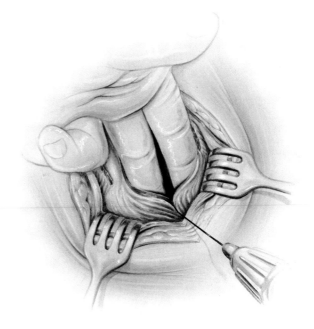

Figure 4. *The peritoneum is carefully pushed medial bluntly and the external oblique, internal oblique and transverse muscles are undermined and stretched, notched by the diathermy needle for a few centimetres. By strict adherence to the visualized line extending from the 12th rib, the incision follows a zone free of vessels and nerves.*

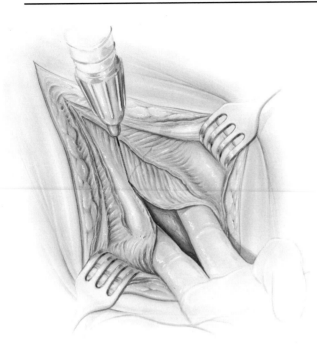

Figure 5. *Cutting of the intercostal muscle along the upper rim of the 12th rib.*

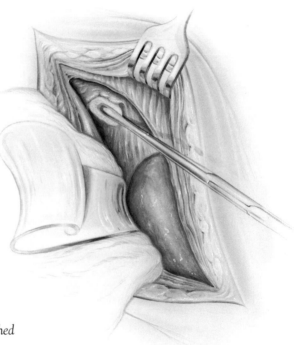

Figure 6. *The pleural fold at the diaphragm is carefully pushed cranial bluntly.*

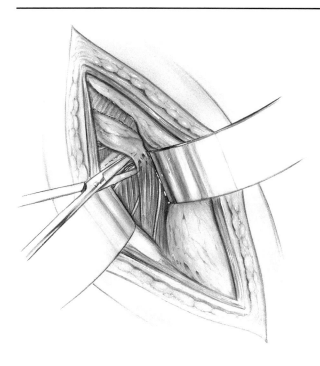

Figure 7. *In severe adherence of the pleura, the dissection is performed partly by spreading the end of the scissors perpendicular to the pleural fold. The vessels and the nerve are landmarks and should be preserved.*

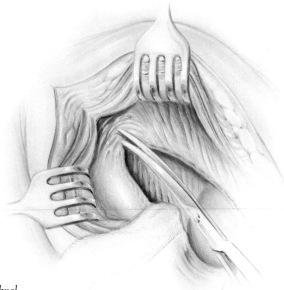

Figure 8. *Blunt (finger tip) or sharp division of the costovertebral ligament.*

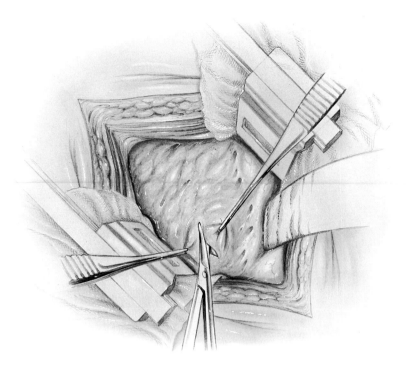

Figure 9. *Insertion of the wound retractor and incision of Gerota's fascia parallel to the axis of the kidney, with preservation of the fat capsule for later reconstruction.*

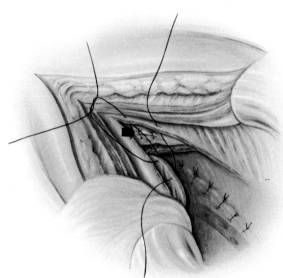

Figure 10. *After removal of the retractor, placement of a drainage tube, small pleural defects can be closed primarily.*

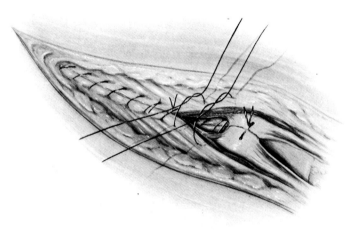

Figure 11. *Closure of the wound layer by layer.*

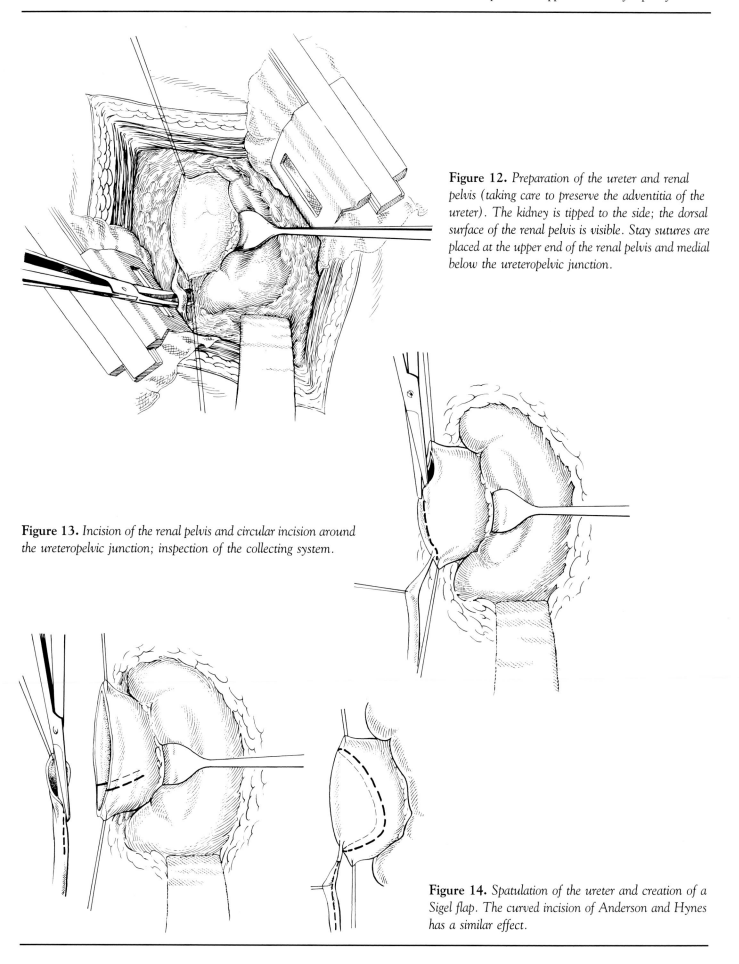

Figure 12. *Preparation of the ureter and renal pelvis (taking care to preserve the adventitia of the ureter). The kidney is tipped to the side; the dorsal surface of the renal pelvis is visible. Stay sutures are placed at the upper end of the renal pelvis and medial below the ureteropelvic junction.*

Figure 13. *Incision of the renal pelvis and circular incision around the ureteropelvic junction; inspection of the collecting system.*

Figure 14. *Spatulation of the ureter and creation of a Sigel flap. The curved incision of Anderson and Hynes has a similar effect.*

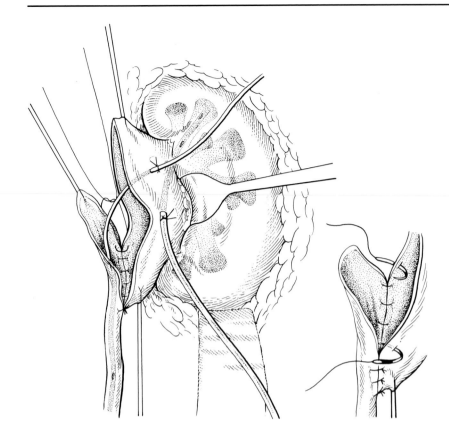

Figure 15. *Anastomosis of the renal pelvis and the ureter; the knots are placed outside.*

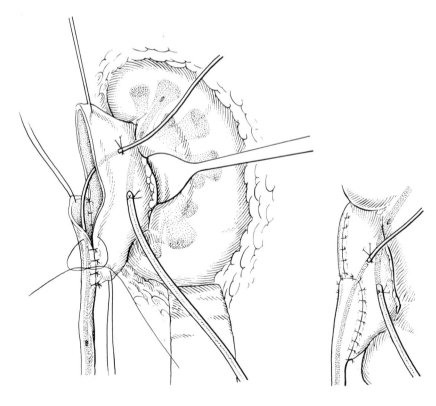

Figure 16. *After completion of the anastomosis the renal pelvis is closed by either interrupted or running sutures, covering the anastomosis with the renal fat capsule. If this is not sufficient, a tension-free flap of omentum majus can be used.*

Surgical Reinterventions on the Kidney

S. Roos, J. Fichtner, S.C. Müller[a], R. Hohenfellner
Department of Urology,
University of Mainz School of Medicine,
Mainz, Germany
[a]*University of Bonn, Bonn, Germany*

Indications

- Pyeloplasty failure

- Tumor recurrence after organ-sparing operations for renal cell carcinoma (RCC) and organ-sparing resections of the renal pelvis for transitional cell carcinoma (TCC)

Diagnosis

Recurrent obstruction of the ureteropelvic junction (UPJ)

- Lasix renography (MAG 3) with split renal function: evidence of a relevant UPJ obstruction with at least 25–30% of normal renal function

- Intravenous pyelography (IVP) for localization and determination of the length of the UPJ obstruction

- Eventually antegrade pyelography (via intermediate percutaneous nephrostomy) or retrograde pyelography

Tumor relapse

- IVP

- Computed tomography (CT) or magnetic resonance imaging (MRI)

- Intra-arterial digital subtraction angiography (DSA) to determine the exact location, tumor size and vessel supply

- Renography (MAG 3) if the efficiency of the contralateral kidney is unknown

- In solitary kidney, information about possible removal of the second kidney and consecutive dialysis

Instruments

- Standard instruments for kidney surgery

- Instruments for vascular surgery

- Magnifying glasses

- PVC stents

- Doppler probe

- Sterile crushed ice (in case of clamping the renal vessels)

Approach

A supracostal incision (Figure 1) one rib above the former incision is used to avoid injury to the kidney adherent to the scar. Extension can easily be achieved by rib resection, separation of the diaphragm or paramedian extension.

Operative technique step by step (Figures 2–13)

- Removal of a nephrostomy if present because it is not suitable as a guideline

- Supracostal incision

- Use of the psoas muscle as a guideline for preparation of the retroperitoneum

- Preparation of the peritoneum medially – usually easy to do in the height of the crossing of the ureter with the iliac vessels

- Identification of the ureter and fixation with a loop

- Preparation of the usually flimsy ureter between the adventitia and scar tissue with a fine right-angled Overholt forceps in the direction of the kidney

- Preparation of the renal pelvis

- Placement of stay sutures at the upper renal pelvis and near the ureteropelvic junction

- Section of the ureter at the ureteropelvic junction

- Preparation of the ureter beyond the iliac vessels to assure a tension-free anastomosis

- Incision of the renal pelvis according to Sigel to provide more length for the anastomosis

- Spatulation of the ureter widely beyond the poststenotic dilated area

- Ureteropelvic anastomosis of the backwall (6/0 monofilament resorbable suture) by single stitches, with the knots on the external side

- Insertion of a 6 Fr ureteric stent through a separate incision of the renal pelvis

- Insertion of a pyelostomy/nephrostomy into the lower calices (to avoid irritation of the anastomosis)

- Anastomosis of the front wall

- Insertion of a 21 Fr drainage tube

Helpful hints

- The use of free peritoneal patches and the greater omentum should be considered in the surgical strategy

- Preparation of the ureter near to the renal pelvis should be performed as dorsally as possible to avoid lesions of the renal capsule

- In long ureteral stenoses, downward mobilization of the kidney can render tension-free anastomosis of the renal pelvis and ureter possible

- For exact mucosal adaptation, magnifying glasses are recommended

- The anastomosis area is wrapped with a free peritoneal patch with the serosa towards the renal pelvis. This preserves the mobility of the ureter and avoids adhesions to the psoas muscle and the lower kidney pole

- Where there is pressure necrosis due to stones or defects due to resection (e.g. TCC of the renal pelvis), a free peritoneal patch can be used to reconstruct the renal pelvis

- The perirenal fat can be supplemented by greater omentum

Intraoperative complications

A number of organs can be injured during surgery, especially if there is extensive mobilization of the kidney. These lesions should be repaired as follows:

- Large bowel and duodenum: seromuscular closure. Duodenal lesions require an additional covering of fibrin-glued free peritoneal patch and insertion of a gastric tube

- Liver: surface-gluing with fibrin, infrared laser coagulation, application of a collagen fleece

- Spleen: fibrin-gluing. Large capsular lacerations may necessitate splenectomy

- Pancreas: inverted sutures with nonresorbable atraumatic material. Additional covering with free peritoneal patch and fibrin-gluing. The extent of the lesions may make partial pancreatic resection and adaptation to a small bowel loop necessary (Roux-en-Y)

- Caval vein: isolation with Satinsky forceps to avoid voluminous bleeding. Closure with a running atraumatic suture (e.g. 5/0 polyglyconate)

- Bleeding from lumbar or adrenal veins: clamping with vessel clips

- Adrenal bleeding: ligation or suture. If the bleeding does not stop the organ should be removed

- Renal vessels: exact reconstruction with 6/0 monofilament suture. Clamping the renal vessels with vascular clamps is possible for 30 minutes. In rare cases when ischemia must

be prolonged, the use of sterile crushed ice around the kidney is appropriate

Postoperative care

- The drainage tube can be removed within the first 6 days after the operation if the drainage is insignificant

- The ureteral stent is removed between days 10 and 12

- The pyelostomy/nephrostomy allows pressure measurements to be taken. If the pressure is less than $15 cmH_2O$, the pyelostomy/nephrostomy should be closed and IVP carried out 20 minutes after contrast media administration. Subsequent radiography even placing the patient in a prone position may be necessary. If the IVP is normal, the pyelostomy/nephrostomy may be removed

Postoperative complications

- If the continuous pressure values are above $20 cmH_2O$, the patient will be discharged with the pyelostomy/nephrostomy *in situ*. Measurement will be repeated within 14 days on an outpatient basis

- Antiphlogistics can force the fading of edema

- Obstructing clots of blood at the UPJ can be removed by ureteral catheterization

- Drainage or more than 50 ml of urine is mostly caused by positioning the drainage tube too close to the anastomosis, and usually stops if the drainage is tube is moved 1–2 cm

- Pseudocystic urinoma appears after ineffective drainage. Paralytic ileus and a palpable mass in the lower abdomen can be caused by this complication. A urinoma should be drained guided by ultrasonography or CT. In addition the ureter should be splinted with a double-J catheter

- Bleeding from the renal parenchyma can be stopped by supraselective embolization

Special problems

If a normal ureteropelvic anastomosis is not possible because of inflammatory changes in the renal pelvis and ureter, a ureterocalicostomy to the lower pole of the kidney may be considered. This method works best in hydronephrotic kidneys with rarefied parenchyma. For more successful anastomsis the parenchyma is resected in a wedgeshape. If preoperative evaluation reveals a long ureteric defect, bowel preparation (e.g. 2–3 L Golytely's solution) is recommended to make a ureteric substitution with small bowel feasible. Autologous kidney transplantation into the contralateral iliac fossa in combination with a pyelocystostomy is the ultimate technique to solve the problem of otherwise inoperable defects of the ureter.

References

1. Campbell SC, Novick AC, Streem SB, Klein E, Licht M. Complications of nephron sparing surgery for renal tumors. *J Urol* **151** (1994) 1177–80.
2. Elem B. Preliminary nephrostomy and total ileal replacement of both ureters in advanced bilharzial obstructive uropathy. *Br J Urol* **63** (1989) 453–6.
3. Floyd JW, Hendren WH. Reoperative pyeloplasty: experience with 22 cases. *J Urol* **143** (1990) 275–9.
4. Hohenfellner R. Sekundär- und Mehrfacheingriffe an der Niere. *Akt Urol* **11** (1980) 123–9.
5. Kavoussi LR, Albala DM, Clayman R. Outcome of secondary open surgical procedure in patients who failed primary endopyelotomy. *Br J Urol* **72** (1993) 157–60.
6. Müller SC, Hradec J, Riedmiller H, Hohenfellner R. Problematik wiederholter rekonstruktiver Eingriffe am Nierenbecken und Harnleiterabgang. *Akt Urol* **15** (1984) 325–35.
7. Novick AC, Jackson CL, Straffon RA. The role of renal autotransplantation in complex urological reconstruction. *J Urol* **143** (1990) 452–7.
8. Ross JH, Streem SB, Novick AC, Montie J. Ureterocalicostomy for reconstruction of complicated pelviureteric junction obstruction. *Br J Urol* **65** (1990) 322–5.
9. Steinbach F, Stöckle M, Müller SC *et al.* Conservative surgery of renal cell tumors in 140 patients: 21 years of experience. *J Urol* **148** (1992) 24–9.
10. Waters WB, Herbster G, Jablokov VR, Reda DJ. Ureteral replacement using ileum in compromised renal function. *J Urol* **141** (1989) 432–6.

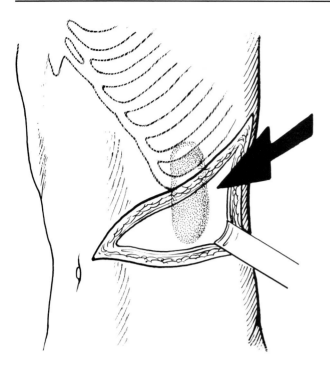

Figure 1. *Supracostal incision and section of the costovertebral ligament one rib above the former incision.*

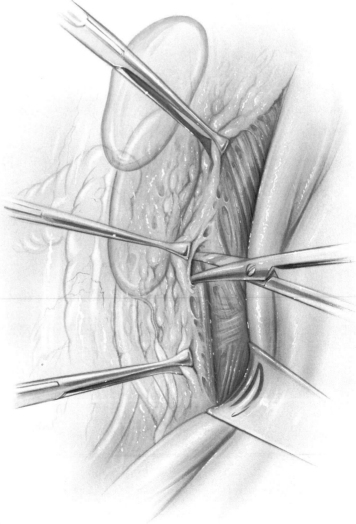

Figure 2. *Complete mobilization of the kidney with its perirenal fat. The psoas muscle serves as a guideline.*

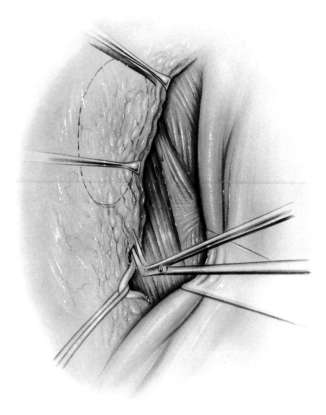

Figure 3. *Identification of the ureter at the entrance to the scar tissue. The ureter is marked with a loop. Further preparation to the renal pelvis.*

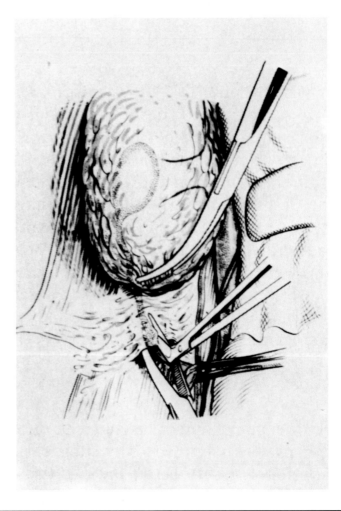

Figure 4. *Preparation of the ureter between the adventitia and scar tissue.*

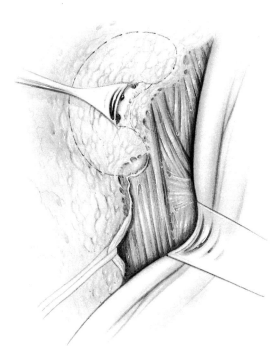

Figure 5. *Preparation of the ureter at the lower kidney pole and of the renal pelvis as dorsally as possible to avoid lesions of the renal capsule.*

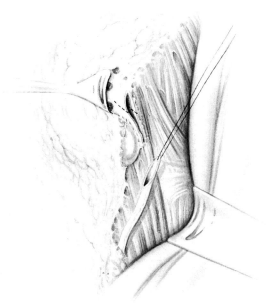

Figure 6. *Section of the ureter at the ureteropelvic junction and fixation with a stay suture.*

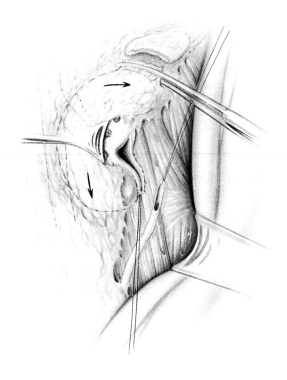

Figure 7. *Section of the upper kidney suspension to render tension-free anastomosis possible. Parallel incisions of the renal pelvis.*

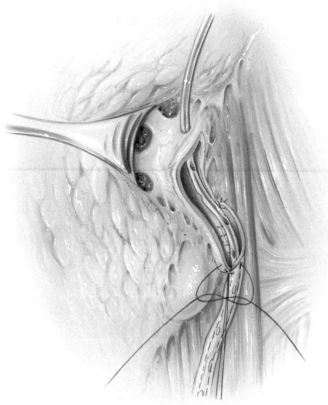

Figure 8. *Suture of the back wall of the renal pelvis and insertion of a ureteric stent. Two holes of the stent stay in the renal pelvis.*

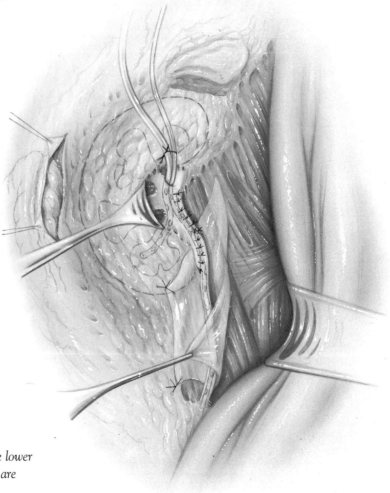

Figure 9. *Insertion of a pyelostomy into the lower caliceal group. The renal pelvis and ureter are wrapped with a free peritoneal patch.*

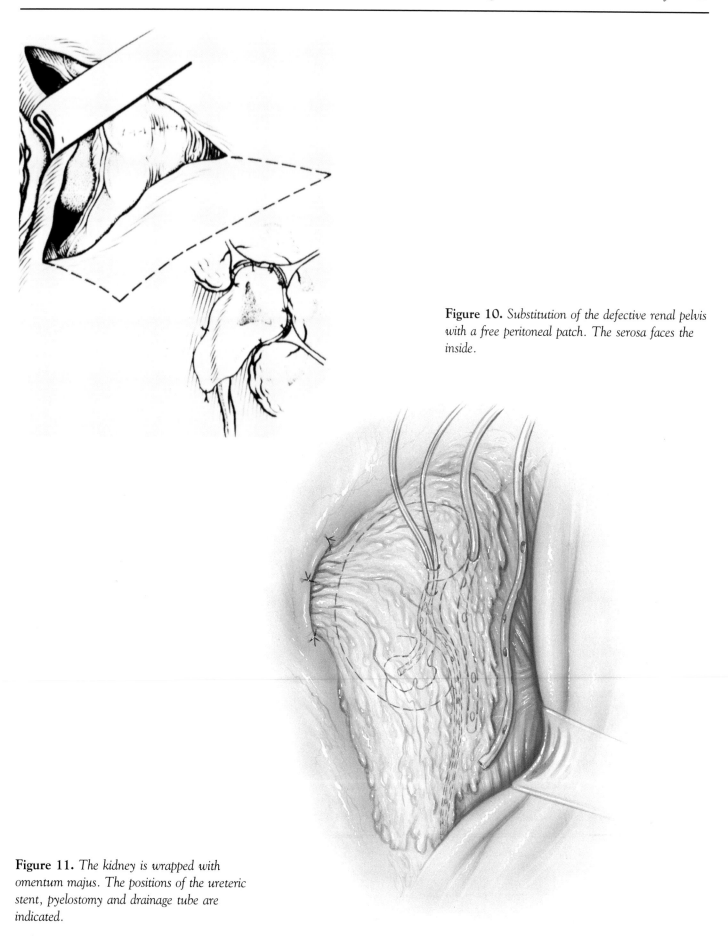

Figure 10. *Substitution of the defective renal pelvis with a free peritoneal patch. The serosa faces the inside.*

Figure 11. *The kidney is wrapped with omentum majus. The positions of the ureteric stent, pyelostomy and drainage tube are indicated.*

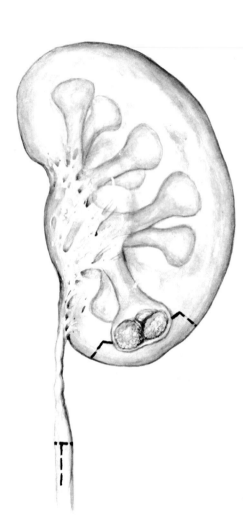

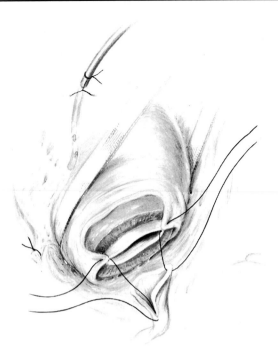

Figure 12. *(b) Stay sutures between the lower calix and the ureter to prepare the anastomosis. Insertion of a nephrostomy.*

Figure 12. *(a) Section lines for ureterocalicostomy (broken lines) with dilated calix. Wedge-shaped resection of the parenchyma at the lower kidney pole.*

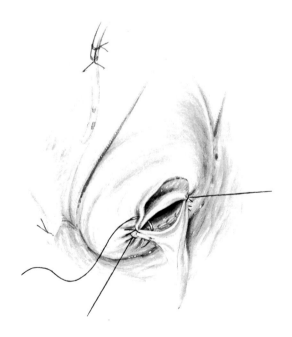

Figure 12. *(c) Anastomosis with single stitches (e.g. 6/0 monofilament resorbable suture). The knots have to be placed externally to prevent stone formation at the sutures.*

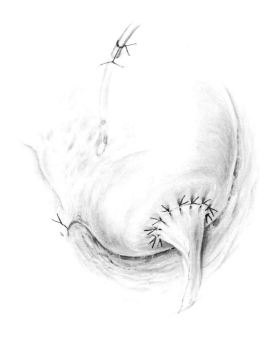

Figure 12. *(d) Complete circular closure of the tension-free anastomosis between the lower calix and the ureter. (From Eckstein HB, Hohenfellner R, Williams DJ. Surgical Pediatric Urology, Thieme, Stuttgart, 1977.)*

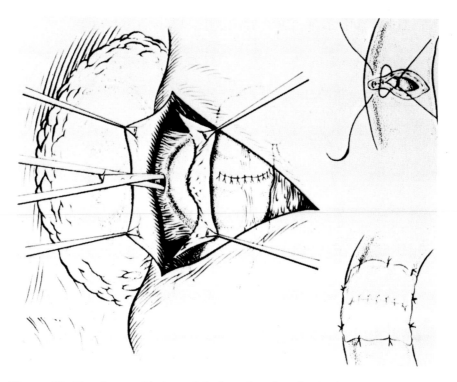

Figure 13. *For closure of lesions of the large bowel or the duodenum a seromuscular suture is recommended (e.g. 4/0 polyglyconate). Duodenal defects should additionally be covered with a free peritoneal graft.*

Radical Nephrectomy

L. Giuliani
Department of Urology,
University of Genova, Italy

Comment

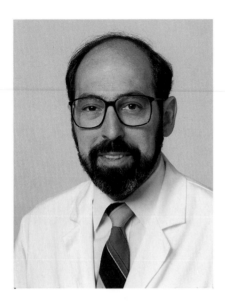

This chapter provides a thorough and well-illustrated description of the technical aspects of radical nephrectomy by an acknowledged expert in this field. The concept of radical nephrectomy was originally popularized by Robson *et al.*[1] and encompasses the basic principles of early ligation of the renal artery and vein, removal of the kidney outside Gerota's fascia, removal of the ipsilateral adrenal gland, and performance of a complete regional lymphadenectomy from the crus of the diaphragm to the aortic bifurcation.

Although radical nephrectomy remains the gold standard for surgical treatment of localized renal cell carcinoma (RCC), there is controversy concerning the need for some of these practices in all patients. Performance of a perifascial nephrectomy is of undoubted importance in preventing postoperative local tumor recurrence, because approximately 25% of localized RCCs will manifest perinephric fat involvement. Preliminary renal arterial ligation remains an accepted practice; however, in large tumors with abundant collateral vascular supply, it is not always possible to achieve complete preliminary control of the arterial circulation. It has now been well demonstrated that removal of the ipsilateral adrenal gland is not routinely necessary unless the adjacent upper portion of the kidney is involved with RCC.[2]

Finally, the need for a complete regional lymphadenectomy in all cases remains controversial. Although this allows more accurate staging of RCC, the therapeutic value of this information is limited because there is no effective form of systemic treatment for patients with advanced disease. The therapeutic merits of lymphadenectomy itself have not been conclusively shown, although data from Professor Giuliani's group suggest that a subset of patients with micrometastatic lymph node involvement may benefit[3]. At present, the need for routine complete lymphadenectomy in all cases is unresolved and there remains a divergence of clinical practice among urologists with respect to this aspect of radical nephrectomy.

With nonmetastatic RCC involving the inferior vena cava (IVC), 5 year survival rates of 47–68% have been reported following complete surgical excision. Accurate preoperative information regarding the complete extent of an IVC tumor thrombus is essential to determine the appropriate operative approach, and magnetic resonance imaging now provides an excellent noninvasive method for obtaining this information.[4] We continue to perform preoperative renal arteriography to detect arterialization of an IVC thrombus. When this is observed, renal arterial embolization 2–3 days before surgery can promote shrinkage of the thrombus, which facilitates its removal.

In surgical removal of an IVC thrombus, it is essential to obtain control of the vena cava above the thrombus to prevent intraoperative embolization of a tumor fragment. This is most challenging with thrombi that extend to the intrahepatic or suprahepatic portion of the IVC. If the right atrium is not involved, temporary occlusion of the intrapericardial IVC can be performed with simultaneous occlusion of the porta hepatis and superior mesenteric artery.[5] However, the maximum period of safe ischemia with occlusion of these vessels is only 20 minutes. In our experience, this amount of time is often insufficient to perform complete removal of friable and adherent thrombi together with vena caval reconstruction. We have employed cardiopulmonary bypass (CPB) with deep hypothermic circulatory arrest (DHCA) in over 90 patients with vena caval thrombi, and we believe that this is the preferred approach for removal of an intrahepatic or suprahepatic IVC thrombus for several reasons.[6] Because formal isolation and control of the distal IVC is not necessary, extensive retrohepatic or intrapericardial caval dissection is avoided. There is no need for mobilization of the liver, occlusion of the porta hepatis, ligation of multiple lumbar veins, or occlusion of the contralateral renal vessels. CPB with DHCA allows direct visual inspection of the entire vena caval and atrial lumen in a completely bloodless field, which facilitates removal of friable or adherent pieces of thrombus. The risk of sudden massive intraoperative hemorrhage or distal tumor thrombus embolization is lessened. Finally, this approach allows up to 60 minutes of safe ischemia for the performance of vena caval thrombectomy or resection and appropriate caval reconstruction.

References

1. Robson CJ, Churchill BM, Anderson W. The results of radical nephrectomy for renal cell carcinoma. *J Urol* **101** (1969) 297–301.
2. Robey EL, Schellhammer PF. The adrenal gland and renal cell carcinoma: is ipsilateral adrenalectomy a necessary component of radical nephrectomy? *J Urol* **135** (1986) 453–5.
3. Giuliani L, Giberti C, Martorama G, Rovida S. Radical extensive surgery for renal cell carcinoma: long-term results and prognostic factors. *J Urol* **143** (1990) 468–73.
4. Goldfarb DA, Novik AC, Lorig R *et al.* Magnetic resonance imaging for assessment of vena caval tumor thrombi: a comparative study with vena cavography and CT scanning. *J Urol* **144** (1990) 1100–3.
5. Skinner DG, Pritchett TR, Lieskovsky G *et al.* Vena caval involvement by renal cell carcinoma: surgical resection provides meaningful long-term survival. *Ann Surg* **210** (1989) 387–92.
6. Novick AC, Kaye MC, Cosgrove DM *et al.* Experience with cardiopulmonary bypass and deep hypothermic circulatory arrest in the management of retroperitoneal tumors with large vena caval thrombi. *Ann Surg* **212** (1990) 472–6.

A.C. Novick, Cleveland, USA

Radical nephrectomy

Introduction

In my experience, all renal tumors are operable; however, limitations are set by the condition of the patient, expectation of life and unacceptable operative risk.

Radical tumor nephrectomy should achieve the following:

- Optimal surgical approach
- Ligation of the renal artery without opening Gerota's fascia
- Lymphadenectomy
- Complete tumor excision, perhaps including resection of a tumor infiltrating the vena cava
- Excision of distant metastases if possible

Operative technique step by step

Surgical approaches (Figure 1–4)
- Abdominal incision for unilateral radical nephrectomy – from the xiphoid process down near the umbilicus and then laterally and transversocaudally up to the middle axillary line, a few centimeters above the iliac crest – has the following advantages: the renal artery is ligated without opening Gerota's fascia; mechanical manipulations on the tumor are avoided; visualization is excellent; the approach to the renal vessels is optimal; and the large vessels are exposed from the bifurcation of the aorta up to the diaphragm
- Thoracoabdominal incision: for caval thrombus and infiltration of the inferior vena cava
- Transversal laparotomy – horizontal or slightly cr",ioconvex with the summit in the middle between the umbilicus and the sternum and on the lateral side to the anterior axillary line – for bilateral renal carcinoma. As in the chevron approach, the incision can be extended cranially
- Mercedes approach: for large bilateral renal cell carcinomas with exploration of the supracolic and subdiaphragmatic region

Exploration of the renal artery (Figures 5–8)
- Movement of the greater omentum and the transverse colon upward, and the short bowel to the right side
- Exploration of Treitz's ligament and, after incision of the posterior parietal peritoneum, preparation of both renal arteries without manipulation of the kidneys
- In cases with a high origin of the renal artery or in patients with a large tumor crossing the midline, a supracolic approach with partial mobilization and caudal displacement of the transverse colon may be advantageous
- Incision of Treitz's ligament and mobilization of the ascending part of the duodenum, and preparation of the superior mesenteric artery
- Opening of the preaortic retroperitoneal space and ligation of the inferior mesenteric artery
- Exploration of the left renal vein (passing over the aorta) and the left renal artery posterior to the vein
- Securing of the right renal artery, posteriorly to the right renal vein by vessel loops with careful retraction of the aorta and vena cava (with special care in obese patients and those with fixed lymph nodes or venous collateral circulation)
- Exact exploration of the origin of the renal artery by preaortocaval and interaortocaval lymph node dissection

(with care when the superior mesenteric artery origin is more anterior)

Right radical nephrectomy (Figures 9–12)

- Right paracolic incision along the white line of Toldt

- Mobilization of the hepatic flexure and ascending colon

- Exploration of the anterior lamina of the renal fascia and the duodenum

- Sharp mobilization and medial retraction of the descending and horizontal parts of the duodenum until the primary incision of the posterior parietal peritoneum is reached

- Where complete exploration of the right retroperitoneum is mandatory, the ascending colon and the complete duodenum including the pancreas and the superior mesenteric artery are mobilized in the cranial direction: the median incision of the posterior peritoneum for exploration of the arteries is extended caudolaterally to the ileocecal region, continued around the cecum and joined to the incision along the ascending colon

- Ligation of the ureter and testicular vessels near the iliac artery and resection of the testicular vessels up to the great vessels

- *En bloc* removal of the kidney, adrenal gland, perirenal fat and Gerota's fascia after ligation of the adrenal vessels

- Marking of the arterial stump with a suture for lymphadenectomy

Left radical nephrectomy (Figures 13–15)

- Paracolic incision along the white line of Toldt in cases with upper pole tumors including tumors of the phrenicocolic ligament

- Mobilization and retraction to the medial side of the descending colon and, if necessary, of the left colic flexure. This space, posterior to the vessels of the colon, is prepared until the initial incision of the posterior parietal peritoneum is reached

- Ligation of the ureter and testicular vessels near the iliac vessels; ligation of the renal vein

- Complete removal of the specimen with para-aortic lymphadenectomy

Complications of radical nephrectomy are treated as follows:

- Spleen: small lesions are treated conservatively; larger ones necessitate splenectomy

- Laceration of the pancreas: repair using nonabsorbable suture material

- Laceration of the common bile duct: repair with drainage

- Liver: lacerations at the surface are oversewn: deep lacerations with injury of the bile ducts need partial resection with drainage

- Duodenum: lesions are oversewn with interrupted sutures; hematomas are opened to check for bleeding; the seromuscularis is closed with interrupted sutures

Lymphadenectomy allows:

- Exact staging (pN-stage)

- Complete local excision of the tumor

- Prevention of local recurrence

- Better prognosis

Right-sided tumor (Figure 16)

- Start of the interaortic lymphadenectomy 2 cm cranial to the renal artery: this should also be done in cases with adherent lymph nodes to guarantee a safe approach to the renal artery

- Lateromedial approach with retraction of the ascending colon to the medial site which has, in my opinion, a higher risk of bleeding (of the vena cava)

- Removal of the paracaval and renal sinus lymph nodes together with the tumor

- Removal of the interaortocaval and retrocaval lymph nodes, from the diaphragm down to the bifurcation of the aorta until the anterior longitudinal ligament is reached

- Identification of the cisterna chyli and careful ligation or clipping of the lymphatic vessels to prevent the development of chylous ascites

- In patients with macroscopic lymph node metastasis mobilization of the vena cava by ligation of the lumbal veins and resection of the celiac ganglion, the ipsilateral sympathetic trunk, the contralateral aortic lymph nodes and the ipsilateral lymph nodes in the region of the common iliac artery

In cases with macroscopic normal lymph nodes, resection of the sympathetic ganglia and nerves is not necessary

Left-sided tumor (Figure 17)

- Dissection of the preaortic lymph nodes and the lymph nodes in the renal sinus

- Ligation of the renal artery, mobilization of the descending colon and division of the renal vein

- Lymphadenectomy of the para-aortic nodes with or after radical nephrectomy

- Lymphadenectomy from the diaphragm down to the bifurcation of the aorta. After ligation of the infrarenal lumbar veins and mobilization of the aorta, lymphadenectomy can be extended to the retroaortic and interaortocaval nodes without risk of ischemia of the spinal cord

- Depending on the lymph node stage the left sympathetic trunk is resected

- At the end of the lymphadenectomy, the longitudinal ligament, the crus of the diaphragm and the psoas fascia should be completely visible

In cases of high cranial lymph node metastasis, the supracolic approach may be advantageous

Inferior vena caval tumor thrombus (Figure 18)

Preoperative magnetic resonance tomography is carried out to determine the size of the tumor. The approach and operative strategy depend on the extent of the thrombus. The aims of the operative strategy are:

- Complete removal of the tumor thrombus

- Avoidance of intraoperative tumor dissemination

- Low operative morbidity and mortality rate

Perirenal tumor thrombus (Figures 19 and 20)

- Anterior transperitoneal surgical approach

- Ligation of the renal artery and ureter

- Mobilization of the vena cava distal and proximal to the thrombus

- In cases with a small nonobstructive thrombus, resection of a part of the vena cava using a curved Satinsky venous clamp

- In cases with a large or obstructing thrombus, clamping of the opposite renal vein and the vena cava distal and proximal to the thrombus, incision of the vena cava, extraction of the tumor thrombus and partial resection of the vena cava

Infrahepatic vena caval tumor thrombus (Figure 21)

- Transperitoneal anterior approach or thoracoabdominal approach (which is preferable in cases with a high infrahepatic thrombus)

- Incision of the right triangular ligament and of the coronary ligament of the liver, and rotation of the liver to the medial site

- Exposure and control of the retrohepatic vena cava

- Incision of the parietal peritoneum of the mesentery of the small bowel from medial to the cecum up to Treitz's ligament

- Division of the inferior mesenteric vein

- Shift of the small bowel to the medial site

- Ligation of the renal artery and clamping of the opposite renal vein and artery, as well as of the vena cava caudal and cranial to the tumor thrombus

- Cavotomy and *en bloc* resection of the thrombus together with a cuff of the vena cava, the kidney and the ipsilateral adrenal gland

Intrahepatic vena caval tumor thrombus (Figures 22–25)

- Right-sided kidney tumor: thoracophrenoabdominal approach (8th or 9th intercostal space)

- Left-sided kidney tumor: anterior abdominal approach with a median sternotomy

- Control of the diaphragmal or intrapericardial part of the vena cava by vessel loops (tourniquets) to prevent pulmonary embolism

- Incision of the right triangular ligament and of the coronary ligament of the liver, and rotation of the liver to the medial site

- Exposure of the retrohepatic vena cava: in cases with portal hypertension and reduced blood flow via the hepatic veins or in those with an obstructive tumor thrombus, collateral venous drainage especially in the falciform process and the round ligament of the liver occurs, and traction of the vena cava and of the large hepatic veins should be avoided

- Exposure of the bare area of the liver and the liver veins; if necessary, maximal rotation of the liver by ligation of the caudal hepatic veins

- Pringle procedure (reduction of the blood flow to the inferior vena cava): preparation of the porta hepatitis and clamping of the portal vein (maximum 30 minutes)

- Preparation of the intrapericardial inferior vena cava, portal vein, the artery and vein of the opposite kidney, all hepatic veins and the inferior vena cava after ligation of the lumbar veins

- Clamping of the portal vein and the artery of the opposite kidney

- Occlusion with tourniquets of the vein of the opposite kidney and the intraepicardial and infrarenal vena cava

- Clamping of the large hepatic veins (to prevent tumor embolism) for a short time only (to minimize venous backflow and arterial hypotension followed by severe cardiac arrhythmia)

- Cavotomy, partial resection of the vena cava and *en bloc* resection of the tumor, kidney, adrenal gland, perirenal fat and Gerota's fascia

- Closure of the cavotomy with a running suture (5/0 Prolene, Ethicon, Edinburgh, UK)); release of the distal tourniquet, before knotting the suture, to displace air through the open corner suture

- Opening of the intrapericardial vena cava, hepatic vein, and ipsilateral renal vein, renal artery and portal vein

- Normally not more than 15 minutes are required; in cases with involvement of the hepatic veins and secondary thrombosis (Budd–Chiari syndrome) blunt dissection may be difficult and more time is required

Suprahepatic vena caval tumor thrombus (Figure 26)

- Right-sided kidney tumor: thoracophrenoabdominal approach (5th intercostal space)

- Left-sided kidney tumor: chevron approach combined with a median sternotomy

- Incision of the diaphragm down to the hiatus of the vena cava (taking care to avoid the phrenic nerve)

- Exposure of the retrohepatic vena cava, mobilization of the kidney outside the fat capsule, precise hemostasis before heparinization, and placement of ascending aortic and right atrial venous cannulas as well as one distal to the thrombus

- Hypothermia to a core temperature of 18°C; for protection of the CNS, the head is packed in ice

- Incision of the vena cava and the right atrium; removal of the thrombus

The advantages of this approach are that the operative field is bloodless and there is no risk of tumor dissemination during the operation.

In about 20% of cases the thrombus infiltrates the vena cava. Depending on the extent of infiltration, partial resection or complete resection of a segment of the vena cava is necessary. In cases with right-sided renal tumor and obstruction of the vena cava, sufficient collateral circulation of the left side develops (as indicated on preoperative venography). In these patients the left renal vein is ligated. If the collateral circulation is not yet sufficient, temporary hemodialysis may be necessary.

In cases of left-sided renal tumor (in which there is commonly no sufficient collateral circulation) or those with inadequate collateral drainage, reconstruction is necessary (Figures 27 and 28). Splenorenal shunt, protocaval anastomosis, temporary femorojugular shunt, renal autotransplantation or other techniques may be used.

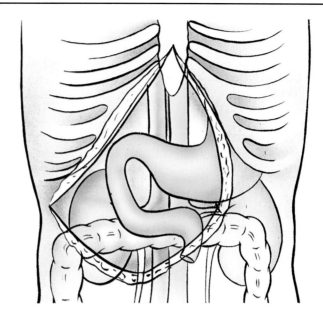

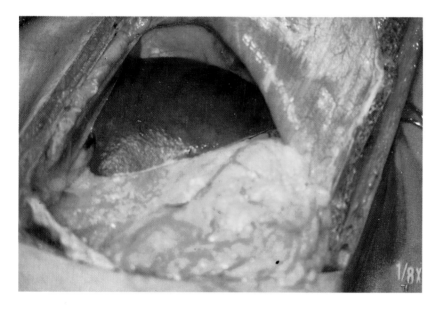

Figure 1. *Right-sided epigastric subcostal flap approach: incision from the xiphoid process near the umbilicus and then to the lateral side up to the middle axillary line, a few centimeters above the iliac crest.*

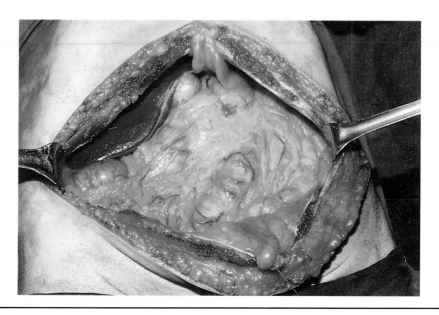

Figure 2. *Chevron incision.*

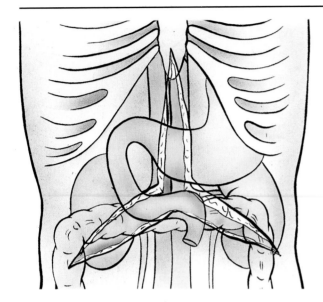

Figure 3. *Mercedes approach: excellent exposition of the subdiaphragmal and supracolic region, suitable in patients with bilateral renal tumors.*

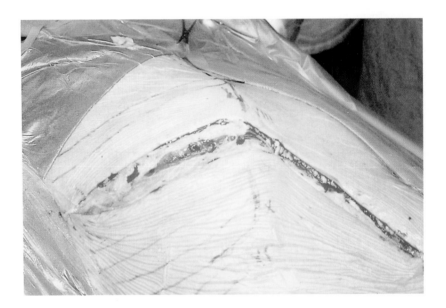

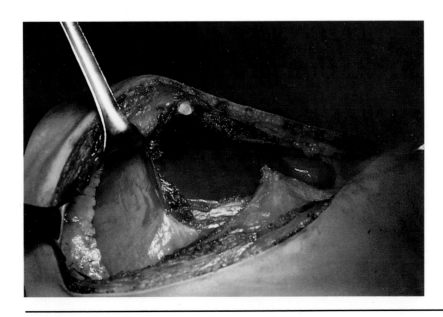

Figure 4. *Thoracophrenoabdominal approach, especially suitable in right-sided tumors with a tumor thrombus above the hepatic veins.*

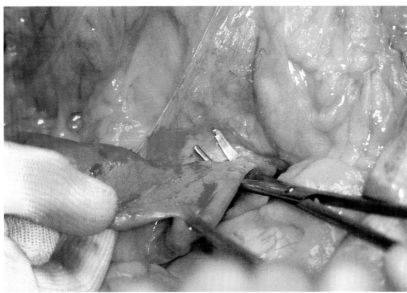

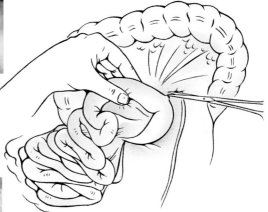

Figure 5. *Exposition and division of Treitz's ligament.*

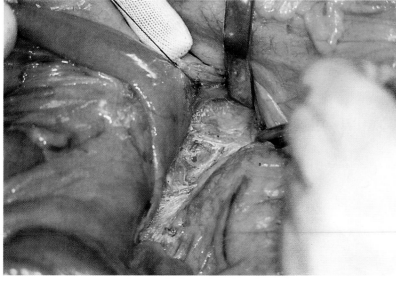

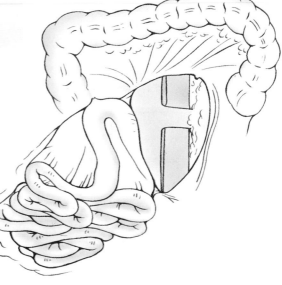

Figure 6. *Exploration in the medial retroperitoneal space by mobilization of the ascending duodenum including the mesenteric root.*

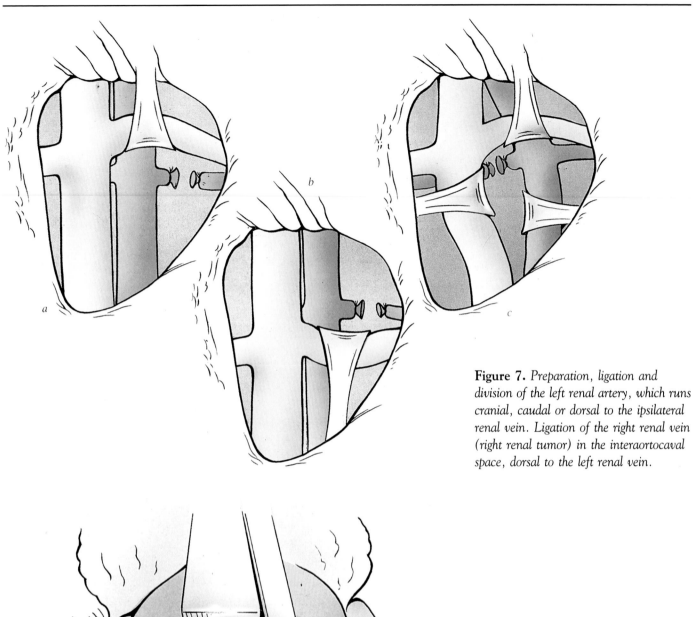

Figure 7. *Preparation, ligation and division of the left renal artery, which runs cranial, caudal or dorsal to the ipsilateral renal vein. Ligation of the right renal vein (right renal tumor) in the interaortocaval space, dorsal to the left renal vein.*

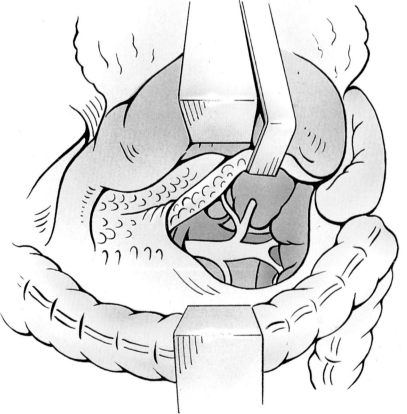

Figure 8. *Supracolic approach to the renal vessels, indicated if access is difficult owing to tumor crossing the middle line or an extremely high opening of the renal artery. Retraction of the caudal margin of the pancreas and the stomach to the cranial side and of the transverse colon to the caudal side.*

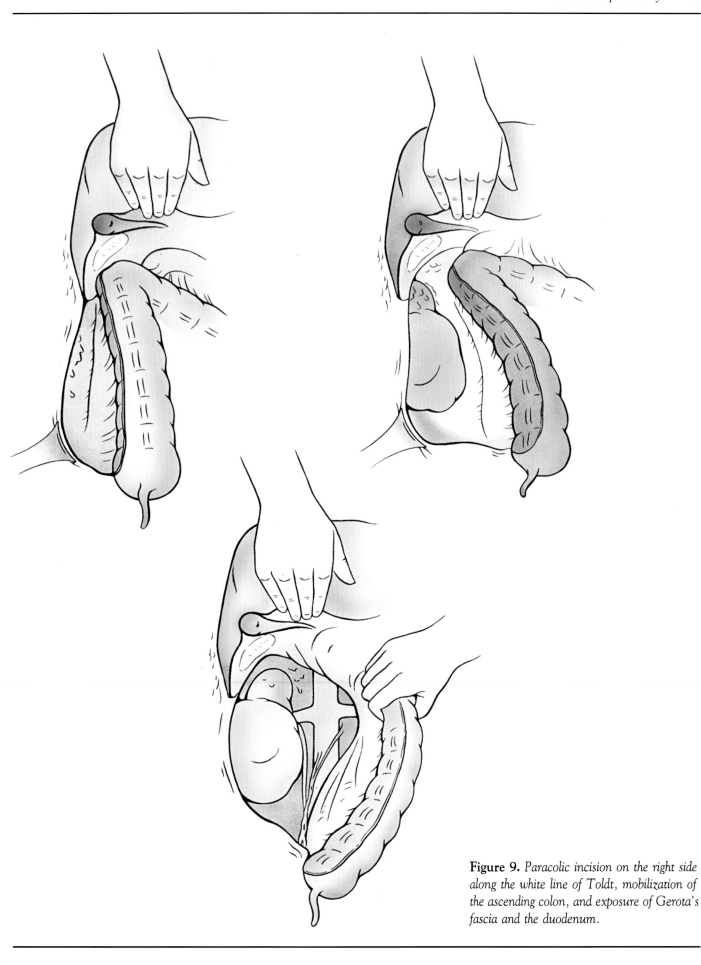

Figure 9. *Paracolic incision on the right side along the white line of Toldt, mobilization of the ascending colon, and exposure of Gerota's fascia and the duodenum.*

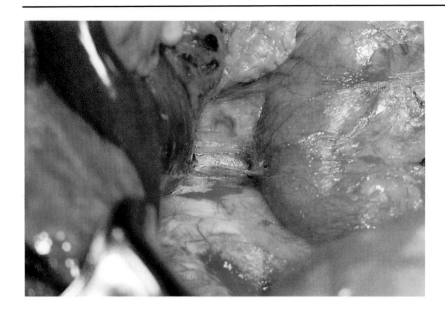

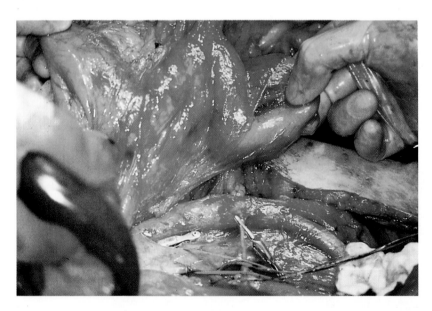

Figure 10. *Mobilization of the descending and horizontal duodenum after identification of the common bile duct.*

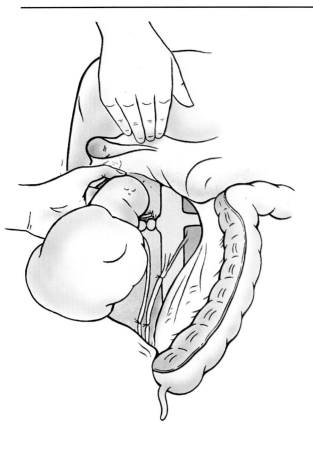

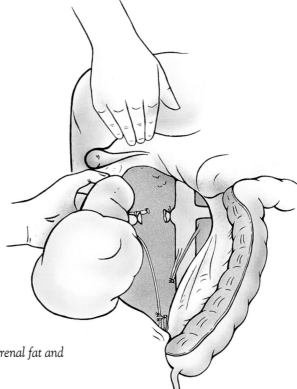

Figure 11. *Ligation and division of the right renal vein, ureter and testicular vessels at the level of the iliac vessels, with additional resection of the testicular vessels at their opening to the large vessels.*

Figure 12. En bloc *removal of the kidney, adrenal gland, perirenal fat and Gerota's fascia.*

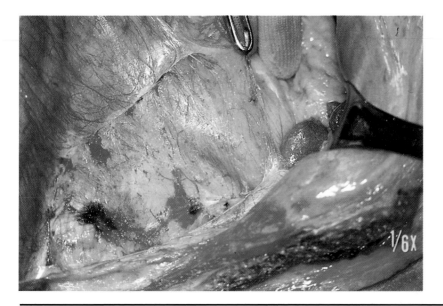

Figure 13. *Left paracolic incision along the white line of Toldt.*

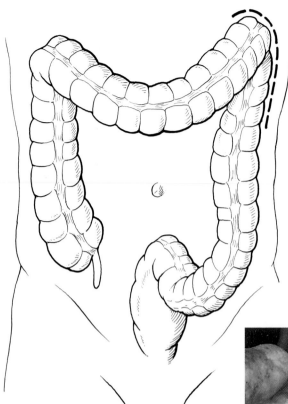

Figure 14. *Mobilization of the descending colon. In advanced or upper pole tumors, expansion of the incision including the phrenocolic ligament.*

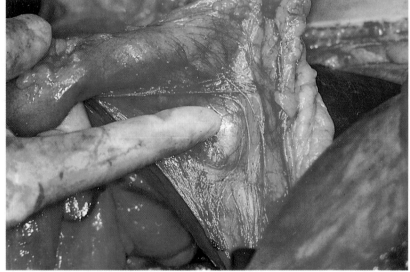

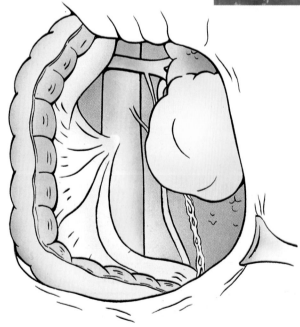

Figure 15. *Medial retraction of the descending colon, exposure of the renal bed, preparation of the ureter and testicular vessels, and ligation at the level of the iliac vessels. Ligation of the renal vein close to the vena cava and removal of the excised material, if possible with the para-aortic lymph nodes.*

Lymphadenectomy

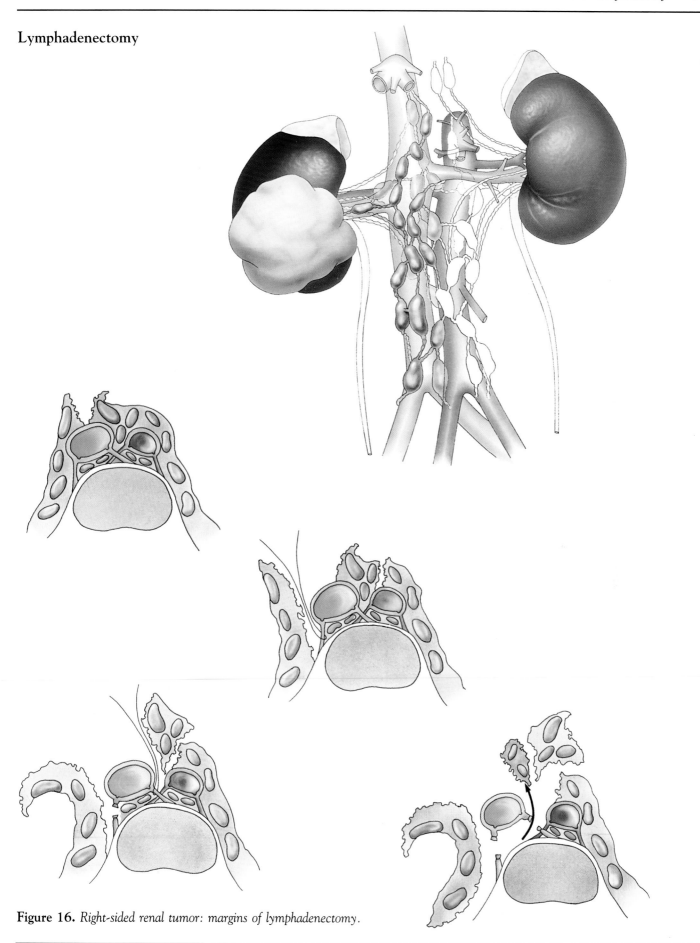

Figure 16. *Right-sided renal tumor: margins of lymphadenectomy.*

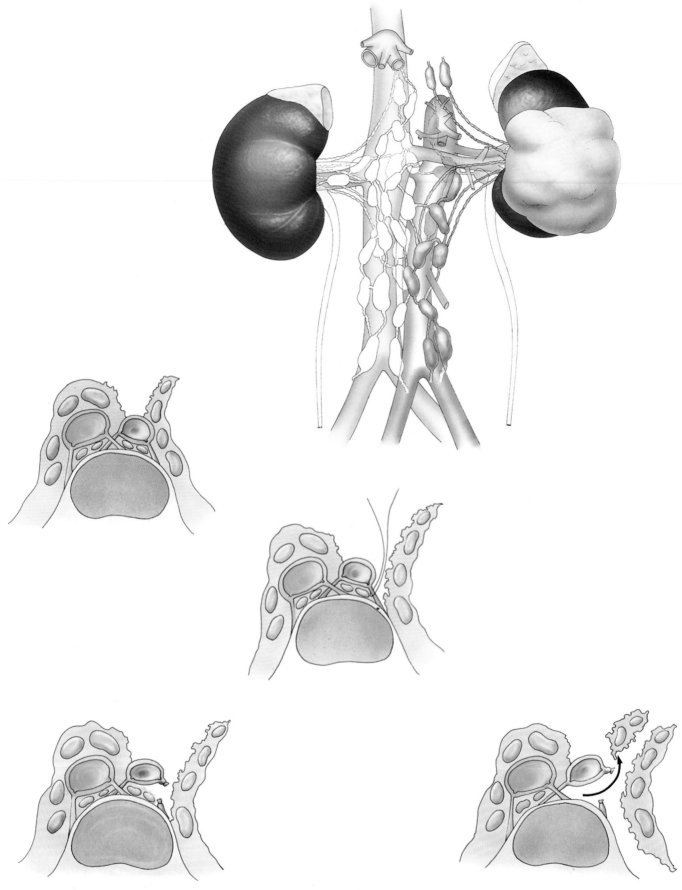

Figure 17. *Left-sided renal tumor: margins of lymphadenectomy.*

Vena cava tumor thrombus

Figure 18. *Classification of the extent of the thrombus: 1, supradiaphragmal (A, intracardial; B, intrapericardial); 2, infradiaphragmal (a, retrohepatic; b, infrahepatic; c, the level of the renal vein).*

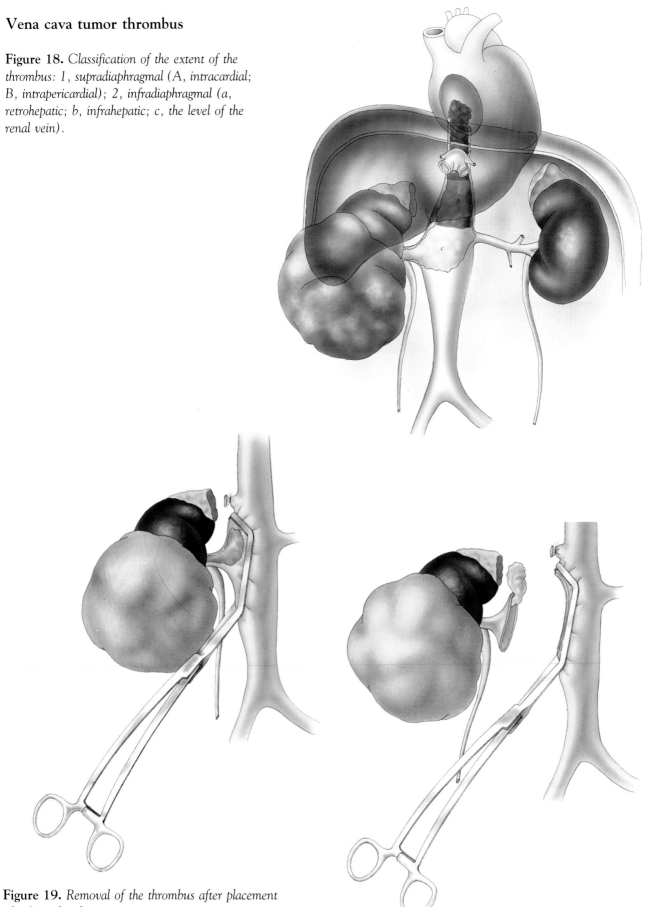

Figure 19. *Removal of the thrombus after placement of a Satinsky clamp.*

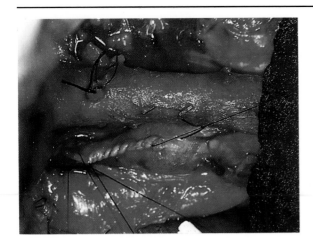

Figure 20. *Closure of the cavotomy by a running suture.*

Infrahepatic tumor thrombus

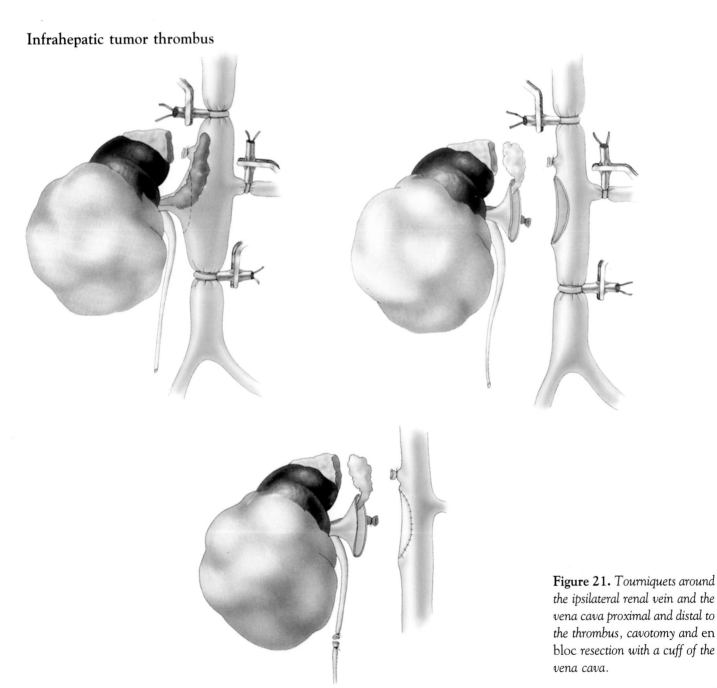

Figure 21. *Tourniquets around the ipsilateral renal vein and the vena cava proximal and distal to the thrombus, cavotomy and en bloc resection with a cuff of the vena cava.*

Retrohepatic vena cava thrombus

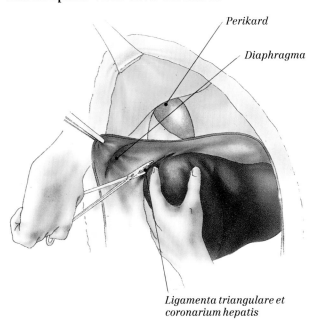

Perikard

Diaphragma

Ligamenta triangulare et coronarium hepatis

Figure 22. *Incision of the right triangular ligament and the coronary ligament of the liver.*

Figure 23. *Medial rotation of the right lobe of the liver. Exposure of the bare area of the liver and the retrohepatic vena cava.*

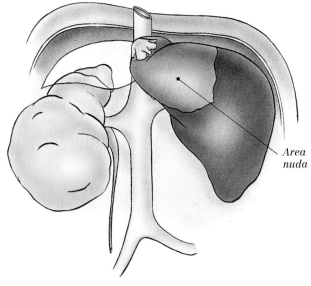

Area nuda

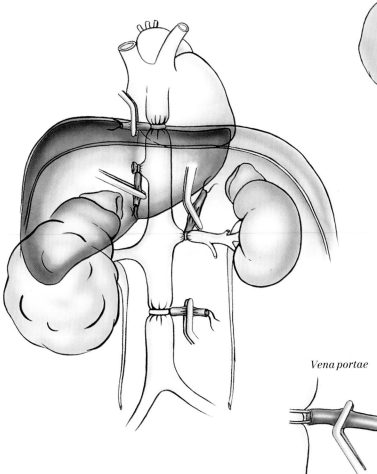

Vena portae

Figure 24. *Complete control of the tumor thrombus by occlusion of the intrapericardial and distal segments of the vena cava, the hepatic veins, the portal vein and the ipsilateral renal vein with tourniquets.*

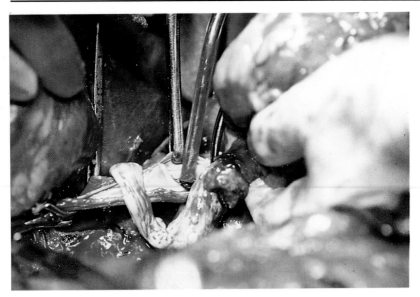

Figure 25. *Cavotomy and removal of the tumor thrombus.*

Supradiaphragmatic vena cava thrombus

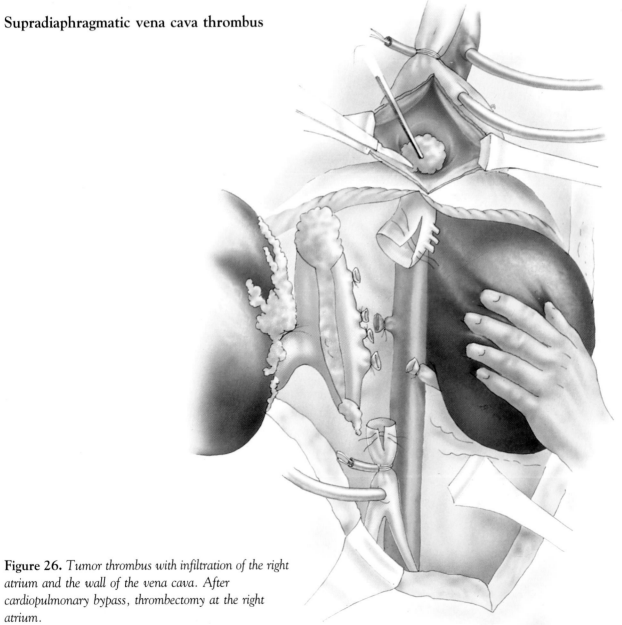

Figure 26. *Tumor thrombus with infiltration of the right atrium and the wall of the vena cava. After cardiopulmonary bypass, thrombectomy at the right atrium.*

Reconstruction of the contralateral
venous renal blood flow

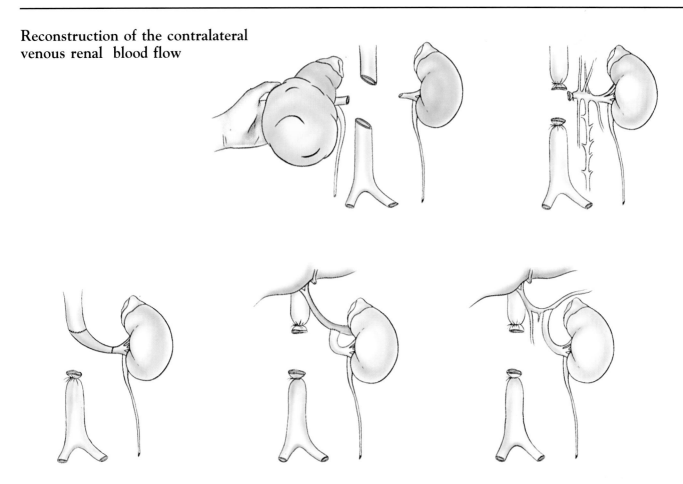

Figure 27. *After right-sided nephrectomy: ligation of the renal vein, autologous implant, portorenal anastomosis or splenorenal shunt.*

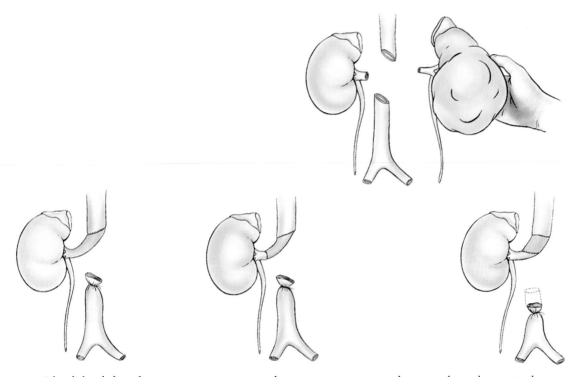

Figure 28. *After left-sided nephrectomy: vena cava–renal vein anastomosis, autologous or heterologous implant or autologous implant from the infrarenal vena cava.*

Renal Cell Carcinoma: Intrarenal Anatomy for Nephron-Sparing Operations

F.J.B. Sampaio
Biomedical Center, Department of Anatomy,
State University of Rio de Janeiro,
Rio de Janeiro, Brazil

Introduction

A comprehensive understanding of the anatomy of each kidney region to be operated on is a prerequisite to expeditious and safe conservative surgery to treat renal carcinoma, enabling total lesion removal and optimal preservation of the remaining parenchyma. This knowledge is especially important in managing large lesions, in which single enucleation is not feasible.[1,2]

Materials and methods

We analyzed 274 three-dimensional polyester resin corrosion endocasts of the intrarenal structures (arteries, veins and pelviocaliceal system) obtained from fresh adult cadavers, according to the technique described previously.[3–5]

Intrarenal anatomy of the arteries and the collecting system

Superior pole resection

In about 90% of cases, the superior pole had three arteries that would be involved in its resection:

- The superior segmental artery (apical artery), which is not in close relationship to the upper infundibulum and usually arises from the anterosuperior segmental artery, progressing to the uppermost region of the superior pole

- Two other arteries (one anterior and the other posterior), which are in close relationship to the ventral and the dorsal surfaces of the upper infundibulum (Figure 1)

Technique
- Isolation and ligation of the superior (apical) segmental artery must be the first step of superior pole resection, and is a very simple procedure because this vessel often has a proximal origin (Figure 1a)

- The second and the most refined step of the procedure must be management of the artery related to the posterior surface of the upper caliceal infundibulum. This vessel arises from the posterior division of the renal artery (posterior segmental artery or retropelvic artery, Figure 1b). The posterior segmental artery may give off two or even three branches related to the dorsal aspect of the superior pole (Figure 2). Therefore, nephron-sparing surgery in this region requires careful sinus dissection to identify, skeletonize and spare the posterior segmental artery before ligature of its branch(es) related to the posterior surface of the upper infundibulum

- Afterward, the ligature of the artery related to the anterior surface of the upper infundibulum may be performed easily

When a superior polar artery is present (6.8%), nephron-sparing surgery in the superior pole is simple because identification and ligation of this vessel are very easy (Figure 3). If, after ligation, the ischemic line of demarcation outlines an area that contains the lesion to be excised with an adequate healthy tissue margin, resection is readily performed (Figure 3). In this case, it is not necessary to be concerned about the posterior segmental artery, because when the superior polar artery is present it supplies both the anterior and the posterior aspects of the superior pole.

Hazard
The posterior segmental artery was close to the upper infundibulum or to the junction of the pelvis with the upper calix in about 60% (Figure 4a), and therefore is at great risk during the handling of the upper collecting system. Resection of the superior pole is unacceptable without gaining access to the posterior segmental artery (retropelvic artery) and achieving its total skeletonization; this artery may describe an arc that contacts the upper infundibulum, and in these cases blind resection of the superior pole may determine the total lesion of this vessel (Figure 4b). Injury to the posterior segmental artery may be associated with destruction of a large area of the remaining renal parenchyma (in some cases, the area supplied by the posterior segmental artery corresponds to about 50% of functioning renal tissue).[1]

Inferior pole resection
In the inferior pole, there are two possibilities.

In 63%, the arterial supply to the inferior pole (both front and back) arose from the inferior segmental artery. This vessel, which comes from the anterior division of the main renal artery, passes in front of the ureteropelvic junction and. after entering the inferior pole, divides into an anterior and a posterior branch. The anterior branch is related to the anterior surface of the lower infundibulum. The posterior branch progresses under the neck of the lower calix to reach the posterior aspect of the kidney (Figure 5a). In these cases, the posterior segmental artery stops before reaching the lower infundibulum, leaving its posterior surface free of arteries (Figure 5b). Both anterior and posterior aspects of the inferior pole are therefore supplied by a single anterior artery (the inferior segmental artery; Figure 5). With this arterial pattern, the dissection and previous occlusion of the segmental artery may outline an anterior and a posterior ischemic area that contains the lesion to be removed with an adequate healthy tissue margin. In this case, inferior pole resection can be carried out with no additional difficulties.

In 37%, the anterior branch related to the lower infundibulum arose from the inferior segmental artery and the posterior branch was an extension of the posterior segmental artery (retropelvic artery, Figure 6). In these cases, the anterior aspect of the inferior pole is supplied by the anterior branch and its posterior aspect is supplied by the posterior branch. Therefore, an addition to isolating and ligating the inferior segmental artery, it is important to dissect the inferior portion of the posterior segmental artery to ligate this vessel safely at a level just above the area to be removed. This will avoid injury to the inferior portion of the posterior segmental artery when deepening the incision to remove the inferior pole.

When an inferior polar artery is present (5%), the procedure will be easier because this artery can be easily identified and ligated (Figure 7). In addition, the inferior polar artery usually supplies both anterior and posterior aspects of the inferior pole.

Mid-zone resection
The artery to the mid-zone arose from the anterior division of the renal artery, and in 64% this artery coursed horizontally on the anterior surface of the renal pelvis (Figure 8a). In some cases, rather than having a defined artery (Figure 8a), the mid-kidney receives secondary division branches from arteries of other regions (Figure 8b). The arterial pattern will be determined before operation by selective angiography. The posterior segmental artery (retropelvic artery) must also be identified and protected from injury.

In mid-kidney resection, the collecting system is of utmost importance because in this region the caliceal arrangement is the most complex. In 37%, the calices draining the mid-zone are independent of both the superior and the inferior caliceal groups (Figure 9a). With this collecting system anatomy, the mid-kidney resection will not present additional difficulties, because the calices can be removed in this area with no risk of injuring the superior and inferior caliceal groups. In 63%, the calices of the mid-zone are dependent on the superior or the inferior or both caliceal groups (Figure 9b). In these cases, partial resection of the mid-kidney will require much care to preserve adequate caliceal drainage to the remaining poles. In the mid-kidney, because of its particular arterial and caliceal distribution, the wedge resection technique will be appropriate (Figure 10a).

Dorsal kidney in mid-zone resection
The dorsal kidney is supplied by the posterior segmental artery (retropelvic artery), which is a direct extension of the posterior division of the main renal artery. Within the kidney substance, the retropelvic artery usually describes an arc, and from its convexity three constant branches emerge and may be identified (superior, middle and inferior; Figure 2). The superior branch was discussed with the superior pole. The inferior branch, which is an extension of the retropelvic artery, was described with the inferior pole.

The middle branch is involved in mid-kidney resection. This artery supplies the middle portion of the posterior segment and may interdigitate with the anterior branches of the mid-kidney. In mesorenal resection, after identifying and ligating the anterior branches related to the mid-kidney as described previously, the surgeon must skeletonize the posterior segmental artery and penetrate the parenchyma to locate and ligate its middle subdivision branch (Figure 10b). Afterward, the resection will be carried out preserving the main trunk of the posterior segmental artery and the superior and inferior subdivision branches.

Intrarenal anatomy of the veins and the collecting system

The intrarenal veins have no segmental organization and anastomose freely. In more than 50% there are three major trunks that form the main renal vein at the hilum. The intersegmental anastomosis can be ligated and divided without hindering partial nephrectomy. Ligation of a vein will not result in vascular disturbance of infarction because the collateral venous channels will provide adequate drainage. This fact is important during hilar dissection because the surgeon may perform the ligature of as many tributaries of the major venous trunks as necessary, enabling ample exposure of the renal arteries that usually lie in a deep plane within the hilum.

Superior pole
The superior caliceal group is involved by two venous plexuses, from which the originated veins course parallel to the anterior and posterior surfaces of the upper infundibulum (Figure 11a). These veins, which are also approximately parallel to the anterior and posterior arterial branches, can be controlled easily during superior pole resection.

Inferior pole
In 50% of cases, the venous drainage of the inferior caliceal group also originated from two plexuses: one anterior and the other posterior. In the other 50% there was only the anterior plexus. These veins also course close to the arteries of this region and can be ligated early during inferior pole resection.

Dorsal kidney
In 70% there was a posterior (retropelvic) vein (Figure 11b) that coursed on the back of the kidney collecting system either to drain into the renal vein or to empty directly into the vena cava. In superior pole or in mid-kidney resection, the retropelvic vein (if present) must be ligated early to provide adequate and comfortable access to control the posterior segmental artery. Early identification and ligation of

the retropelvic vein will provide a bloodless field for the safe management of the posterior segmental artery.

References

1. Sampaio FJB. Anatomical background for nephron-sparing surgery in renal cell carcinoma. *J Urol* **147** (1992) 999–1005.
2. Sampaio FJB. Anatomische Grundlagen der organerhaltenden Nierentumorchirurgie. *Akt Urol* **24** (1993) 1–4.
3. Sampaio FJB, Mandarim-de-Lacerda CA. 3-dimensional and radiological pelviocaliceal anatomy for endourology. *J Urol* **140** (1988) 1352–5.
4. Sampaio FJB, Aragão AHM. Anatomical relationship between the intrarenal arteries and the kidney collecting system. *J Urol* **143** (1990) 679–81.
5. Sampaio FJB, Aragão AHM. Anatomical relationship between the renal venous arrangement and the kidney collecting system. *J Urol* **144** (1990) 1089–93.

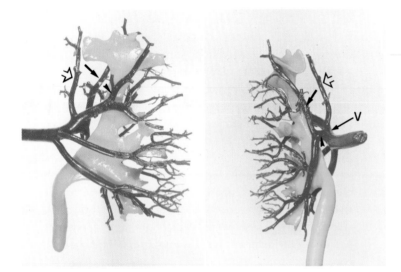

Figure 1. (a) Ventral view of the left kidney. The upper pole is supplied by three arteries: the superior segmental artery and two additional arteries that run ventral and dorsal to the infundibulum.
(b) Dorsolateral view: ventral branching of the renal artery. The superior branch of the posterior segmental artery lies close to the infundibulum.

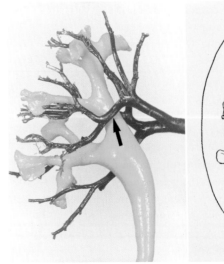
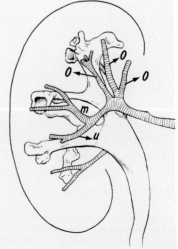

Figure 2. (a) The posterior segmental artery runs in a curve and crosses the infundibulum. (b) Branching of the posterior segmental artery into three vessels: the upper, middle and lower artery branches.

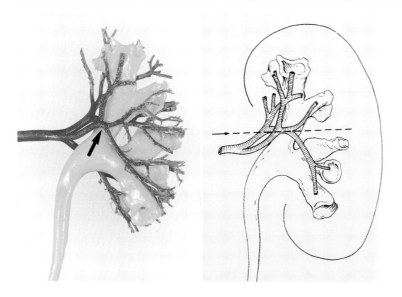

Figure 4. (a) Curved course of the posterior segmental artery. (b) Resection of parenchyma along the dotted line would result in injury to the posterior segmental artery. To prevent this, the vessel should be identified before the planned surgery.

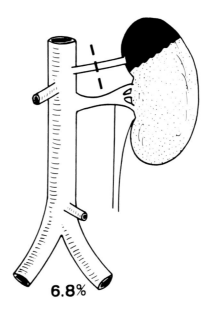

6.8%

Figure 3. Supply of the upper pole by a separate artery from the abdominal aorta. After ligature, resection of the upper pole along the demarcation line.

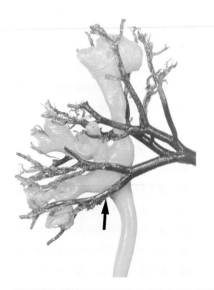

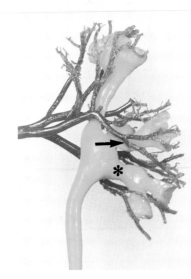

Figure 5. (a) Arterial supply of the lower pole by an anterior and posterior branch of the inferior segmental artery. (b) The posterior segmental artery (retropelvic artery) does not reach the lower pole.

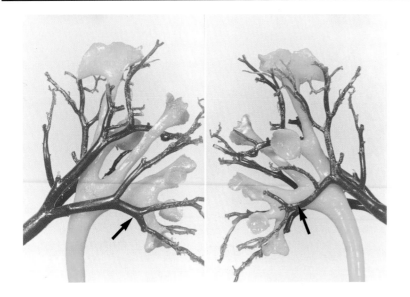

Figure 6. *The anterior aspect of the lower pole (arrows) is supplied by the inferior segmental artery; the lower branch of the posterior segmental artery (arrow) runs to the dorsal parenchyma.*

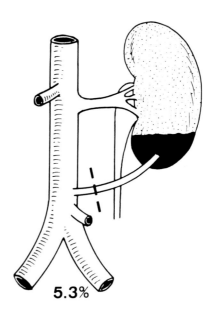

Figure 7. *Lower pole artery with ischemic area after ligation.*

5.3%

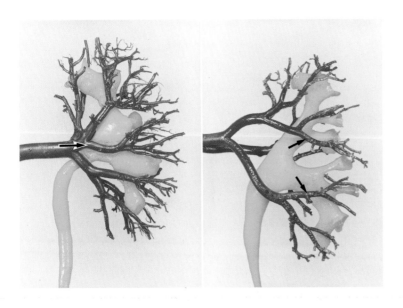

Figure 8. *(a) Supply of the mid-kidney region by a separate artery (arrow), crossing the renal pelvis. (b) The hilar region is supplied by branches of neighboring segments (arrows).*

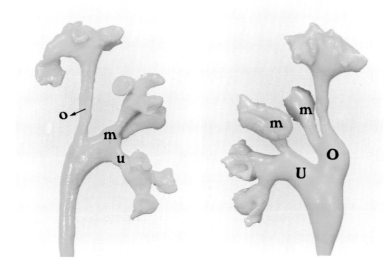

Figure 9. *(a) The upper (o), middle (m) and lower (u) calyces drain independently to the renal pelvis. (b) There is no separate middle calyceal area: the middle calyx drains to both the upper and the lower calyces.*

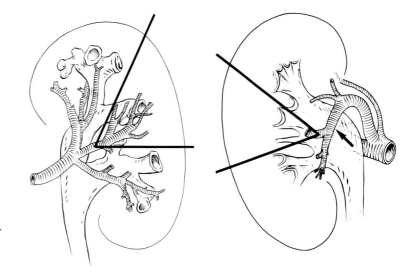

Figure 10a,b. *Because of the special anatomic features, wedge resection is especially useful in the mid-kidney. Only the middle branch of the posterior segmental artery should be ligated.*

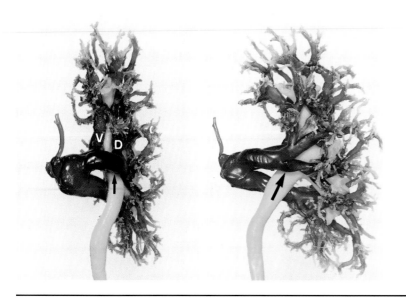

Figure 11. *(a) Ventral (V) and dorsal (D) vein plexuses enclose the anterior infundibulum. (b) The retropelvic vein crosses the pelvis at the middle aspect (arrow).*

Partial Nephrectomy for Renal Cell Carcinoma

A.C. Novick
Department of Urology,
Cleveland Clinic Foundation,
Cleveland, Ohio, USA

Indications

Accepted indications for partial nephrectomy to treat renal cell carcinoma (RCC) include situations in which radical nephrectomy would render the patient anephric with subsequent immediate need for dialysis. This encompasses patients with bilateral RCC, RCC involving a solitary functioning kidney, or unilateral RCC and a functioning opposite kidney when the opposite kidney is affected by a condition that might threaten its future function. A growing number of centers are now also performing partial nephrectomy in selected patients with small unilateral RCCs and a completely normal contralateral kidney.

General considerations

Patients undergoing partial nephrectomy for RCC should be studied before operation with renal arteriography to delineate the main renal artery and its branches. Figure 1 illustrates the normal renal arterial supply. The kidney has four constant vascular segments, which are termed apical, anterior, posterior and basilar. Each of these segments is supplied by one or more major arterial branches. All segmental arteries are end-arteries with no collateral circulation; therefore, all branches supplying tumor-free parenchyma must be preserved to avoid devitalization of functioning renal tissue.

The normal renal venous anatomy (for the left kidney) is depicted in Figure 2. The renal venous drainage system differs significantly from the arterial blood supply in that the intrarenal venous branches intercommunicate freely between the various renal segments. Ligation of a branch of the renal vein, therefore, will not result in segmental infarction of the kidney because the collateral venous blood supply will provide adequate drainage. This is important clinically as it allows safe surgical access to tumors in the renal hilus by ligation and division of small adjacent or overlying venous branches. This allows major venous branches to be completely mobilized and freely retracted in either direction, to expose the tumor, with no vascular compromise of uninvolved parenchyma.

During partial nephrectomy, every attempt should be made to minimize intraoperative ischemic renal damage. Patients should be well hydrated before operation to ensure optimal renal perfusion in the operating room. Important general intraoperative measures include prevention of hypotension during anesthesia, administration of mannitol, and avoidance of traction or excessive manipulation of the renal vessels.

When the renal circulation is temporarily interrupted, additional specific protection from ischemic renal failure is indicated. Local hypothermia is currently the most effective technique and can allow safe tolerance of up to 3 hours of renal arterial occlusion. We use ice slush cooling for surface renal hypothermia because of its relative ease and simplicity. An important caveat with this method is to keep the entire kidney covered with ice slush for 10–15 minutes immediately after occluding the renal artery and before commencing the partial nephrectomy. This amount of time is needed to obtain core renal cooling to a temperature (15–20 °C) that optimizes *in situ* renal preservation. During excision of the tumor, invariably large portions of the kidney are no longer covered with ice slush and, in the absence of adequate prior cooling, rapid rewarming and ischemic injury can occur.

When performing partial nephrectomy for RCC after excision of all gross tumor, the surgeon should verify absence of malignancy in the remaining portion of the kidney during the operation by frozen section examinations of biopsies obtained at random from the renal margin of excision. It is unusual for such biopsies to demonstrate residual tumor but, if so, additional renal tissue must be excised. Intraoperative ultrasonography is helpful in achieving accurate tumor localization and thereby in facilitating complete tumor removal.

Operative techniques

A variety of surgical techniques are available for performing partial nephrectomy in patients with RCC. All of these techniques require adherence to basic principles of early vascular control, avoidance of ischemic renal damage, complete tumor excision with free margins, precise closure of the collecting system, careful hemostasis, and closure or coverage of the renal defect with adjacent fat, fascia, peritoneum or oxidized cellulose.

It is usually possible to perform partial nephrectomy for RCC *in situ*. We employ an extraperitoneal flank incision through the bed of the 11th or 12 rib for all of these operations. This incision allows the surgeon to operate on the mobilized kidney almost at skin level and provides excellent exposure of the peripheral renal vessels.

In *in situ* partial nephrectomy for RCC, the kidney is mobilized inside Gerota's fascia; however, the perirenal fat around the tumor is left undisturbed. For small peripheral renal tumors, temporary occlusion of the renal artery may not be necessary. In most cases, however, partial nephrectomy is most effectively performed after temporary renal arterial occlusion. This not only limits intraoperative bleeding but, by reducing renal tissue turgor, also improves access to intrarenal structures. We believe that it is important to leave the renal vein patent throughout the operation. This decreases intraoperative renal ischemia and, by allowing venous back-bleeding, facilitates hemostasis by enabling identification of small transected renal veins.

Segmental polar nephrectomy

In patients with cancer confined to the upper or lower pole of the kidney, partial nephrectomy can be performed by isolating and ligating the segmental apical or basilar arterial branch while allowing unimpaired perfusion to the remainder of the kidney from the main renal artery (Figure 3). The apical or basilar artery is dissected away from adjacent structures, ligated and divided. An ischemic line of demarcation will then generally appear on the surface of the kidney and outline the segment to be excised. If this is not obvious, a few millimeters of methylene blue can be directly injected distally into the ligated apical artery to better outline the limits of the involved renal segment. An incision is then made in the renal cortex at the line of demarcation, which should be at least one or two centimeters away from the visible edge of the cancer. The parenchyma is divided by sharp and blunt dissection, and the polar segment is removed.

The collecting system is carefully closed and small transected blood vessels on the renal surface are ligated. The argon beam coagulator can be useful for achieving hemostasis on the transected renal surface. The edges of the kidney are then reapproximated as an added hemostatic measure with simple interrupted 3/0 chromic sutures.

Wedge resection

Wedge resection is an appropriate technique for removing peripheral tumors on the surface of the kidney, particularly larger ones. Because these lesions often encompass more than one renal segment, and because this technique is generally associated with heavier bleeding it is best to perform wedge resection with temporary renal arterial occlusion and surface hypothermia (Figure 4).

During a wedge resection, the surgeon removes the tumor with a 1–2 cm surrounding margin of grossly normal renal parenchyma. After the tumor resection is completed, the collecting system is closed and transected blood vessels on the renal surface are secured. The kidney may be closed on itself by approximating the transected cortical margins with simple interrupted 3/0 chromic sutures, after placing a small piece of oxidized cellulose at the base of the defect. Alternatively, a portion of perirenal fat may simply be inserted into the base of the renal defect as a hemostatic measure and sutured to the parenchymal margin.

Major transverse resection

A transverse resection is done to remove large tumors that extensively involve the upper or lower portion of the kidney (Figure 5). This technique is performed under surface hypothermia after temporary occlusion of the renal artery. Major branches of the renal artery and vein supplying the tumor-bearing portion of the kidney are identified in the renal hilus, ligated and divided. After the renal artery is occluded, the parenchyma is divided leaving a 1–2 cm margin of grossly normal tissue around the tumor. If possible, the renal defect is

sutured using one of the techniques described above. If this cannot be done without tension or without distorting the renal vessels, a piece of peritoneum or perirenal fat is sutured in place to cover the defect.

Complications

The incidence of complications after partial nephrectomy for RCC has decreased with improvements in operative technique. In patients with a solitary kidney, ischemic renal failure requiring dialysis can occur; this is usually a temporary condition. Postoperative occlusion of the renal artery or vein is another potential cause of renal failure, but is rarely encountered. Immediate or delayed bleeding from the partial nephrectomy site can occur and may require re-exploration. Careful intraoperative attention to hemostasis is mandatory to prevent this complication. A urinary fistula can occur after major tumor resections in which the collecting system has been entered. Most such fistulas resolve spontaneously with conservative management provided that ureteral obstruction is not present.

Patient survival

Survival after partial nephrectomy for RCC parallels that reported for radical nephrectomy and is related to the pathologic stage of the excised tumor. We observed a 5-year disease-specific survival rate of 87% in 216 patients treated with partial nephrectomy. The corresponding survival figure for pathologic stage 1 tumors was 94%, which was significantly better than for higher-stage RCCs. Similar survival statistics have been reported by others. We also observed an improved disease-specific survival rate in patients with unilateral RCC compared with patients with either synchronous or asynchronous bilateral RCC. The survival advantage for unilateral RCC was still apparent when considering only stage 1 tumors, suggesting a true prognostic advantage for unilateral RCC independent of local tumor stage.

Postoperative follow-up

Patients who undergo partial nephrectomy for RCC must be followed closely for recurrence of malignancy. Local tumor recurrence is of particular concern and had been reported in 4–10% of patients. Computed tomography is presently the most accurate method of detecting local recurrences and should be performed at 6-month intervals after operation to ensure prompt detection. Patients who develop a local recurrence with no signs of metastasis may be considered for secondary surgical treatment. In some cases, another partial nephrectomy can be performed with preservation of renal function. If this is not technically possible, total nephrectomy with initiation of chronic dialysis and subsequent renal allotransplantation is an alternative.

References

1. Licht MR, Novick AC. Nephron-sparing surgery for renal cell carcinoma. *J Urol* 149 (1993) 1–7.
2. Licht MR, Novick AC, Goormastic M. Nephron-sparing surgery in incidental versus suspected renal 1 cell carcinoma. *J Urol* **152** (1994) 39–42.
3. Morgan WR, Zincke H. Progression and survival after renal-conserving surgery for renal cell carcinoma: experience in 104 patients and extended follow-up. *J Urol* **144** (1990) 852–7.
4. Novick AC, Streem SB. Long-term follow-up after nephron sparing surgery for renal cell carcinoma in von Hippel–Lindau disease. *J Urol* **147** (1992) 1488–90.
5. Novick AC. Renal hypothermia: *in vivo* and *ex vivo*. *Urol Clin North Am* **10** (1983) 637–44.
6. Novick AC. Partial nephrectomy for renal cell carcinoma. *Urol Clin North Am* **14** (1987) 419–33.
7. Robson CJ, Churchill BM, Anderson W. The results of radical nephrectomy for renal cell carcinoma. *J Urol* **101** (1969) 297–301.
8. Novick AC, Gephardt G, Guz B, Steinmuller D, Tubbs RR. Long-term follow-up after partial removal of a solitary kidney. *N Engl J Med* **325** (1991) 1058–68.
9. Moll V, Becht E, Ziegler M. Kidney preserving surgery in renal cell tumors: indications, techniques and results in 152 patients. *J Urol* **150** (1993) 319–23.
10. Steinbach F, Stockle M, Muller SC *et al.* Conservative surgery of renal cell tumors in 140 patients: 21 years of experience. *J Urol* **148** (1992) 24–9.

Vascular anatomy

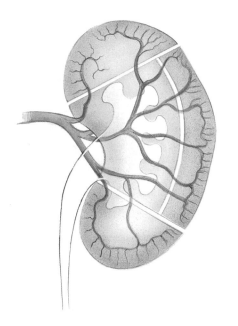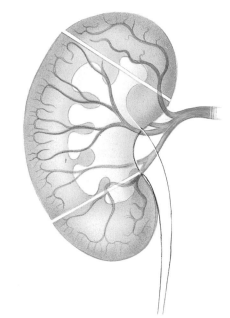

Figure 1. *Normal renal artery supply and four vascular segments of the kidney, as shown in anterior (left) and posterior (right) projections.*

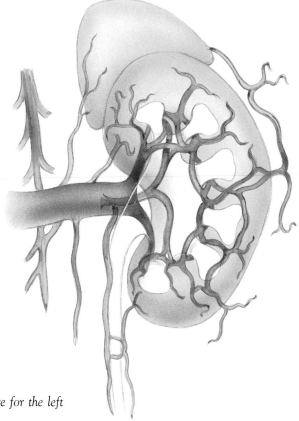

Figure 2. *Normal renal venous drainage, shown here for the left kidney.*

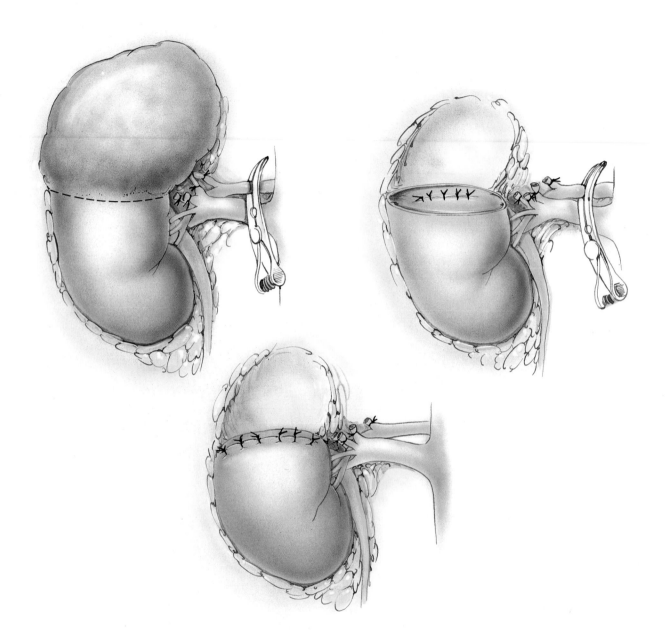

Figure 3. *Segmental (apical) polar nephrectomy with primary ligation of apical arterial and venous branches. Methylene blue can be injected into the arterial branch to delineate the line of demarcation.*

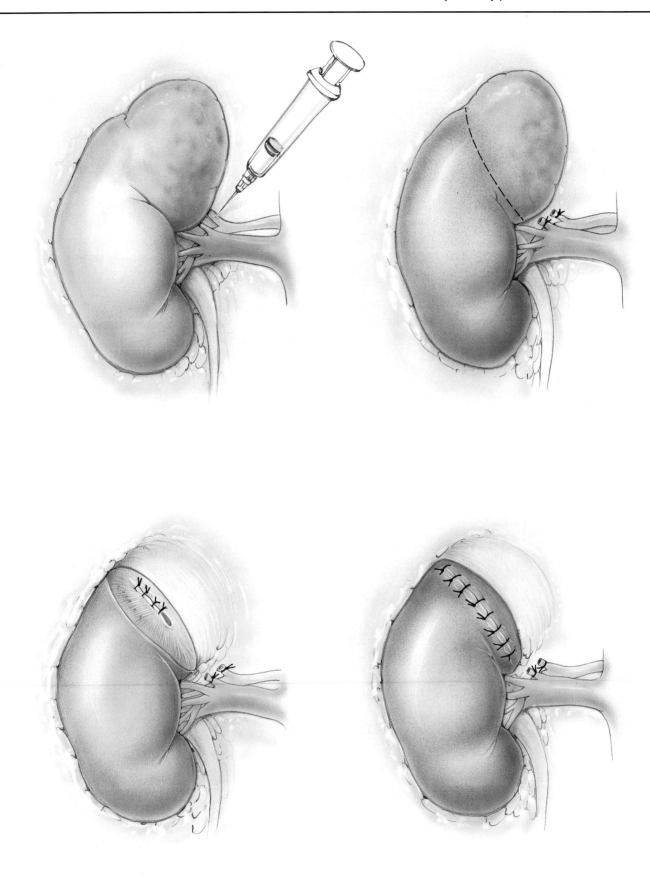

Figure 3. continued

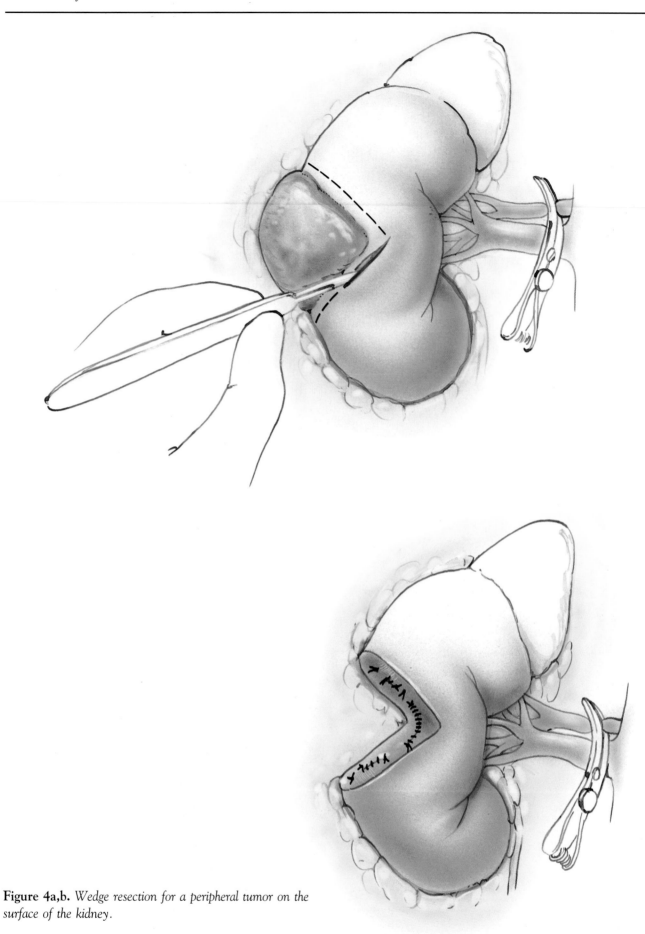

Figure 4a,b. *Wedge resection for a peripheral tumor on the surface of the kidney.*

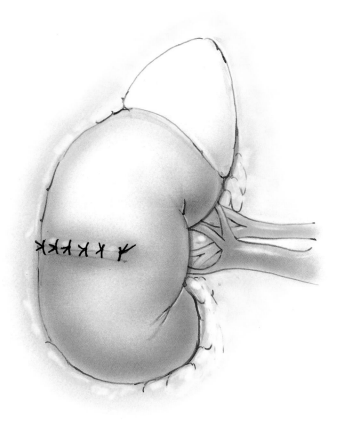

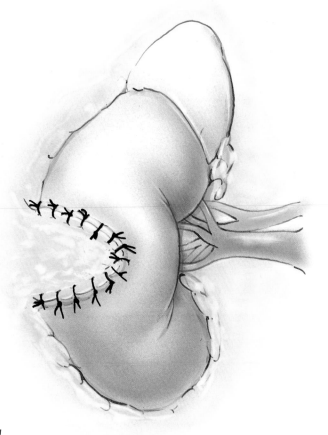

Figure 4. *The renal defect may be closed on itself (c) or covered with perirenal fat (d).*

'Work bench' resection

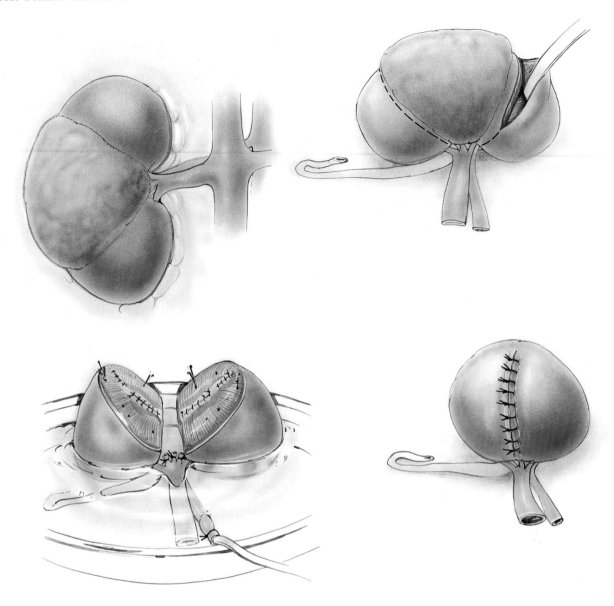

Figure 5. *Extracorporeal partial nephrectomy of a large central tumor. Intermittent renal perfusion to identify blood vessels. Closure of the parenchymal defect.*

Modified Enucleation of Renal Tumors

F. Steinbach[a], R. Stein, M. Stöckle[b],
R. Hohenfellner
Department of Urology,
University of Mainz School of Medicine,
Mainz, Germany
[a]*University of Kiel, Kiel, Germany*
[b]*University of Magdeburg, Germany*

Introduction

During 'modified tumor enucleation' the tumor is removed together with the pseudocapsule and an additional layer of parenchyma.[1]

The renal tumor compresses the surrounding parenchyma (like the skin of an onion), which results in a concentric space outside the pseudocapsule. The tumor resection in this layer is usually complete.

Advantages

- Excellent intraoperative diagnosis by frozen section examinations of multiple biopsies from the surrounding parenchyma
- Minimal loss of parenchyma – of great importance in patients with multiple tumors, solitary kidney or bilateral tumors
- Wound repair with clamping of the artery and cooling of the kidney, with the option of re-resection or nephrectomy in cases with positive margins, without time pressure on the pathologist
- Minimal blood loss by clamping the tumor vessel

Indications

See Novick[3] and Marshall *et al.*[2] In patients with synchronous bilateral renal cell carcinomas, the kidney with the better chance for parenchyma-sparing surgery is operated on first and the other 6–8 weeks later.

Diagnostics

- After the initial ultrasonography, which usually detects the tumor, computed tomography (CT) and magnetic resonance imaging (MRI) are of equal value. At the end of the CT examination a conventional radiograph of the abdomen documents the morphology of the collecting system
- Special indications for MRI include allergic reaction to a contrast medium and tumor thrombus of the renal vein or inferior vena cava
- Renal angiography may be used in cases of a central or large renal tumor for planning the operative strategy

Operative risks

- Where there is an imperative indication (anatomically or functionally solitary kidney), ischemic renal failure and temporary dialysis
- Complete renal failure and permanent dialysis

This is a relatively new operative method; long-term follow-up studies are lacking.

Special instruments and materials

- Suture material: 5/0 polyglyconate (e.g. Maxon, Davis and Geck, Gosport, UK) for closure of the collecting system, 4/0 polyglyconate for closure of the renal capsule
- Hemostatic oxidized cellulose
- Ice slush for cooling
- Vessel loops and bulldog clamps
- Infrared-sapphire coagulator or argon beam laser

Surgical approach

- Supracostal, extraperitoneal flank approach through the bed of the 11th or 12th rib[4]

Operative technique step by step

- After opening Gerota's fascia the kidney is completely mobilized, the perirenal fat tissue is left untouched at the surface of the tumor, and the kidney is inspected for other tumors
- In cases with expected large parenchymal defects, a peritoneal patch is taken (Figure 1) and the peritoneum is closed again. This patch is later used to cover the defect
- The renal vessels are prepared and secured by vessel loops
- Clamping of the renal artery is not routinely performed in small peripheral tumors. Indications for clamping include central position, and a diameter of more than 5–6 cm
- If more than 15–20 minutes of ischemia will be necessary, the parenchyma must be protected by local hypothermia starting after occluding the renal artery (ice slush)
- A circumferential incision of the renal capsule is made at a distance of 4–7 mm from the tumor. Using a brain spatula the tumor is bluntly enucleated outside the pseudocapsule with a small surrounding margin of parenchyma (Figure 2). Small vessels are coagulated and larger vessels are oversewn. The base of the tumor is clamped by an Overholt clamp and ligated (Figure 3)
- Frozen section examination confirms the complete tumor resection. If there is a positive margin, nephrectomy is performed in all patients with a normal contralateral kidney, and re-resection otherwise
- Bleeding vessels are secured with a purse-string ligature (5/0 monofilament suture). Opened calices are closed with interrupted or uninterrupted sutures
- Additionally an infrared coagulator or argon beam laser is used for coagulation (Figure 4). The suture of the renal capsule is important for the hemostasis

- The whole kidney is covered with oxidized cellulose and the remaining fat capsule is closed (Figure 5)

Intraoperative ultrasonography

Ultrasonography is indicated in tumors that are not visible on the renal surface. An accurate determination of the location and of the tumor diameter is possible.

Complications

- Temporary ischemic renal failure (requiring hemodialysis)
- After bleeding: in patients with a stable circulatory system, angiography and percutaneous treatment; re-exploration if this fails
- Urinary fistula, diagnosed by determination of the creatinine levels from the drainage fluid; without ureteral obstruction, most fistulas resolve spontaneously; in cases with dilatation, drainage by urethral catheter
- Urinoma, diagnosed by ultrasonography and CT: control examinations and antibiotic treatment, followed by re-exploration if there is enlargement

Postoperative care

- Removal of the drainage step by step between days 4 and 5 (depending on the secretion)

- Removal of the skin sutures on day 7 or 8
- Documentation of renal function and intact collecting system by intravenous pyelography

Oncological control examinations

- Ultrasonography at 6-month intervals
- CT at 12-month intervals

References

1. Blackley SK, Lagada L, Woolfitt RA, Schellhammer PF. *Ex situ* study of the effectiveness of enucleation in patients with renal cell carcinoma. *J Urol* **140** (1988) 6–10.
2. Marshall FF, Taxy JB, Fishman EK, Chang R. The feasibility of surgical enucleation for renal cell carcinoma. *J Urol* **135** (1986) 231–4.
3. Novick AC. Nierenteilresektion beim Nierenzellkarzinom. *Akt Urol* **24** (1993) Operative Techniken, chapter 1.5.
4. Steinbach F, Riedmiller H, Hohenfellner R. Suprakostaler Zugangsweg und Nierenbeckenplastik. *Akt Urol* **21** (1990) Operative Techniken, chapter 11.1.

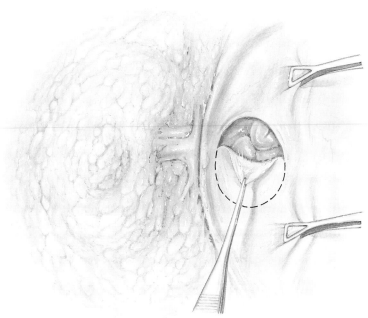

Figure 1. *Preparation of a peritoneal patch to cover the defect produced by excision of larger renal tumors.*

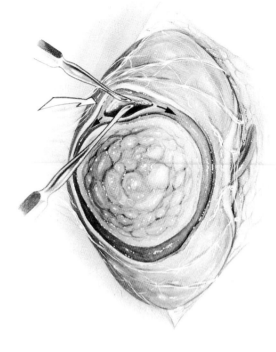

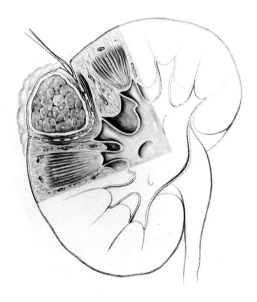

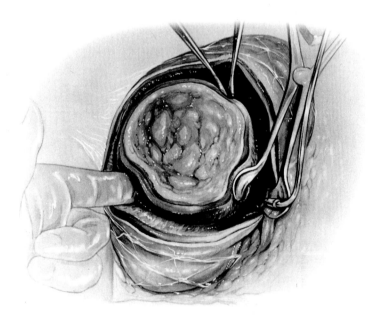

Figure 2. *After the vessels are surrounded by vessel loops, a sharp incision of the renal capsule 4–7 mm away from the tumor, followed by blunt enucleation with brain spatulas outside the pseudocapsule.*

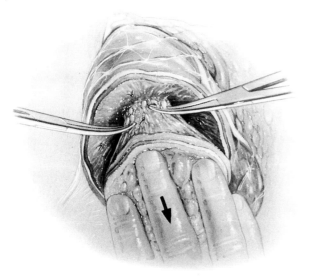

Figure 3. *Ligation of the tumor base and frozen section examination of the tissue.*

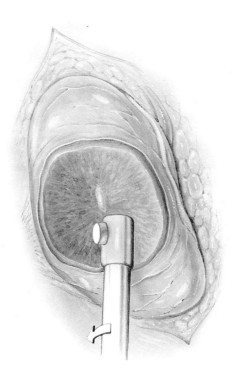

Figure 4. *Coagulation of the tumor bed with the infrared-sapphire coagulator or argon beam laser.*

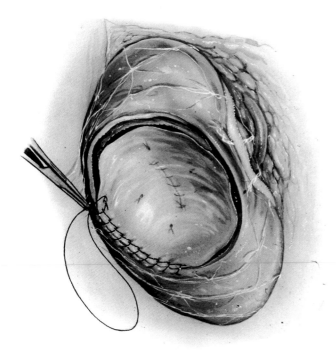

Figure 5. *Closure of the parenchymal defects. Defects left by small tumors can be closed by adaptation of the renal capsule. Larger defects are closed using the renal fat capsule or a peritoneal patch.*

Organ-Preserving Surgery of Kidney Tumors in situ During Ischemic Preservation

M. Kallerhoff, B. Schorn,[a] M. Hermanns,
G. Zöller, R.-H. Ringert
*Departments of Urology and [a]Thoracic and Cardiovascular Surgery,
University of Göttingen,
Göttingen, Germany*

Introduction

An interesting alternative to 'workbench' surgery, described by A.C. Novick, is the resection of tumor during ischemia. Perfusion with histidine–tryptophan–ketoglutarate (HTK) solution (Table 1) makes preservation of the kidney (and other organs) possible during *in situ* operation. *In situ* application of Euro-Collins or University of Wisconsin (UW) solution should be avoided because of their high potassium content (about 120 mM).

Table 1. Composition of histidine–tryptophan–ketoglutarate solution*

Na$^+$ (mM)	15
K$^+$ (mM)	10
Ca^{2+} (mM)	—
Mg^{2+} (mM)	4
Cl$^-$ (mM)	50
Tryptophan (mM)	2
K$^+$ α-ketoglutarate (mM)	1
Histidine/histidine hydrochloride (mM)	180/18
Mannitol (mM)	30
Osmolarity (Mosmol/L)	310
pH at 8°C	7.3
PO$_2$ at 37°C	200

*Custodiol, Dr Franz Köhler, Chemie GmbH, Neue Bergstraße 3–7, D-64665 Alsbach-Hähnlein, Germany.

Patient selection

If an organ-preserving operation for cancer of the kidney is intended, the patient has to be free of normal risks and of the danger of injury to neighboring organs. The operation carries a risk of secondary hemorrhage, secondary nephrectomy and postoperative renal sufficiency. Dialysis should be available.

Operative technique

The patient is placed in the overstretched dorsal decubitus position (Figure 1). The abdomen is opened with a large horizontal epigastric incision, and the ascending or descending colon is mobilized, revealing the kidney and the renal artery and renal vein up to the aorta and vena cava, respectively (Figure 2). At the end of preparation the kidney is fixed only on the vessels and the ureter. The perirenal capsule should be saved to cover the resected area of the kidney. During preparation a solution of 5% glucose is infused

continuously to attain a good level of substrate before ischemia starts. About 20 minutes before the protective perfusion with HTK solution starts furosemide (20 mg i.v.) is given to obtain a forced diuresis. The washout of the osmotic gradient in the kidney makes the following homogeneous perfusion with the HTK solution easier. Also 20 minutes in advance 2500 units of heparin are given intravenously.

The aorta is exposed 5–10 cm distal to the insertion of the renal artery and fixed over a distance of 5 cm by two threads (Figure 3). Between these two threads an intramural purse-string suture of 5–7 mm diameter is fixed by 4/0 Prolene 1(Ethicon, Edinburgh, UK) and armed by an ebonite valve-tube. The aorta is clamped with two aortic clamps or a Satinsky clamp, and a puncture incision into the aorta is made and widened with an Overholt clamp. An 8 Fr perfusion catheter is then introduced into the aorta. The incision is sealed by the ebonite valve-tube and the aortic clamps are removed. The catheter is introduced into the renal artery with the right hand while the artery is pulled cranial by two fingers of the left hand. For homogeneous perfusion of the whole kidney the catheter must be placed securely in the renal artery – *not* in any vascular branches. Perfusion can then be started, and continued for 10 minutes with the HTK solution, cooled to 4°C. A perfusion pressure of about 120–180 cmH$_2$O and an 8 Fr catheter provides a flow of 150–200 ml/min. Influx of the solution into the circulation should be avoided because of the high volume (1.5–2 L within 10 minutes) and the 10 μM potassium content. The tourniquet round the renal artery is tightened after introduction of the catheter (Figure 4). The renal vein is pinched shut and an incision is made in it on the side of the vena cava, through which the perfusing solution can flow out and be suctioned off. At the end of perfusion the renal clamps are removed and the venotomy is closed by a soft clamp or a small bulldog clamp (Figure 6). The kidney should be bloodless during the whole ischemic period.

Tumor resection

After perfusion the kidney is pale and cool. Ischemia may be maintained for a maximum of 2 hours. (This time can be prolonged to 4 hours by extreme cooling.) The renal adipose capsule is opened and the tumor resected (Figure 7). Good visualization and the long renal tolerance for ischemia allow safe work. After resection, test biopsies of the tumor base to confirm the adequacy of the resection are taken (Figure 8). Vessels which are visibly opened on the resected area are clotted or stitched, and the pelvis of the kidney is nearly always opened and has to be closed. The insertion of a double-J catheter is normally unnecessary. Because of the bloodlessness and dryness of the surface, fibrin, gluten and a collagen patch can then be located in the wound cavity, and the border of the kidney can be stuck together by manual compression. An adapting suture of the renal fat further protects against bleeding (Figure 9). Deep sutures of the parenchyma should, if possible, be avoided because of the associated loss of parenchyma. After restoration of the circulation by removing the clamps on the renal vein, ureter and renal artery (Figure 10), any vessels which are still bleeding can be located and closed with stitches. Only exceptionally should a Vicryl net (Ethicon) be used, because the compression may impair renal blood flow. Normally, covering the kidney with the renal fat is sufficient. The kidney is returned to its original position, drainage is adjusted and the retroperitoneum is closed by adapting sutures. The wound is closed in layers.

Postoperative treatment

- Postoperative supervision because of the possibility of secondary hemorrhage

- Good diuresis by furosemide and dopamine in 'renal' doses

- Control of creatinine excretion and urine volume daily

Discussion

The perfusion catheter was first used in the Seldinger technique. Because, in one case, the catheter caused closure of the renal artery, in following patients the catheter was introduced via the inferior mesenteric artery. However, because of the danger of ischemia, this technique was discontinued. In one case the renal artery was directly punctured instead, but after good function obtained initially there was a thrombosis. Later, the safer procedure of direct puncture of the aorta was used: one bleeding renal vein and one secondary hemorrhage required nephrectomy in two patients.

Our experience indicates that the *in situ* operation with ischemic protection, in the hands of an experienced surgeon, is an acceptable approach for organ-preserving renal tumor surgery.

Acknowledgment

This work was supported by the Deutsche Forschungsgemeinschaft, SFB 330 Organprotektion, Göttingen.

References

1. Bretschneider HJ, Helmchen U, Kehrer G. Nierenprotektion. *Klin Wochenschr* **66** (1988) 917–27.

2. Gschwend JE, dePetriconi R, Maier S, Kleinschmidt K, Hautmann RE. Continuous *in situ* cold perfusion with histidine tryptophan ketoglutarate solution in nephron sparing surgery for renal tumors. *J Urol* **154** (1995) 1307–11.

3. Kallerhoff M, Hölscher M, Kehrer G, Kläss G, Bretschneider HJ. Effects of preservation conditions and temperature on tissue acidification in canine kidneys. *Transplantation* **39** (1985) 485–9.

4. Kallerhoff M, Blech M, Kehrer G et al. Nierenfunktionsparameter nach Ischämiebelastung unter der Euro-Collins Lösung oder unter der Kardioplegischen Lösung HTK nach Bretschneider. *Urologe* (A) **26** (1987) 96–103.

5. Kallerhoff M, Blech M, Kehrer G et al. Effects of glucose in protected ischemic kidneys. *Urol Res* **16** (1987) 215–22.

6. Kallerhoff M, Blech M, Isemer FE et al. Metabolic, energetic and structural changes in protected and unprotected kidneys at temperatures of 1°C and 25°C. *Urol Res* **16** (1988) 57–62.

7. Kallerhoff M, Blech M, Götz L et al. A new method for conservative surgery: experimental and first clinical results. *Langenbecks Arch Chir* **375** (1990) 340–6.

8. Kehrer G, Blech M, Kallerhoff M, Langheinrich M, Bretschneider HJ. Contribution of amino acids in protective solutions to postischemic functional recovery of canine kidneys. *Res Med* **189** (1989) 381–96.

9. Novick AC. Nierenteilresektion beim Nierenzellkarzinom. *Akt Urol* **24** (1993) Operative Techniken, chapter 1.5.

10. Pichlmayer R, Grosse H, Hauss J, Gubernatis G, Lamesch P, Bretschneider HJ. Technique and preliminary results of extracorporal liver surgery (bench procedure) and of surgery on the *in situ*-preserved liver. *Br J Surg* (1990) 21–6.

11. Preusse CJ, Schulte HD, Bircks W. High volume cardioplegia. *Ann Gynaecol* **76** (1987) 39–45.

12. Timmons SL, Ward R, deVere White RW. *In situ* perfusion. *World J Urol* **8** (1990) 55–7.

13. Wickham JEA. Conservative renal surgery for adenocarcinoma: the place of bench surgery. *Br J Urol* **47** (1975) 25–36.

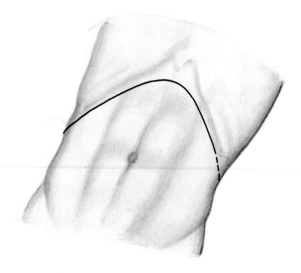

Figure 1. *Extended supine position and wide oblique upper abdominal incision with extension to the operated side.*

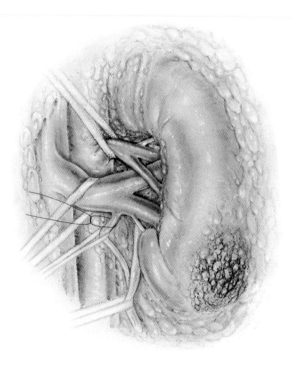

Figure 2. *Total dissection of the renal vessels up to the aorta and vena cava.*

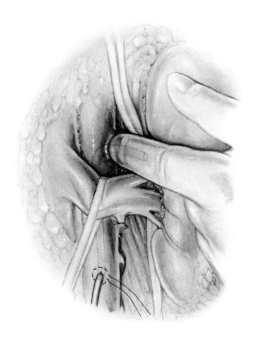

Figure 3. *Dissection of the aorta 5–10 cm distal to the renal artery. A purse-string suture with a diameter of 5–7 mm is prepared with 4/0 Prolene. After placement of two aortic clamps or one Satinsky clamp the aorta is incised and an 8 Fr perfusion catheter is inserted into the aortic lumen with an Overholt clamp and secured with the previously placed suture after advancement up to the level of the renal artery.*

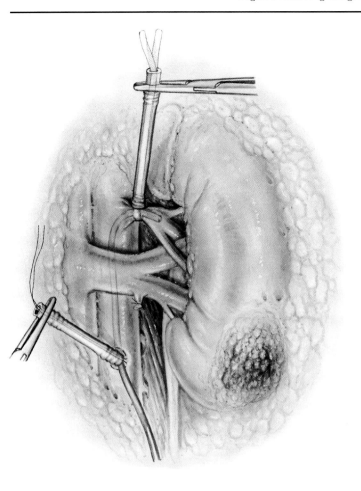

Figure 4. *After insertion of the catheter into the renal artery the tourniquet around the artery is tied.*

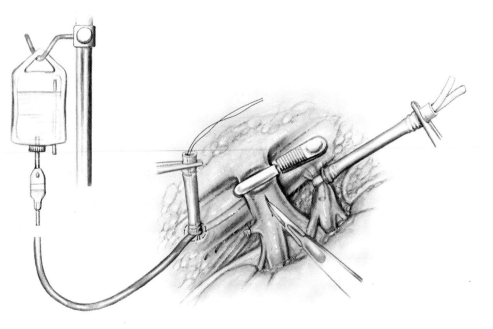

Figure 5. *After initiation of perfusion, incision of the renal vein and suction of the solution.*

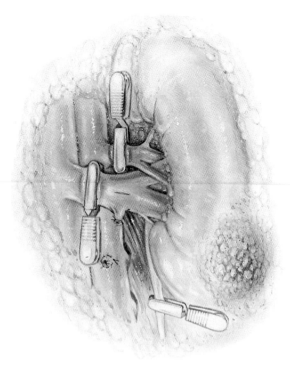

Figure 6. *Placement of a bulldog clamp on the renal artery proximal to the perfusion catheter and a clamp on the vena cava and ureter, and closure of the purse-string suture.*

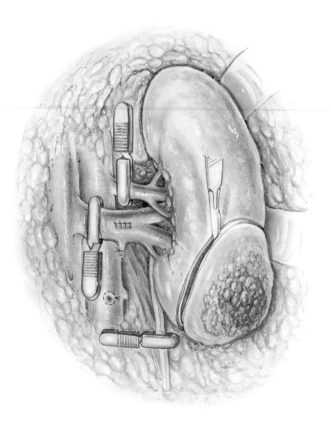

Figure 7. *After closure of renal vein defect, tumor resection begins.*

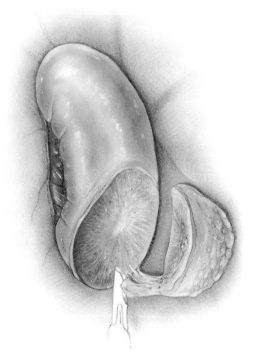

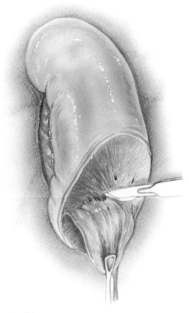

Figure 8. *(a) Complete resection of the tumor. (b) Excision of additional tissue from the margin for histologic evaluation.*

Fig. 8 (b)

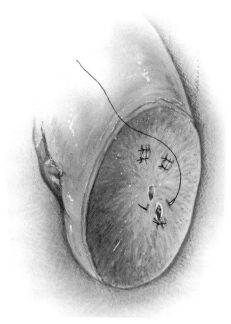

Figure 9. *(a) Selective coagulation and/or ligation of bleeders.*

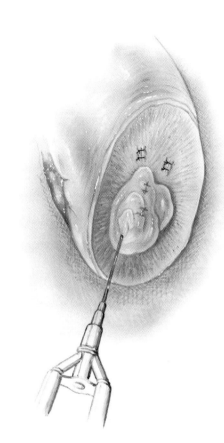

Figure 9. *(b) Optional additional fibrin application.*

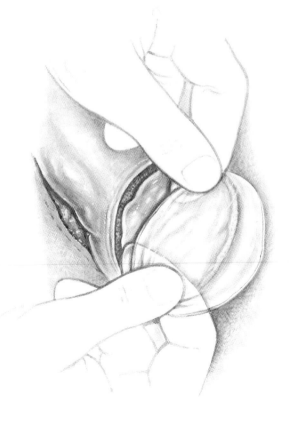

Figure 9. *(c) Optional application of a collagen net.*

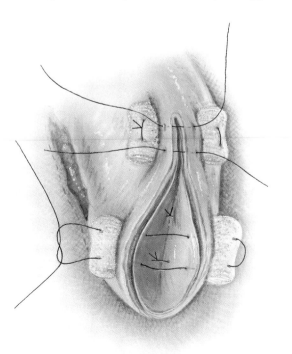

Figure 9. *(d) Adapting renal capsule sutures.*

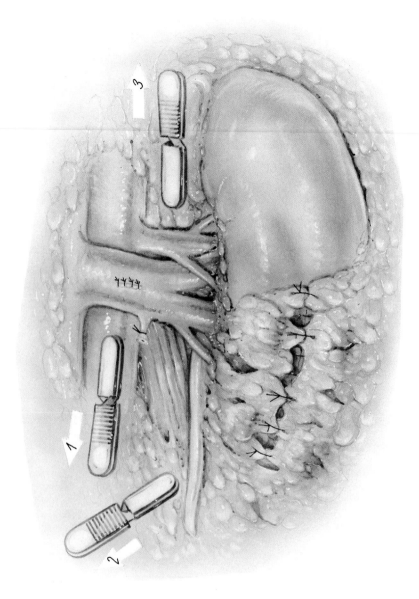

Figure 10. *Removal of the vessel clamps in the following order: vein, ureter, artery.*

Renal Exploration after Trauma

J.W. McAninch, P.R. Carroll
Department of Urology,
University of California School of Medicine,
San Francisco, USA

Introduction

The kidney is a well-protected organ, lying high in the retroperitoneum between the abdominal viscera and the back muscles. Because of this position the incidence of associated organ injury in patients with renal trauma is high. In patients with suspicion of renal trauma (gross hematuria, microscopic hematuria associated with shock) complete staging is required, including excretory urography, computed tomography and angiography.

Indications for exploration

Less than 10% of blunt renal trauma cases require operation; penetrating renal injury (knife or gunshot), on the other hand, requires exploration in up to 76% of cases.

Absolute indications
- Expanding upper retroperitoneal hematoma or pulsating hematoma indicating persistent bleeding (consistent with major parenchyma or renal vessel laceration)

Relative indications
- Urinary extravasation (laceration of the renal pelvis, from extension of parenchymal laceration into the renal collecting system or from avulsion of the ureteropelvic junction from the renal pelvis by blunt trauma; extravasation from a renal fornix without parenchymal or renal pelvic injury)

    Small degree of extravasation (intracapsular) often subside spontaneously. Extensive extravasation may also subside spontaneously, but requires careful monitoring because of the risk or urinoma. Patients with evidence of infection in the urine of the injured kidney require surgical drainage. Conservative therapy carries a risk of retroperitoneal fibrosis due to chemical irritation to local tissue by long contact with urine, and requires careful follow-up.

- Nonviable tissue

    Large areas of nonviable tissue associated with parenchymal laceration can lead to persistent extravasation and abscess formation as tissue necrosis occurs, requiring surgical intervention. Renal tissue that has partial viability along the margins of the injury can result in hypertension.

- Incomplete staging (in patients whose clinical condition demands that the abdomen be explored immediately by one-shot (large bolus) intravenous urography on the operating table; in poorly opacified kidneys where the extent of injury is indeterminate)

- Arterial thrombosis

Blunt renal trauma may result in a thrombosis of the renal artery or segmental branches resulting in infarction (after 12 hours the chance of salvage is remote). If diagnosis of main renal artery thrombosis is delayed, nephrectomy may be necessary when laparotomy is performed for other reasons; there is no need for immediate nephrectomy as the single indication for exploration. Nephrectomy may be necessary in the follow-up period if the kidney atrophies and hypertension develops.

Segmental renal artery thrombosis in the absence of parenchymal injury (intact renal capsule) requires careful follow-up. If it is associated with parenchymal injury and heavy bleeding, surgical exploration will be needed.

Operative technique step by step

- Midline transabdominal approach: ready access to the kidneys and exploration of the abdominal contents for associated injury

- Excessive renal bleeding: immediate renal exploration

- No severe renal bleeding: repair of injury to other organs

- Exposure of the retroperitoneum: lifting of the small bowel from the abdomen

- Retroperitoneal incision over the aorta just above the inferior mesenteric artery; in cases with large retroperitoneal hematoma (no easy identification of the aorta) incision medial to the inferior mesenteric vein, an important landmark

- Dissection through the hematoma to the aorta and then superiorly to the left renal vein, crossing the aorta anteriorly

- Preparation of the left and right renal artery and placement of vessel loops around both arteries and veins (Figure 2) – no clamping unless renal bleeding demands it

- Complete exposure of the kidney (identification of all injuries) (Figures 3 and 4); incision of the retroperitoneum lateral to the colon, entering the hematoma

- Cooling with ice slush if warm ischemia time exceeds 60 minutes

Debridement
- Removal of all nonviable tissue (Figure 5); active bleeding indicates viability even though the cut margin may look somewhat 'dusky'

- Preservation of the renal capsule (if possible) for later reconstruction

- Evaluation of all viable tissue after debridement: approximately 30% of one kidney will provide sufficient function to avoid dialysis

Hemostasis
- Ligation of blood vessels within the renal parenchyma (Figure 6) with 4/0 chromic sutures (monofilamentous and absorbable)

  Large veins coursing within the parenchyma may be ligated without worry because of the well-developed intrarenal collateral circulation. Segmental and intralobar artery ligation may result in distal parenchymal infarction.

- Application of hemostatic agents (e.g. absorbable collagen) to the cut surface aid in hemostasis

Collecting system closure
- Water-tight closure of the collecting system with a running 4/0 chromic suture

- Exclusion of extravasation: retrograde injection of methylene blue into the renal pelvis and careful inspection for leaks along the repair

Defect coverage
- Renal capsule: ideal to cover the cut parenchymal surface (mostly destroyed)

- Pedicle flap of omentum sutured to the parenchymal margins (Figure 7): excellent vascular and lymphatic supply

- Free grafts of peritoneum

Partial nephrectomy
- Control of the blood vessels and exposure of the complete kidney

- Partial nephrectomy if the upper or lower pole is extensively damaged

- Bleeding control: manual compression is often sufficient (no need to clamp the artery)

- Sharp removal of devitalized tissue, ligation of bleeding vessels and closure of the collecting system (4/0 chromic suture)

- Defect coverage: renal capsule or pedicle flap of omentum

Renorrhaphy
- Injury of the mid-portion of the kidney (Figure 8): removal of all nonviable tissue (if necessary down into the collecting system)

- Approximation of the parenchymal margins with interrupted absorbable 3/0 sutures placed through the capsule for strength, avoiding the parenchyma as much as possible (Figure 9)

- Tying of sutures over an absorbable gelatin sponge bolster (to add strength to the repair and provide hemostasis) (Figure 10)

- Large or multiple defects (approximation difficult): coverage by a pedicle flap of omentum

- Unstable coverage: placement of an absorbable mesh around the kidney

Vascular injuries (Figure 11)
- Injury to the main renal vein: clamping of the renal artery and renal vein (back flow from the vena cava); repair with 5/0 vascular sutures

- Injuries to segmental veins (usually lacerations): vessels ligation (there is no fear of renal damage)

Follow-up examination

- Functional data: renal scans

- Anatomic information: computed tomography and intravenous urography

Exploration of renal vessels and kidney

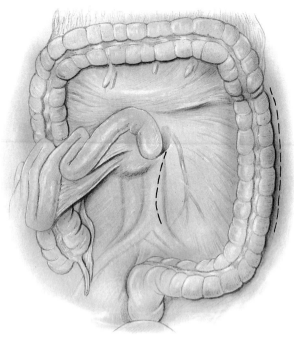

Figure 1. *Retroperitoneal incision over the aorta medial to the inferior mesenteric vein.*

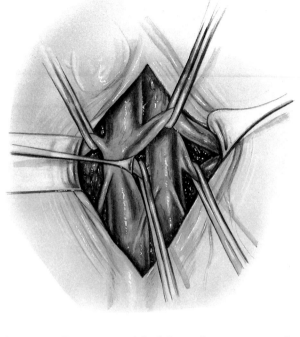

Figure 2. *Preparation of the left renal vein, crossing the aorta anteriorly, and both renal arteries, placing vessel loops around both renal veins and arteries.*

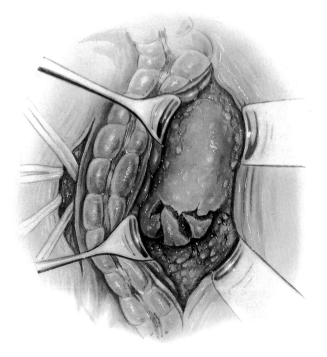

Figure 3. *Laterocolic incision of the peritoneum and exploration of the left kidney.*

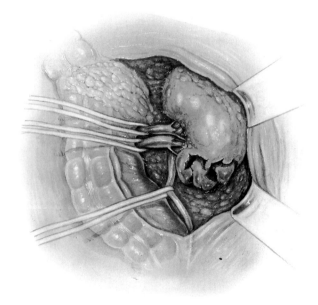

Figure 4. *Careful exploration of the complete kidney to discover all renal injuries.*

Renal polar injuries

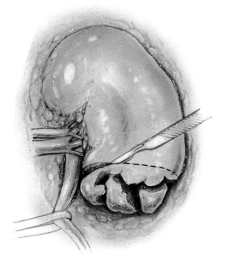

Figure 5. *Sharp removal of nonviable tissue.*

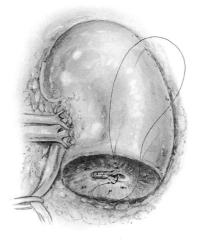

Figure 6. *Ligation of the bleeding vessels and closure of the collecting system.*

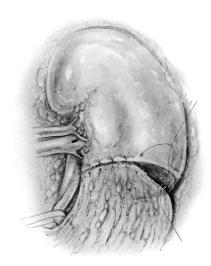

Figure 7. *Defect covered with omental pedicle flap.*

Injuries of the mid-portion

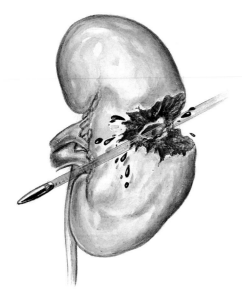

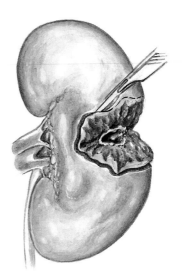

Figure 8. *Typical injury in the mid-portion of the kidney: debridement of all nonviable tissue. Bleeding margins indicate viable parenchyma.*

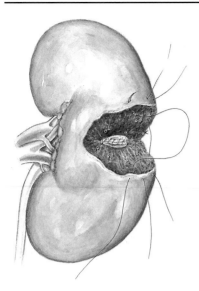

Figure 9. *Approximation of parenchymal margins (3/0 chromic sutures).*

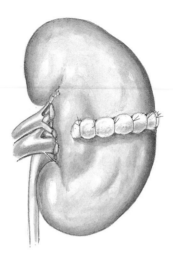

Figure 10. *Sutures are tied over a gelatin sponge bolster.*

Injuries of renal vessels

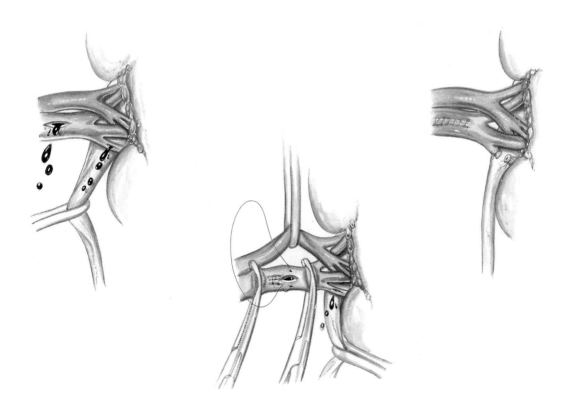

Figure 11. *Clamping of the renal artery and vein; closure of the main renal vein; ligation of segmental veins.*

Living Donor Nephrectomy

K. Tanabe, K. Takahashi, H. Toma
Department of Urology,
Kidney Center,
Tokyo Women's Medical College,
Tokyo, Japan

Introduction

Living donor nephrectomy is very different from the other nephrectomies such as radical nephrectomy. The two most important objectives of living donor nephrectomy are:

- To maintain good renal function
- To keep donors absolutely safe because they are *volunteering* to undergo a major surgical procedure

Indications

- The donor should have two kidneys
- Both kidneys should have normal function
- There should be no kidney disease (glomerulonephritis, polycystic kidney disease, etc.)
- The donor should have no active infectious disease
- The donor should have no active malignant disease

Preoperative examination

- Physical examination
- Laboratory assays: complete blood count, blood glucose level, liver function, serum electrolytes, transmissible disease (hepatitis, human immunodeficiency virus, human T-cell lymphotrophic virus 1, cytomegalovirus, syphilis)
- ECG, chest radiography, lung function tests
- Blood tests (creatinine, blood urea nitrogen), urinalysis (especially proteinuria, hematuria), urine culture, creatinine clearance
- Intravenous pyelography, ultrasonography of the kidneys, angiography (aortography or digital subtraction angiography)

Instruments

- Standard instruments for kidney and vessel operations

Operative technique step by step

Site of the kidney
- Usually the left kidney is used (it has a longer renal vein than the right and the vascular anastomosis is easier to transplant into the right iliac fossa)

- If there is some functional difference between the two kidneys, the better kidney should be left in the donor
- If one of the kidneys has multiple renal arteries, the kidney with a single artery or the smaller number of renal arteries should be removed

Approach to the kidney
- Transperitoneal or retroperitoneal approach: many surgeons prefer the retroperitoneal approach because of the lower incidence of intraperitoneal complications such as spleen injury
- Place the patient in the semilateral position at an angle of about 45° (Figure 1). This position gives better visualization of the great vessels and renal vessels than the complete lateral position
- Skin incision (Figure 2) starting with a posterior axillar incision over the 11th rib and toward the rectus muscle, extended by a pararectal incision up to 3–5 cm below the umbilical level to provide good visualization of the ureter. For good visualization of the upper pole of the kidney, the 11th rib (5–7 cm) is usually removed

Dissections of the ureter
- The ureter is dissected distally as near to the bladder as is feasible (Figure 3), but usually enough urethral length is obtained at the level of the iliac vessels. The most important point of this procedure is to keep the feeding vessels of the ureter intact. (I think the ureter should be dissected first because: the urine flow is then visible during later procedures that are harmful to kidney function, such as renal vessel dissection; it is easy to mobilize the kidney; and the kidney can be removed immediately if there are unexpected problems, such as major bleeding from vessels.)

Dissection of the kidney
- Start to dissect the kidney from the lower pole and extend the dissection toward the upper pole (Figure 4): this always gives very good direct visualization during the whole procedure. After dissection of the lower and middle pole, the kidney becomes more movable and can easily be pulled down to visualize the upper pole
- Gerota's fascia is removed by making an incision down to the kidney capsule and dissecting the areolar tissue adhesions of Gerota's capsule free from the underlying renal capsule (Figure 5). An assistant retracts the Gerota's fascia against the renal capsule, and the operator cuts the areolar tissue with an electric knife. (This method allows the surgeon to see the color and feel the tension of the

kidney, which reflect renal blood flow. Arterial spasm may occur during the dissection of vessels, and the change of color and consistency of the kidney will indicate this immediately.)

Dissection of renal vessels

- Dissection of the renal vessels should be started at the anterior surface of the renal vein because there are no tributaries

- On the left side, we usually divide the adrenal vein, gonadal vein and lumbar vein to reveal a sufficient length of renal vein (Figure 6). All tributaries should be dissected by suture-ligation. The color and consistency of the kidney and the urine output from the divided ureter should be monitored

- Drip mannitol during the vascular dissection and for 10 minutes after dissection to maintain good renal blood flow and prevent vascular spasms

- Small arterial branches (3 mm or more) in the upper pole may be sacrificed but in the lower pole the branches should be saved to feed the ureter

- When removing the kidney, we prefer to ligate the renal artery as close to the aorta as possible and then to place an arterial suture immediately distal to this point for additional hemostasis. If there are three renal arteries, the smallest should be divided first to reduce the possibility of tubular necrosis

- The renal vein is divided in the same way

Graft irrigation

- The removed kidney should be immersed in slushed ice as soon as possible and irrigated with appropriate solution

(e.g. Euro-Collins). It is most important to check for, and remove, any thrombus in the renal artery before irrigation; otherwise, the thrombus will be pushed into the renal artery by the irrigation solution and may cause renal infarction. Also take care not to injure the intima by cannulation

Reconstruction of renal vessels

- Large and small arteries: if there are two renal arteries, the smaller vessel should be anastomosed to the larger one (end-to-side anastomosis) (Figure 7)

- Two renal arteries of the same size: we usually use a conjoined anastomosis technique, spatulating the two arteries for about 5 mm and joining them to form one artery (Figure 8)

- For other difficult cases (Figures 9 and 10) the internal iliac artery of the recipient can be used

Skin closure

- After meticulous hemostasis of the kidney bed, the muscle and skin are closed in the usual manner

Complications

The most frequent complication is pneumothorax. After operation, we usually check by chest radiography.

Postoperative follow-up

Donors should be followed routinely. We see them at 1 month, 3 months, 6 months, 1 year, and every year thereafter.

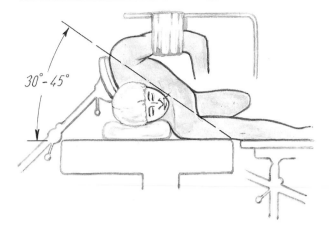

Figure 1. *The semilateral position with an angle of about 45°.*

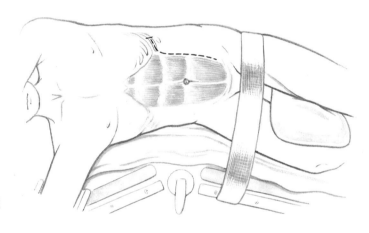

Figure 2. *Skin incision: a posterior axillar line over the 11th rib and toward the rectus muscle, and a pararectal incision up to 3–5 cm below the umbilical level to provide good visualization of the ureter. To achieve good visualization of the upper pole of the kidney, the 11th rib (5–7 cm) is usually removed.*

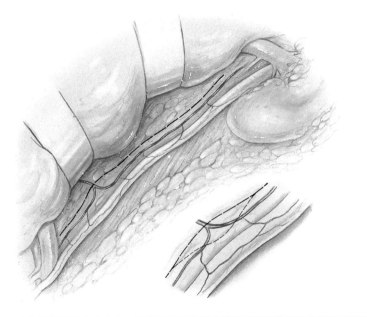

Figure 3. *It is most important to keep the vessels feeding the ureter intact. For this purpose, vessels feeding the ureter from the iliac artery should be severed close to the iliac vessels, to avoid cutting the ureteral feeding arcade from the renal hilum.*

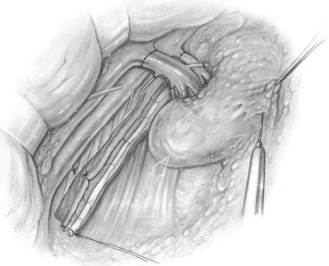

Figure 4. *Dissection of the kidney starts from the lower pole and extends toward the upper pole. This direction always gives very good direct visualization during the whole procedure.*

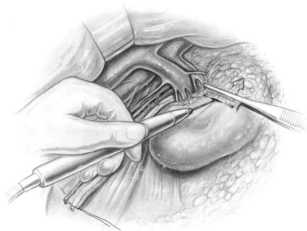

Figure 5. *Gerota's fascia is removed by making an incision down to the kidney capsule and dissecting the areolar tissue adhesions of Gerota's capsule free from the underlying renal capsule.*

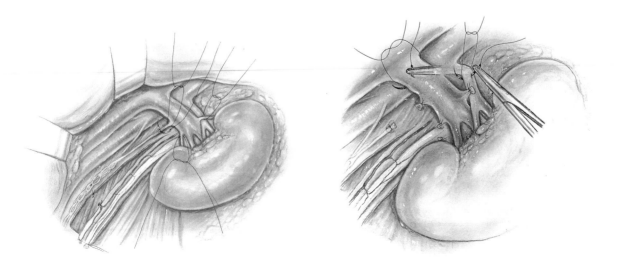

Figure 6. *Division of the adrenal vein, gonadal vein and lumbar vein. All tributaries should be dissected by suture-ligation, because ligation with clips could dislocate and may cause massive bleeding. After dissection of the vein, the renal artery can be identified and easily dissected as close to the aorta as possible. The renal vein is divided in the same way.*

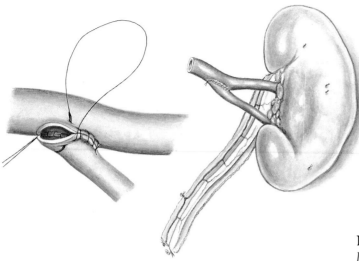

Figure 7. *End-to-side anastomosis of a small renal artery to a larger one.*

Figure 8. *Conjoined anastomosis of two renal arteries of the same size. The arteries are spatulated for about 5 mm and joined to form one artery.* ▶

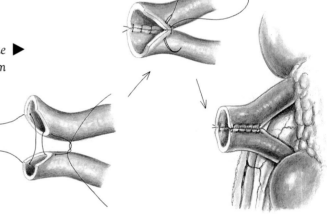

Figure 9. *End-to-end and end-to-side anastomosis to the recipient's hypogastric artery. When the long renal artery cannot be used for some reason and the lower pole small branch has to be saved, the donor's hypogastric artery can be used for extension of the main renal artery and side-to-end anastomosis of a small branch.*

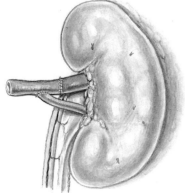

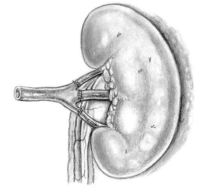

Figure 10. *Reconstruction of multiple short renal arteries: the hypogastric artery usually has three or four branches, which can be used for anastomosis of multiple short renal arteries.*

Cadaver Donor Nephrectomy

J. Leissner[a], J. Fichtner, M. Stöckle
Department of Urology,
University of Mainz School of Medicine,
Mainz, Germany
[a]University of Kiel, Kiel, Germany

Introduction

Cadaver donor nephrectomy can be performed either in isolation or as part of multiple organ recovery. A completed diagnostic procedure for brain death is obviously a prerequisite. Brain death is defined as an irreversible loss of brain function while artificial respiration maintains vital parameters. Legal requirements vary from country to country: in Germany, two physicians, independent of the transplantation team, must confirm the brain death clinically and with additional imaging and neurophysiologic methods. Additionally, the consent of the patient (e.g. by donor card) or the relatives is necessary.

In addition, the donor kidney must fulfill the following criteria:

- Absence of vascular or autoimmune kidney disease

- Absence of potentially transmittable disease

- Absence of bacterial kidney infections, which may occur after long-term bladder catheterization or central venous catheterization

- Normal kidney function (no kidney failure or crash kidney); an elevated serum creatinine level is acceptable provided there is evidence of prerenal failure (e.g. lack of intravenous fluid)

- Angiography of the renal vessels is not necessary, and is contraindicated because high-dose contrast medium and intimal lesions after intubation of the renal arteries may cause renal failure

Instruments

- Modified balloon catheter with blind ending tip and several outlets between the base of the catheter and the balloon

- Iced protective solution: Euro-Collins (EC) solution, University of Wisconsin (UW) solution, or histidine–tryptophan–ketoglutarate (HTK) solution

- A second sterile area with iced sodium chloride or Ringer's lactate solution

- Sterile plastic bags for kidney transportation

Operative technique step by step

Bilateral nephrectomy of isolated kidneys has largely been replaced by a careful *en bloc* technique, in which both kidneys with the great vessels will be removed. The latter approach has fewer complications and a higher success rate and, as the preferred technique, is described here.[1,2]

- Exposure: xiphoid-to-pubis midline incision with extension laterally until both axillary lines (Figure 1). The 'rectangles' of the wound are sutured to both iliac crests and the chest wall; retractors are therefore dispensable

- Evisceration: incision of the peritoneal attachments of the right colon, small bowel mesentery and distal duodenum at the ligament of Treitz for cephalad mobilization of the small bowel and right colon as described previously.[3] Keep the intestine on the chest wall. Ligation and dividing of the inferior mesenteric vessels in left colonic mesentery. Cephalad dissection of the ascending colon, small bowel, proximal duodenum and pancreas

- Dissect both ureters at the level of the crossing iliac vessels; sling the ureters with vessel loops. The left ureter can be dissected from either lateral of the left colon, which is advantageous in obese patients, or medial to the left colon. Preserve the mesoureter as it contains the blood supply for the ureter. Failure to do so risks the possibility of ischemic necrosis and urinary extravasation after renal transplantation

  Trick: do not divide the ureters before finishing the *en bloc* preparation. This prevents involuntary ureter lesions and eases preparation; otherwise, large amounts of urine may spill down the abdomen (e.g. in the polyuric phase of kidney failure).

  Dissect and sling the aorta twice with heavy ligatures just above the bifurcation, and slit between ligatures for catheter insertion (or sling the distal aorta and both iliac arteries and slit directly in the bifurcation).

  Ligate and divide both testicular or ovarian arteries, the superior mesenteric artery and the celiac trunk close to the aorta. Sling two ligatures at the proximal aorta just under the diaphragm (Figure 2).

- Ligate and divide the right gonadal vein. Sling two ligations each around the proximal and caudal vena cava

- Insert the modified balloon catheter retrogradely into the aorta via the aortotomy. Inflate the balloon to occlude the aorta above the level of the renal arteries. All catheter outlets must be inside the aortic lumen (Figure 3). Ligate and divide the distal aorta; the upper distal ligation secures the catheter. At this time the iced protective solution, hanging on an intravenous stand, should be connected to the catheter. Continue perfusion until both kidneys are pale and cold: usually 1.5–2 L are necessary

  Ligate but do not divide the proximal aorta, because this often damages the catheter and leads to ineffective perfusion.

Three kinds of protective solution are available. We use EC solution for isolated donor nephrectomy; UW and HTK solutions are favored for multiple organ recovery.[4,5]

Alternatively, the balloon catheter can be inserted from above the renal arteries and inflated in the lower aorta (usually during multiple organ recovery).

• Tie the ligatures at the proximal and distal vena cava. An ordinary noninflated catheter incorporated in the lower ligation may serve for the solution to run off (Figure 4).

• Incise Gerota's fascia ventrally and separate the kidneys with or without the adrenal glands. Surrounding fatty tissue must be preserved from both the kidney and the ureter. Dissection of renal vessels is not necessary; atypic pole arteries should be preserved.

Sharp cephalad dissection of the great vessels is carried out up to the level of the diaphragm. Lumbar veins may be divided without ligation; lumbar branches of the aorta should be clipped for effective ongoing perfusion (Figure 5). Complete the bilateral nephrectomy by dividing both ureters if this has not been done before.

• Remove the mesenteric lymph nodes and spleen for tissue typing and histocompatibility studies. Close the incisions in one layer with heavy interrupted sutures.

• Simultaneous dissect the *en bloc* specimen in a second sterile area. Cold sodium chloride or Ringer's lactate and EC solution are useful. To prevent icy necrosis, avoid direct contact of the tissue with icy fluid or metal (Figure 6). Divide the vena cava lengthwise ventral and dorsal, paying attention to the right renal vein as it is typically significantly shorter than the left. Dissect the left renal vein and place it, together with the vena cava patch, beside the left kidney. Divide the aorta and remove the catheter. Create patches of at least 1 cm for both renal arteries and veins, separating them from the great vessels (Figure 7). Finally, ligate the adrenal vessels and gonadal veins.

Further dissection should be done by the transplantation team according to their specific technique.

Insert the completely dissected and separated kidneys in sterile bags, marking the side of origin.

References

1. Pichlmayr RC, Brölsch CE. Auswahlkriterien und Voruntersuchungen beim potentiellen Organspender. In: Pichlmayr R (ed.) *Transplantationschirurgie*, Vol. III, Berlin: Springer-Verlag (1981) 467–77.
2. Tidow, G, Pichlmayr R. Nierenentnahme beim Spender. In: Pichlmayr R (ed.) *Transplantationschirurgie*, Vol. III, Berlin: Springer-Verlag (1981) 483–92.
3. Steinbach F, Stöckle M, Stein R, Hohenfellner R. Zugangswege für abdominale und pelvine Eingriffe: Mobilisation von Peritoneum und Intestinum. In: Hohenfellner R (ed.) *Ausgewählte urologische OP-Techniken*, Stuttgart: Georg Thieme (1994) 5.1–5.8.
4. Belzer FO, Southard JH. Principles of solid-organ preservation by cold storage. *Transplantation* **45** (1988) 673–6.
5. Hölscher M, Groenewoud AF. Current status of the HTK solution of Bretschneider in organ preservation. *Transplant Proc* **23** (1991) 2334–7.

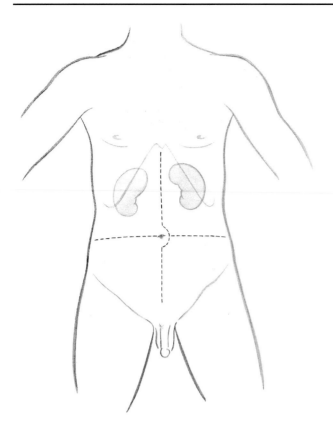

Figure 1. *Xiphoid-to pubis midline incision with extension laterally to both axillary lines.*

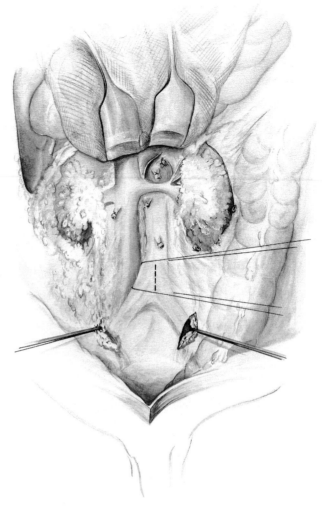

Figure 2. *Dissection and cephalad mobilization of intra-abdominal organs. The following tributaries to the aorta and vena cava are ligated and divided: the celiac trunk, the superior mesenteric artery, the right gonadal vein and artery and the inferior mesenteric vein and artery. Dissection of the left kidney after ligation of the inferior mesenteric vessels and mobilization of the left colon. The aortotomy at the distal aorta is marked. Dissection of both ureters to the level of the crossing of the iliac vessels (the left ureter may be dissected from laterocolic in obese patients).*

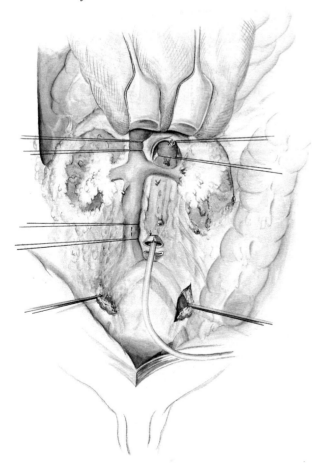

Figure 3. *Insertion of a modified balloon catheter retrogradely via the aortotomy; the inflated balloon occludes the aorta proximal to the renal arteries. Venotomy for insertion of an ordinary catheter to collect the perfusion medium.*

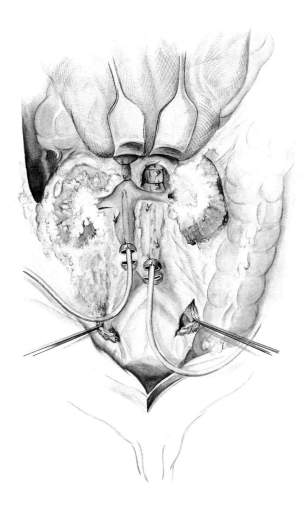

Figure 4. In situ *perfusion of both kidneys with cold protective solution (1.5–2 L). Incision of Gerota's fascia and dissection of both kidneys. Do **not** free the kidneys from the surrounding fatty tissue.*

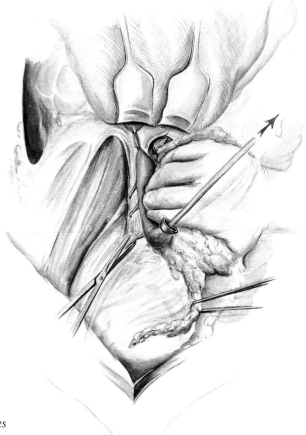

Figure 5. *After mobilization of both kidneys, the lumbar branches are divided and the great vessels are cut off directly in front of the spine. Complete en bloc nephrectomy by cranial dividing of aorta and vena cava.*

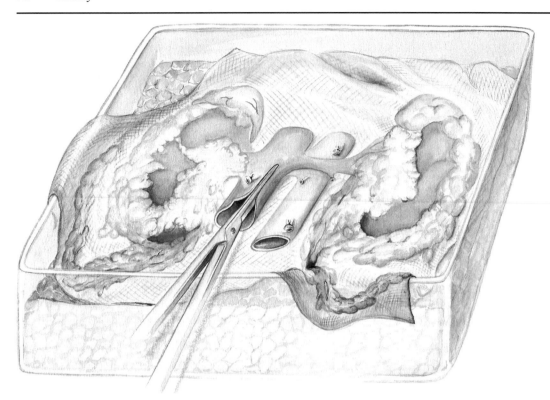

Figure 6. *In a second sterile area for further preparation of the removed kidneys, the kidneys are separated by dividing the aorta and vena cava lengthwise.*

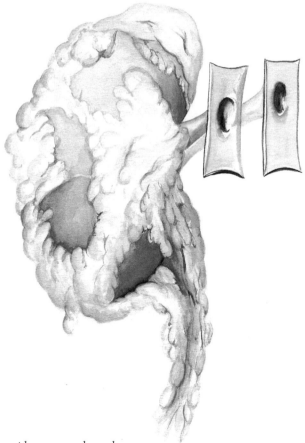

Figure 7. *Completely dissected right kidney with ureter and renal vessels. The surrounding fatty tissue and mesoureter are preserved.*

Kidney Transplantation

K. Tanabe, K. Takahashi, H. Toma
Department of Urology,
Kidney Center,
Tokyo Women's Medical College,
Tokyo, Japan

Introduction

Kidney transplantation to the iliac fossa has the following advantages over orthotopic kidney transplantation:

- Easier operative technique
- Better approach to the transplanted kidney for biopsy, nephrostomy, etc.

Patient selection

- End-stage renal disease
- The recipient should have no active infection
- The recipient should have no active malignancy
- The donor should not have lymphocytotoxic antibodies to donor (T cells)
- The recipient should have no psychosocial problems: after surgery patients need to take long-term immunosuppressive medication, and many patients lose their allograft because of noncompliance
- The recipient should have no active gastrointestinal ulcer; steroids may exacerbate the condition

Preoperative preparation and examination

- Physical examination
- Laboratory assays: complete blood count, urinalysis, urine culture, renal function (creatinine, blood urea nitrogen), blood glucose level, liver function, serum electrolytes, hepatitis, human immunodeficiency virus, human T-cell lymphotrophic virus 1, syphilis, ECG, chest, radiography, lung function tests
- Gastroscopy; control of peptic ulcer if present
- Treatment of dental caries
- Immunologic examination: human lymphocyte antigen (HLA) typing (include DNA typing), lymphocyte cross-match
- VCUG
- Sonography or computed tomography of native kidneys
- Preoperative dialysis in the recipient heparin must be inactivated by protamine
- In an anemic patient, blood transfusion to raise the hematocrit level to 30%

Operative technique step by step

- Oblique or curvilinear skin incision in the right lower quadrant of the abdomen (Figure 1)
- Pararectal incision of the muscle fascia and ligature of the inferior epigastric vessels
- Dissection of the iliac vessels from external iliac vein, from the inguinal ligament to the origin of the internal iliac artery (Figure 2). We do not usually divide the internal iliac vein but, if the kidney is to be located in the right retroperitoneal space rather than the iliac fossa, we divide the internal iliac vein to achieve better mobility
- Venous branches should be double ligated because veins may have high pressure due to vascular clamping during blood vessel anastomosis
- For adults, only the internal iliac artery is dissected because the kidney will be located in the iliac fossa, and so the artery does not need to rotate around the external artery (Figure 3). In a small pelvis (children), or if the kidney should be placed in the retroperitoneal space, the external iliac artery should also be dissected to avoid kinking

Workbench surgery
- The renal vein and artery are dissected free of the connective tissue or fat; the edges of damaged vessels should be removed
- Leakage test: the renal vein is closed with a small vascular clamp, and irrigation solution is instilled through the renal artery (Figure 4). Leakage points should be ligated to prevent bleeding

Renal vein anastomosis
- Total occlusion of the external iliac vein with DeBakey's clamp (Figure 5). The iliac vein (anastomosis site) is picked up with forceps, and an ellipse is cut from the iliac vein equal in length to the diameter of the renal vein. The lumen of the iliac vein is flushed with heparinized saline
- Three stay sutures (5/0 monofilament nylon or Prolene (Ethicon, Edinburgh, UK)) are placed, one at each angle and one at the middle of the posterior wall, thereby triangulating the venous anastomosis opening and preventing suture of the two walls together

- Starting with the inferior stay suture, the external wall of the venous anastomosis is completed with continuous over-and-over sutures, everting the edge. Then, reflecting the kidney laterally, the median wall anastomosis is completed (Figure 6)

Renal artery anastomosis

- End-to-end anastomosis of the renal artery with the internal iliac artery

- Ligation of the distal end of the internal iliac artery

- Application of a bulldog clamp to the origin of the hypogastric artery

- Division of the hypogastric artery at the distal end

- Placement of stay sutures on the anterior and posterior walls

- Completion of the anastomosis with a running suture (Figures 7 and 8)

Ureterovesicostomy

- Ureterovesicostomy is carried out after adequate hemostasis of suture lines in a modified Paquin technique. The anterior wall of the bladder is opened a little lateral to the midline. A retractor is placed into the bladder to expose the trigonal area and the mucosa adjacent to the ureteral orifice. From outside the bladder, a submucosal tunnel is created by a right-angle hemostat (Figure 11)

- The upper aspect of the ureter is incised longitudinally for about 1 cm. The proximal edge of the longitudinal incision is fixed with 5/0 catgut using the full thickness of the ureter and the bladder mucosa (Figure 12)

- Both sides of the distal end of the ureter are fixed using the full thickness of the ureter and the bladder musculature. Then an additional two or three stitches between the stay sutures are added through the full thickness of the ureter and the bladder mucosa (Figure 13)

- The cystostomy is closed using continuous 4/0 plain catgut sutures of the mucosa and muscularis to produce a water-tight closure, including enough tissue to prevent pressure necrosis. Then, using 3/0 chromic catgut, interrupted sutures are placed in the muscularis and perivesical fat

Alternative extravesical ureteroneostomy (Figure 14): the bladder is filled with saline through the urethral catheter, and the bladder muscle incised over 3 cm near the dome on the anterolateral wall. The mucosa bulges forward and an incision 1 cm in length is made in the mucosa at the distal end of the muscle incision. The ureter is spatulated over 1 cm and is anastomosed to the opening of the mucosa with a single suture of 5/0 chromic catgut or interrupted sutures of 4/0 chromic catgut. The ureter is tacked to the bladder at the distal end of the incision through the full thickness of the bladder wall

- The muscle is reapproximated to form a valve mechanism by interrupted 4/0 chromic catgut sutures over 2.5 cm in length, care being taken not to obstruct the ureter

- A cystostomy is created and a bladder catheter is inserted

Postoperative care

- Catheter and cystostomy removal after 1 week

- Follow-up

Surgical tricks

- A pararectal incision of the muscle layer causes less pain and less bleeding than a regular Gibson's incision

- Venous branches should be double ligated because veins may be subjected to high pressure due to vascular clamping during blood vessel anastomosis

- When the pelvis is small (in children) and the graft must be placed in the retroperitoneal space, the external artery should also be dissected to achieve good rotation; otherwise, the artery may be kinked. The internal iliac vein can also be cut to achieve better mobility

- Cadaveric donor kidneys are particularly prone to vascular injury during organ harvesting. For the leakage test, the renal vein is closed with a small vascular clamp and irrigation solution is instilled through the renal artery. Any leakage points should be closed

- If the hypogastric artery is not suitable for anastomosis (because of atherosclerosis, etc.), end-to-side anastomosis should be performed between the renal artery and the external or common iliac artery

- If the recipient is a child, interrupted suture is employed instead of continuous over-and-over suture because the vessel diameter should grow as the patient grows

- The muscular layer of the bladder should be opened adequately to prevent stenosis during ureterovesicostomy

Pediatric recipients

For older children the transplant procedure is the same as for adults if their weight is more than 20 kg. In smaller children, we employ an extraperitoneal approach. The skin incision is carried out up to the costal margin, and the great vessels are approached extraperitoneally (Figure 9). This approach has many advantages: fewer intra-abdominal complications, a less invasive procedure, easy access for graft biopsy, and easy observation by ultrasonography.

The vena cava is dissected over 3–4 cm, ligating and dividing two or three lumbar veins posteriorly. The aorta is dissected in the same manner. Then, using a total occluding clamp to isolate the vena cava, an end-to-side technique with sutures of 5/0 monofilament Prolene is used to anastomose the renal vein. The renal artery is then similarly anastomosed to the aorta (Figure 10). We sometimes anastomose the renal artery around the bifurcation of the aorta, depending on the recipient's size. The renal artery is usually brought in front of the vena cava. Careful observation of the recipient's hemodynamic response on declamping the great vessels is essential.

References

1. Hume DM, Magee JH, Kaufmann HM, Rittenburg MS, Prout GR. Renal homotransplantation in man in modified recipients. *Ann Surg* **158** (1963) 608–44.
2. Starzl TE, Marchioro TL, Morgan WW, Waddell WR. A technique for use of adult renal homografts in children. *Surg Gynecol Obst* **119** (1964) 106–8.
3. Robson AJ, Calne RY. Complication of urinary drainage following renal transplantation. *Br J Urol* **43** (1971) 586–90.

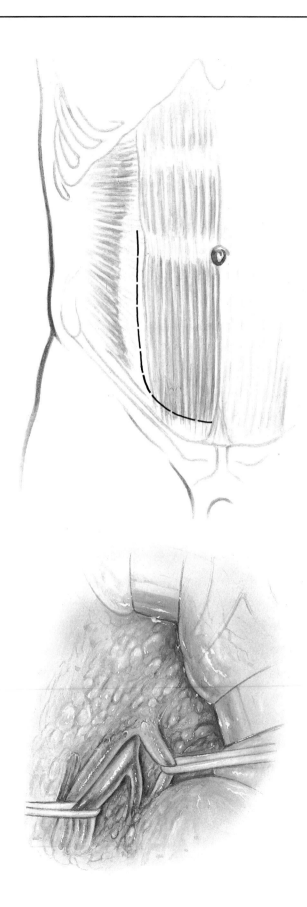

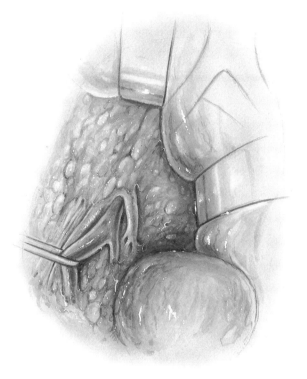

Figure 1. *Incision of the muscle layer: the pelvic space is approached through the pararectal incision sparing the rectus muscle.*

Figure 2. *The external iliac vein dissected from the inguinal ligament to the origin of the internal iliac artery, usually without division of the internal iliac vein. (If the kidney is to be located in the right retroperitoneal space rather than the iliac fossa, we divide the internal iliac vein to achieve better mobility.)*

Figure 3. *For adults we usually dissect only the internal iliac artery because the kidney will be located in the iliac fossa.*

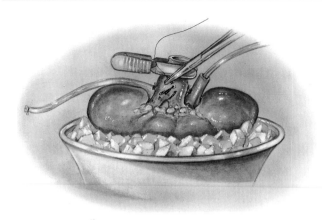

Figure 4. *The renal vein is closed with a small vascular clamp, and irrigation solution is instilled through the renal artery. Leakage points should be closed before transplantation.*

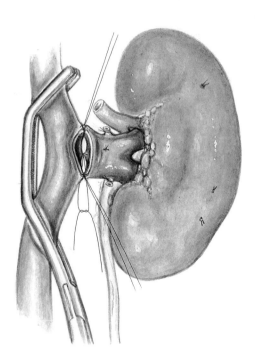

Figure 5. *Total occlusion of the external iliac vein with DeBakey's clamp. The iliac vein is picked up with forceps, and an ellipse is cut from the iliac vein equal in length to the diameter of the renal vein. The lumen of the renal vein is flushed with heparinized saline. Using 5/0 monofilament nylon or Prolene, three stay sutures are placed, one at each angle and one at the middle of the posterior wall, thereby triangulating the venous anastomosis opening and preventing suture of the two walls together.*

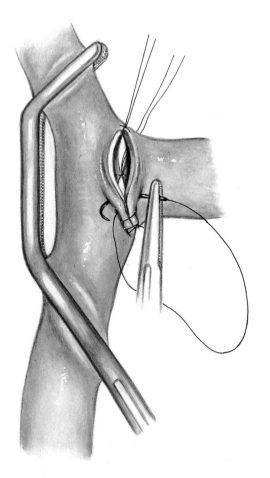

Figure 6. *Starting with the inferior stay suture, the external wall of the venous anastomosis is completed with continuous over-and-over sutures, everting the edge. Then, reflecting the kidney laterally, the median wall anastomosis is completed.*

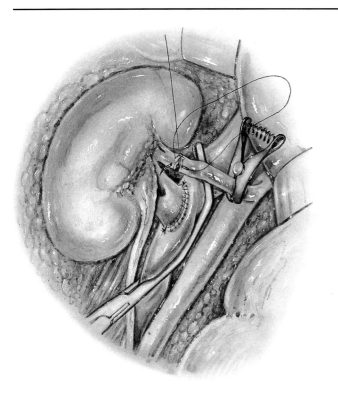

Figure 7. *The most common arterial anastomosis is an end-to-end anastomosis. After ligation of the distal end of the internal iliac artery, a bulldog clamp is applied to the origin of the hypogastric artery and the hypogastric artery divided. Stay sutures should be placed on the anterior and posterior walls, and anastomosis is completed with a continuous over-and-over suture.*

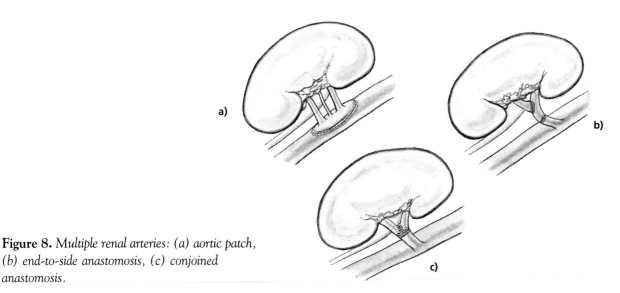

Figure 8. *Multiple renal arteries: (a) aortic patch, (b) end-to-side anastomosis, (c) conjoined anastomosis.*

Kidney transplantation in children

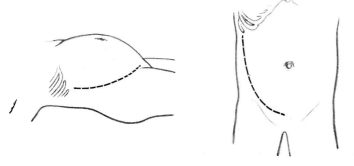

Figure 9. *In children, the skin incision is carried up to the costal margin and the great vessels are approached extraperitoneally.*

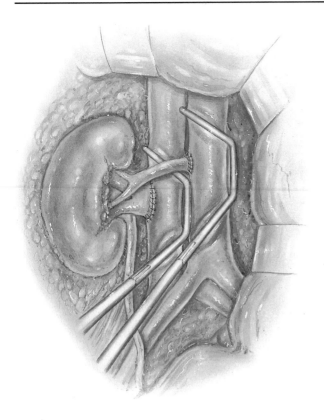

Figure 10. *Vascular anastomosis in pediatric recipients: end-to-side anastomosis to the inferior vena cava and aorta. The vena cava is dissected over 3–4 cm, ligating and dividing two or three lumbar veins posteriorly. The aorta is dissected in the same manner. Then, using a total occluding clamp to isolate the vena cava, and end-to-side technique with sutures of 5/0 monofilament Prolene is used to anastomose the renal vein. The renal artery is then anastomosed to the aorta in a similar fashion. The renal artery is usually brought in front of the vena cava.*

Intravesical ureteroneocystostomy

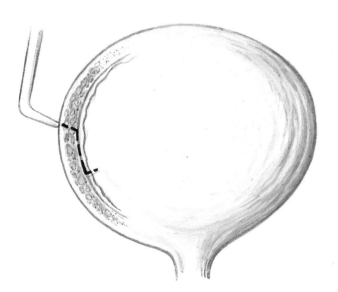

Figure 11. *From outside the bladder, a submucosal tunnel will be created bluntly by right-angle hemostat.*

Figure 12. *The upper aspect of the ureter is incised longitudinally about 1cm. The proximal edge of the longitudinal incision is fixed with 5/0 catgut using the full thickness of the ureter and the bladder mucosa. Both sides of the distal end of the ureter are fixed using the full thickness of the ureter and the bladder musculature. The distal-end sutures are very important in firmly fixing the ureter to the bladder.*
▼

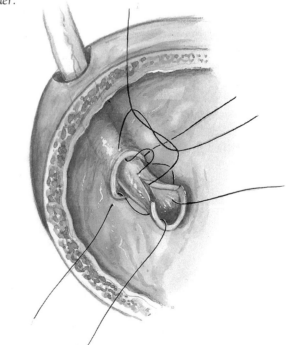

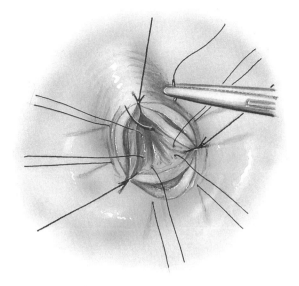

Figure 13. *An additional two or three stitches between the stay sutures have been inserted through the full thickness of the ureter and bladder mucosa.*

Extravesical ureteroneocystostomy

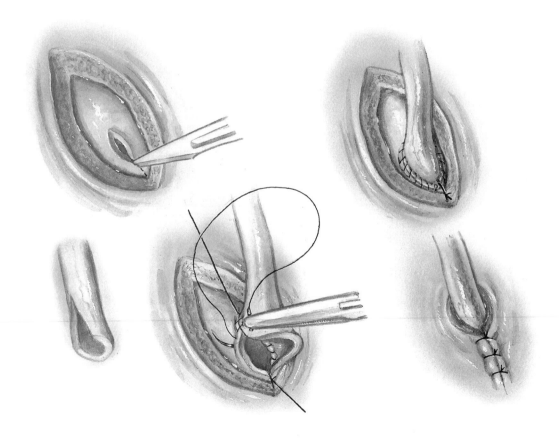

Figure 14. *Extravesical ureteroneocystostomy. The bladder is distended with saline through the urethral catheter. The bladder muscle is incised over 3 cm near the dome on the anterolateral wall. The mucosa bulges forward and an incision 1 cm in length is made in the mucosa at the distal end of the muscle incision. The ureter is spatulated over 1 cm and this is anastomosed to the opening of the mucosa with a single over-and-over suture of 5/0 chromic catgut or interrupted sutures of 4/0 chromic catgut. The ureter is tacked to the bladder at the distal end of the incision through the full thickness of the bladder wall. The muscle is reapproximated to form a valve mechanism by interrupted 4/0 chromic catgut sutures over 2.5 cm in length, care being taken not to obstruct the ureter.*

Nephroureterectomy with Transurethral Ureteral Stripping

S. Roth, H. van Ahlen,
A. Semjonow, L. Hertle
Department of Urology,
University of Münster,
Münster, Germany

Introduction

Nephroureterectomy with complete removal of the ureter is occasionally the treatment of choice for benign kidney disorders such as reflux nephropathy, but is usually the treatment of choice for transitional cell carcinoma of the upper urinary tract. The usual operative technique for open ureterectomy is either a single incision extending from the flank to the ipsilateral lower abdominal quadrant, or two separate smaller incisions, one lumbar and the other lower-abdominal. However, in open distal ureterectomy it is sometimes difficult both to sufficiently expose the distal ureter and to excise the surrounding bladder mucosa, especially in obese patients.

In 1910, Suter[1] and subsequently other urologists[2–4] advocated removal of the ureter using a transvesical approach with intussusception of the ureter into the bladder through insertion of a sutured ureteral catheter during nephrectomy. The idea of total nephroureterectomy without a second skin incision or extensive lumboabdominal wound was first described by H.P. McDonald[5] in 1952. As a first step for subsequent nephroureterectomy via a single flank incision, he proposed transurethral disconnection of the intramural ureter. In 1953, D.F. McDonald became the first urologist to use single-incision nephroureterectomy with ureteral intussusception and transurethral ureteral stripping of the distal ureter.[6] After attachment of the previously inserted ureteral catheter the distal ureter was mobilized as far distally as possible. For this mobilization, D.F. McDonald used a 'Mayo vein stripper'. After suturing of the flank incision the ureter was invaginated into the bladder via traction on the ureteral catheter and then disconnected from the bladder near the ureteral meatus. All later publications and modifications,[1,7,8] including ours, are based on McDonald's basic idea.

To obtain a sufficiently large diameter for invagination, it is necessary to dilate the proximal end of the ureteral stump. In the first two patients on whom we tried this technique the ureteral catheter dislodged without invagination. This gave us the idea for the proposed modification. Traction on a ureteral catheter which had previously been attached to the ureteral stump by means of a kinked ureteral catheter produces ureteral compression. However, this procedure failed in two patients. In one patient on whom this technique was attempted, a dislodgment of the ureteral catheter occurred because the kinked ureteral catheter was not sufficiently ligated to the ureteral stump (see Surgical tricks). In another patient, the ureter was not sufficiently mobilized and the ureteral stripping was incomplete. In both patients we performed open ureterectomy. The last six procedures with transurethral ureteral stripping were performed without difficulty. Whether or not our 'compression' technique is superior to the 'invagination' technique is an open question, which can only be resolved through further experience.

Indications

- Transitional cell carcinoma of the renal pelvis or the proximal ureter
- Atrophic kidney with vesicorenal reflux

Contraindications

- Immobilization of the pelvic ureter due either to an inflammatory process or to prior surgery
- Known or suspected malignant disease in the distal ureter

Instruments

- 5 Fr ureteral catheter (with curved olive tip) with stylet
- Transurethral resectoscope with a Turner-Warwick loop
- Standard instruments for extraperitoneal nephrectomy via a flank incision

Exposure

- Transurethral insertion of the ureteral catheter
- Flank incision for extraperitoneal nephrectomy

Operative technique step by step

- Insertion of a 5 Fr ureteral catheter with curved olive tip halfway up the length of the ureter on the affected side. Alternatively, a ureteral catheter with a Chevassu pattern can be used. It is important to note that, to give the catheter added strength during traction, the stylet should be left in place or reintroduced after positioning of the catheter.

- After placement of a 16–18 Fr Foley catheter in the bladder adjacent to the ureteral catheter, the ureteral catheter is sutured to the indwelling catheter.

- Extraperitoneal nephrectomy is performed via a flank incision (Figure 1). After division of the renal pedicle, the ureter is dissected and the ureteral catheter is pulled distally by the first assistant. To minimize the amount of ureteral tissue that needs to be transurethrally stripped, the ureter should be divided as distally as possible. This point is usually 3–5 cm above the iliac vessels, but can vary depending on the length of the flank incision. The proximal ureter is ligated just cephalad to the catheter tip to prevent escape of infected material or tumor cells during the subsequent removal of the kidney and proximal ureter. After ligation, a small cotton pad is wrapped around the ureter to absorb any intraluminal fluid extravasated during ureteral transection with scissors. This transection is performed just below the ligation and, to decrease the risk of tumor spillage, both ends of the transected ureter are subsequently cauterized.

- To attach the distal ureter to the ureteral catheter, the ureter is pushed downwards so that the tip of the catheter projects 2 cm beyond the severed section. Subsequently, the tip of the catheter is kinked and the kinked tip ligated to the ureter with 3/0 polypropylene sutures, which can be passed through the eyes of the catheter, thus closing the severed ureter. Once this has been accomplished, the previously placed cotton pad can be safely removed. We find it of critical importance that the kinked tip be at least 2 cm in length to prevent it from being dislodged and straightening during stripping.

- Before suturing of the flank incision, it is crucial that the distal ureter be mobilized as far distally as possible and that any tissue connections to the ureter near the iliac vessels be severed.

- This enables the first assistant to safely carry out ureteral compression by gentle traction on the ureteral catheter without risk of injury to the iliac vessels. This also allows for ureteral compression under direct visual surveillance down to the point just below the common iliac vessels.

- After closure of the nephrectomy incision, the patient is again placed in the dorsal lithotomy position. A 24 Fr resectoscope with a Turner-Warwick loop is introduced directly adjacent to the ureteral catheter.

- By means of gentle traction on the ureteral catheter, the previously compressed ureter is pulled against the trigonal bladder wall, thereby causing the bladder to protrude near the orifice. To disconnect the ureter from the bladder wall, the first cuts with the Turner-Warwick loop are made around the ureteral meatus, and 1 cm distant from it, incising the intramural tract until perivesical fat becomes visible around the resected ureter.

- Any bleeding that occurs subsequent to transurethral removal of the ureter can be controlled by means of the coagulating current. During this procedure, care should be taken not to unduly distend the bladder. By thus maintaining a low intravesical pressure, extravasation of irrigating fluid through the resected hole in the bladder is kept to a minimum. Finally, a 20 Fr Foley catheter is inserted into the bladder and the correct catheter position fluoroscopically visualized. The catheter is removed on postoperative day 3–5, after cystography to confirm closure of the hole in the bladder.

Surgical tricks

- Dislodgment and straightening of the ureteral catheter during stripping can be avoided through the use of a double ligature applied to the 2 cm of kinked ureteral catheter (Figure 2b).

- When inserting the Foley catheter at the end of the operation, the surgeon must ensure that the catheter does not accidentally enter the perivesical space through the hole in the bladder wall. The tip of the catheter should be turned to the nonaffected side. The position of the catheter tip can be either fluoroscopically visualized or monitored through low-pressure intermittent bladder irrigation, because the same amount of instilled fluid will always flow out again.

Postoperative care

The catheter is removed on day 3–5 after operation, after cystography to confirm closure of the hole in the bladder. In all cases, the Foley catheter is removed by day 5 if the cystography shows no sign of extravasation.

Acknowledgments

The authors would like to thank Robert Nusbaum for help in writing and Angela Haas for providing the drawings.

References

1. Bub P, Rassweiler J, Eisenberger F. Harnleiterstripping nach transurethraler Ostiumschneidung: eine Alternative zur Ureterektomie. *Akt Urol* **20** (1989) 67–9.
2. Howerton LW, Lich R, Jr, Goode LS, Amin M. Transvesical ureterectomy. *J Urol* **104** (1970) 817–20.
3. Johnson DE, Babaian RJ. Transvesical intussusception (Lich) ureterectomy. *Urology* **13** (1979) 522–4.
4. Mason T. Transvesical removal of diseased ureteral stump. *Surg Gynecol Obstet* **104** (1957) 238.
5. McDonald HP, Upchurch WE, Sturdevant CE. Nephroureterectomy: a new technique. *J Urol* **67** (1952) 804–9.
6. McDonald DF. Intussusception ureterectomy: a method of removal of the ureteral stump at time of nephrectomy without an additional incision. *Surg Gynecol Obstet* **97** (1953) 565–8.
7. Clayman RV, Garske GL, Lange PH. Total nephroureterectomy with ureteral intussusception and transurethral ureteral detachment and pull-through. *Urology* **21** (1983) 482–6.
8. Jacobson JD, Raffnsoe B, Olesen E, Kvist E. Stripping of the distal ureter in association with nephroureterectomy. *Scand J Urol Nephrol* **28** (1994) 45–7.

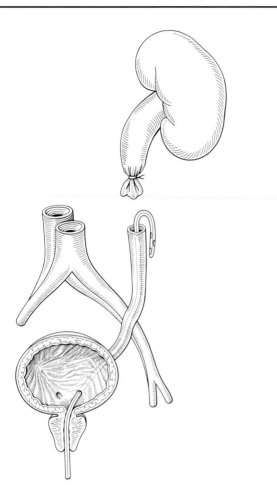

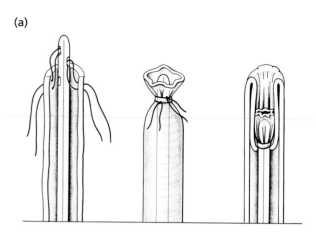

(a)

(b)

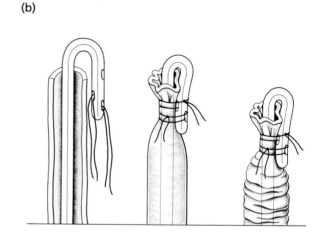

Figure 1. When extraperitoneal nephrectomy is performed via a flank incision, the proximal ureter is ligated just cephalad to the tip of the previously inserted ureteral catheter to prevent escape of infected material or tumor cells. The tip of the catheter is then kinked.

Figure 2. (a) Classic ureteral intussusception technique. (b) Modified ureteral compression technique. It is vital that the kinked tip of the ureteral catheter be at least 2 cm in length, and that it be attached to the ureteral stump with a double ligature, to prevent straightening and dislodgment of the catheter during stripping.

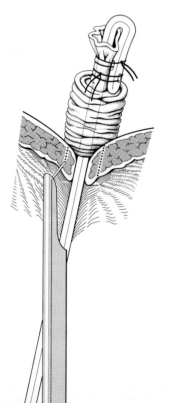

◄ **Figure 3.** Amputation of the redundant ureter. By gentle traction on the ureteral catheter the previously compressed ureter is pulled against the trigonal bladder wall, causing the bladder to protrude near the orifice. The ureter can then be disconnected from the bladder wall. The first cuts with the Turner-Warwick loop are made 1 cm away from and around the ureteral meatus. This incision of the intramural tract is performed until perivesical fat becomes visible around the resected ureter.

Suprainguinal Incision and the Lich–Grégoir Antireflux Operation

H. Riedmiller, J. Leissner[a], F. Steinbach[b]

Department of Urology,
Philipps University Medical School,
Marburg, Germany
[a]University of Mainz, Mainz, Germany
[b]University of Magdeburg, Magdeburg, Germany

Comment

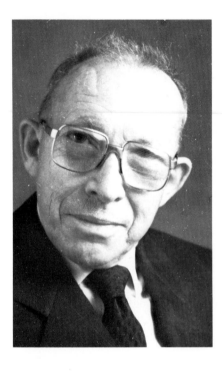

This excellent paper shows the experience and competence of the authors. Undoubtedly an inguinal incision gives wider and easier access to the ureterovesical junction. The simple inguinal incision has the advantage of cutting through aponeurotic formations only, the line of incision following externally the sheath of the rectus muscles. I have used it many times, especially in unilateral cases.

For many years, for esthetic reasons, we have used the Pfannenstiel incision, especially in girls (who represent the majority of cases) and also in bilateral reflux. There is no doubt that with this incision the field is narrower and needs more experience, but there is no convenience in operating on both sides at the same time.

I quite agree with the indications and contraindications. The operation is to be avoided in adults. If the ureter is very large, reimplantation after proper tailoring is indicated. This can be done either with the bladder open or extravesically after resection of the terminal narrow part of the ureter, leaving a small opening in the mucosa at the lower angle of the incision. Fixation of the ureter through the orifice by a single transfixing suture, 0.5–1 cm below, through the thickness of the trigonum, allows safe intravesicalization of the ureteral end. In duplex ureters the operation is the same as for a single one, avoiding opening the sheath and separating the ureters.

I have never left an indwelling catheter, even for a single day, unless the mucosa was accidentally torn.

There is often confusion between the Lich and Grégoir operations. In the Lich operation the vertical incision on the posterior bladder wall is continued by a circular incision all around the implantation, leaving the ureter attached to the bladder only by the mucosa. To achieve this it is necessary to cut the posterior ureteral artery, which comes from the inferior vesical artery and runs through the trigone and upwards into the thickness of the posterior ureteral wall. In an extensive histologic study of the ureterovesical junction, this artery was always present. The Lich incision creates a relative ischemia of the ureteral end. No long series of this operation have ever been published, but I am sure that they would show a certain percentage of stenosis. In the Grégoir operation, the incision goes down to where the ureter normally lies in contact with the bladder wall to avoid kinking and stops exactly at the anterior intramural ureter where, with magnifying glasses, one can easily see the few transverse muscle fibers.

Years ago we used to close the musculature with two layers of 3/0 or 4/0 chromic catgut, but since the introduction of polyglycolic suture material we have used only one suture layer, whether running or interrupted being of no importance.

W. Grégoir, Brussels

Suprainguinal incision

The curved suprainguinal incision (Gibson incision) is the best exposure for dealing with the distal ureter. The incision can be lengthened in both directions if it becomes necessary. Cephalad dissection of the ureter can be carried out to the level of the iliac vessels. Additionally, intraperitoneal inspection can easily be performed using this exposure.

For mobilization of the external peritoneal layers, which are fixed at the internal inguinal ring, dissection and division of the round ligament in female patients is required. In male patients, dissection of the peritoneal from the spermatic cord should be performed to free the peritoneal sac from the abdominal wall.

An important landmark for this incision is the lateral umbilical cord. The ureter is found directly under the cord.

The incision is closed with either running or interrupted sutures of muscle and fascia.

Risks

Retroperitoneal or subfascial hematomas are mostly caused by insufficient ligation or damage to the epigastric vessels.

Suture material

- Polyglycolic acid 3/0 or 2/0 for muscle and fascia
- Polydioxanone 4/0 or 5/0 for peritoneal lesions

Lich–Grégoir antireflux operation

Lich *et al.*, in 1961, described an extravesical approach to create a submucosal tunnel without disturbing the ureterovesical mucosa. The distal ureter is placed between the bladder mucosa and the muscular wall without altering the position of the ureteral orifice. This technique imitates the passive physiologic antireflux mechanism. The Lich–Grégoir operation has a low complication and high success rate, no intraoperative splinting of the ureter is required and the patient can be discharged a few days after the operation.

In our series of 780 cases, 97% were successfully treated with the Lich–Grégoir technique; an overcorrection leading to significant ureterectasis was seen in 0.1% and other major complications were noted in 1%.

Indications

- Noncomplicated vesicoureteral reflux in children before puberty
- Nondilated ureter and kidney on intravenous pyelography (IVP)
- Reflux in duplex ureter (both ureters can be placed in one tunnel)
- Diverticula close to the orifice are not contraindications

Contraindications

- Dilated ureter on preoperative IVP
- Infravesical obstruction
- Age: the operation is not suitable for adults and adolescents
- Combined pathologic findings in which ureterocystoneostomy is required (e.g. ureteral stenosis)

Diagnosis

- Voiding cystography is the method of choice to detect or exclude vesicoureteral reflux. To avoid retrograde manipulation a suprapubic puncture combined with bacteriologic examination of the urine is useful. Additional films should be exposed during and after voiding to exclude infravesical obstruction
- Sonography can be employed to measure renal parenchyma, kidney dilatation and residual urine. Dilated distal ureters during or immediately after voiding are indicative of severe reflux
- IVP should be performed to evaluate ureter morphology
- When decreased kidney function is suspected, isotope (MAG 3) clearance is necessary to evaluate kidney function
- Directly before the operation, cystoscopy shows the location and morphology of the refluxing orifice as well as possible infravesical obstruction

Operative technique step by step (Figures 1–12)

When vesicoureteral reflux on both sides is diagnosed, the ureter with the more pathologic orifice or the side with the higher reflux grade should be operated on first. The contralateral side may be operated on 3 months later to avoid postoperative neurogenic voiding problems. If decreased kidney function has been diagnosed, the antireflux operation in the ureterorenal unit with the better kidney function should be performed first.

- Exposure: suprainguinal incision as described above

- Cranial and medial dissection of the peritoneal sac, dissection of the iliac vessels and exposure of the lateral umbilical cord. The ureter can easily be found directly under the cord. Ligation and dissection of the cord

- Dissection of the ureter from the point of crossing the iliac vessels up to the muscular bladder wall. The mesoureter should be preserved as it contains the arterial and venous blood supply. Blood vessels in the ureterovesical angle can be ligated and divided

- Definitive decision for the Lich–Grégoir technique when the ureter is not dilated

- Placement of two muscular stay sutures perpendicular to the ureterovesical junction. Sutures should be located at the beginning of the bladder dome

- Filling the bladder with 50–100 ml saline via a transurethral catheter. Incision off the detrusor muscle with scissors or scalpel, without violating the mucosa, from the stay sutures to the ureterovesical junction; all muscle fibers must be divided. The length of this new submucosal tunnel should be about 3 cm in children under the age of 2 years and 4 cm in older children. Complete dissection of the ureter should be avoided as dissection of the posterior ureteric artery may cause ischemic lesions of the distal ureter

    A strict perpendicular course of the submucosal tunnel is important to prevent later angulation or kinking of the ureter.

- If the bladder mucosa has been accidentally opened, watertight closure of the mucosa is necessary

- Embedding of the ureter is the preformed submucosal tunnel and closure of the tunnel with interrupted sutures.

The first stitch should be placed directly under the ureterovesical junction to prevent iatrogenic bladder diverticula. The neohiatus must not be too tight as stenosis of the ureter may result

- Paravesical drainage and wound closure as described

Risks

- Angulation and kinking of the ureter during bladder filling because of a horizontal course of the submucosal tunnel

- Remaining detrusor muscle fibers during tunnel preparation

- Tight and narrow ureteral neohiatus

- Ischemia lesions due to complete and circular dissection of the distal ureter

- Development of a diverticulum close to the orifice when complete closure of the detrusor muscle has not been carried out

Special situations

- In cases of duplex ureter, both ureters can be embedded without dividing the Waldeyer fascia in one submucosal tunnel

- A Hutch diverticulum should be freed completely from all muscle fibers and enclosed in the submucosal tunnel when the detrusor muscle is closed

Postoperative care

Paravesical drainage is removed on day 2 or 3 and the transurethral catheter on day 3 or 4. If the bladder mucosa has been opened, the transurethral catheter is removed 2 days later. Renal sonography should be performed after 7 days and control cystography 6 months after the operation. Prophylactic antibiotics can be administered until control cystography excludes persisting reflux.

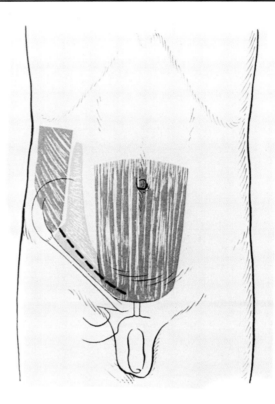

Figure 1. *Skin incision from the anterior superior iliac spine to the pubic symphysis.*

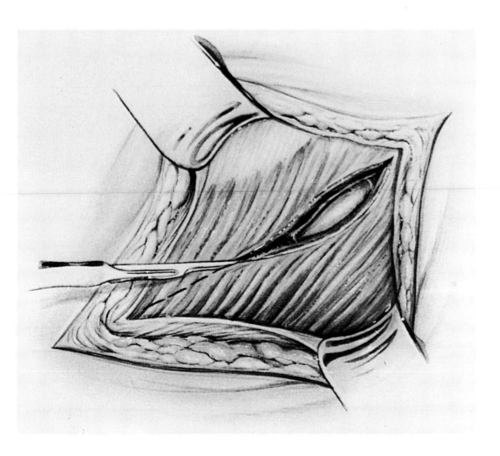

Figure 2. *Parallel incision of the external oblique fascia and division of the internal oblique and transverse muscle by electrocautery.*

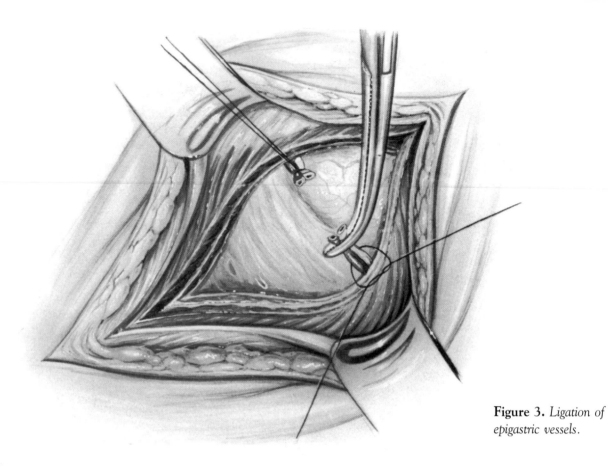

Figure 3. *Ligation of epigastric vessels.*

Figure 4. *Incision of the transverse fascia.*

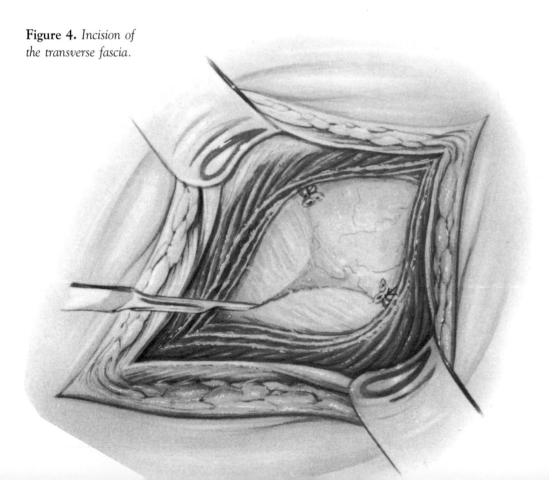

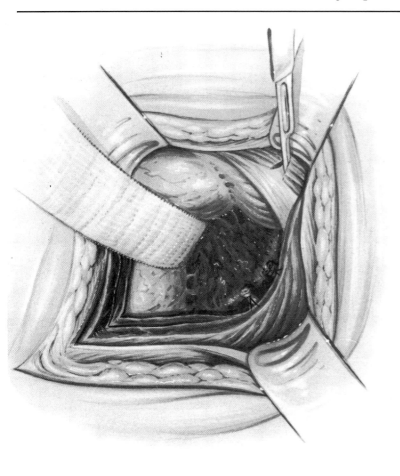

Figure 5. *Blunt dissection of the peritoneal sac after division of the round ligament or preparation of the spermatic cord. Incision of the pyramidalis muscle for better exposure.*

Figure 6. *The lateral umbilical cord is ligated and divided. The ureter is found directly under the cord.*

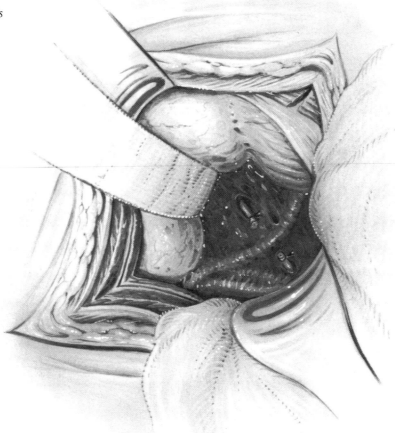

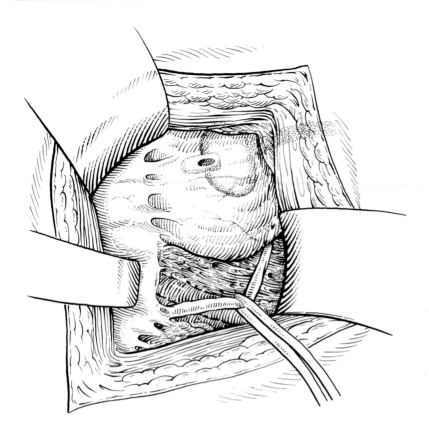

Figure 7. *Dissection of the ureter from the point of crossing the iliac vessels to the ureterovesical junction.*

Figure 8. *Stay sutures perpendicular to the ureterovesical junction. (Move to the contralateral side of the patient to facilitate this.)*

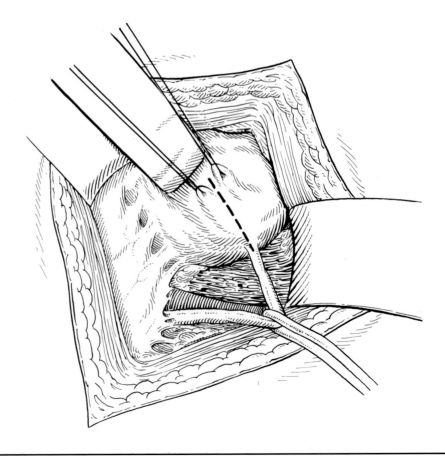

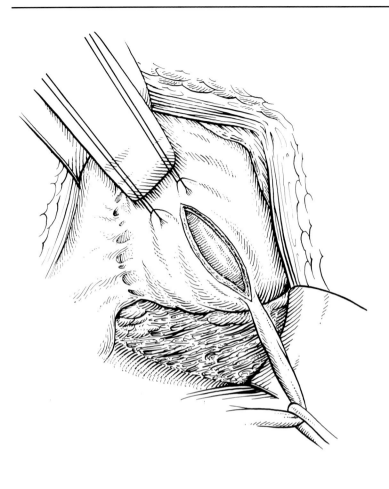

Figure 9. *Incision of the detrusor muscle to the ureterovesical junction, keeping the bladder mucosa intact.*

Figure 10. *Embedding of the ureter in the submucosal tunnel and closure of the tunnel by interrupted suture of the detrusor muscle.*

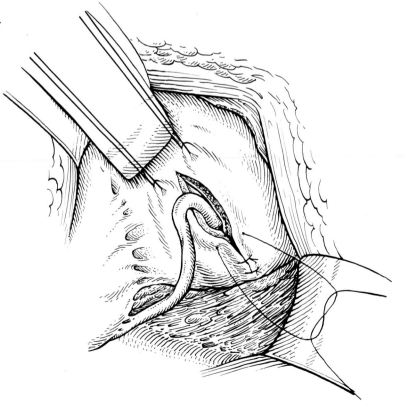

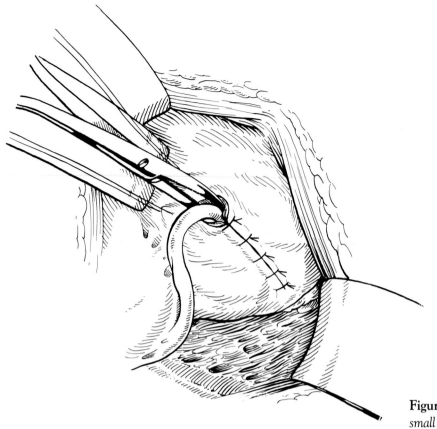

Figure 11. *Checking the width of the neohiatus with a small Overholt clamp.*

Figure 12. *After emptying of the bladder, the distal ureter shows no kinking or angulation.*

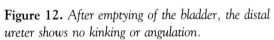

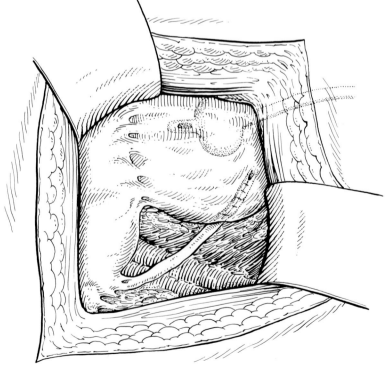

Bladder Reduction Plasty with Doubling of the Detrusor Muscle

M. Fisch, J. Fichtner, R. Hohenfellner
Department of Urology,
University of Mainz School of Medicine,
Mainz, Germany

Comment

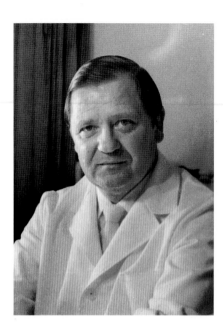

The procedure of detrusor doubling described here has its origin in the same considerations as those on which the cystoplasty presented in 1964 is based. By doubling the bladder wall, it reduces the capacity to normal and strengthens the expulsive force.

The detrusor doubling described here is technically easier, less time-consuming and also less burdensome than the doubling in the cystoplasty of 1964, which practically involves the entire bladder. It is therefore also capable of successfully treating chronic distension of the bladder which, after removal of an obstruction, has not responded in the same way expected. Thus, such an uncomplicated procedure should stand the test of time even in distinct distensions of the decompensated or so-called exhausted bladder, if the bladder wall – as in idiopathic myogenic bladder atony – is not trabeculated. In other cases (such as decompensated exhausted bladder caused by obstructions), idiopathic myogenic atony is based on a primary insufficiency of the bladder muscles and is therefore spontaneously and absolutely irreversible. For this reason the symptoms – large micturition intervals, overlong micturition time, micturition possible only with the support of abdominal muscle pressure and more or less portion by portion – can be traced back to childhood.

Cystoscopy shows an even nontrabeculated pale bladder wall, which upon discharge of the bladder contents floats like a limp mainsail. This corresponds to the cystometric curve, which shows the intentional use of abdominal muscle pressure as unproportionally high peaks compared with the extremely reduced intrinsic tension. Histologically, the bladder muscles are mixed with fibrotic tissue and connective tissue and show almost no ganglia.

In these extreme cases of an idiopathic large limp bladder with residual urine, conduct a comprehensive approximate bisection of the bladder by splitting longitudinally. Practically the entire bladder wall is doubled or multiplied and, by the multiple strengthening of the muscular elements of the entire bladder, the expulsion capability is considerably increased. The concentration of receptors in the bladder wall is also (at least) doubled, and so the sensible life of the bladder is intensified. Furthermore, the bladder assumes a longitudinal–oval form and, due to the ventrofixation, an upright position (which appears to be important for the opening phase of micturition).

Both techniques have their indications and applications. One cannot hope by doubling to obtain a permanent strong elasticity. However, the goal of surgery (reduction of the bladder capacity to normal values, largely residual free emptying with sufficient flow, prevention of new distension of the bladder, and if possible an undisturbed sensibility for micturition without an irritated bladder) is achieved to a great degree by doubling the bladder wall.

Bibliography

1. Binard J, Zoedler D. Treatment of the hypotonic, decompensated urinary bladder. *Int Surg* **6** (1968) 502–6.
2. Brenez J. L'Autoplastie vesicale 'en paletot'. Traitement de la megavessie par l'operation de Zoedler. *J Urol* **75** (1969) 497–502.
3. Losermann ML. Die operative Behandlung der kongenitalen Harnblasenatonie. Dissertation. University of Düsseldorf (1973).
4. Sachse H. Operative Massnahmen bei der idiopathischen Blasenatonie der Frau. *Urologe* **5** (1966) 256–8.
5. Satatoku J, Fukuyama T. An improved procedure of Zoedler operation for atonic bladder. *Acta Urol Jap* **13** (1967) 605–9.
6. Vanwelkenhuyzen P. Traitement operatoire de la megavessie. *Acta Urol Belg* **36** (1968) 235–8.
7. Wienhöwer R. Operative Behandlung der Blasenatonie. *Vortrag Nordrh Ges Urol Rheydt* (1973).
8. Zoedler D. Zur operativen Behandlung der Blasenatonie. *Z Urol* **57** (1964) 743–8.
9. Zoedler D. Traitement operatoire de la vessie atonique. *Acta Urol Belg* **33** (1965) 143–7.
10. Zoedler D. Zur Atonie der Harnblase. *Verh Dt Ges Urol* **21** (1965) 129.

D. Zoedler, Düsseldorf

Bladder reduction plasty with doubling of the detrusor muscle

Introduction

Bladder reduction plasty is indicated in rare cases with enlarged bladder capacity without or after treatment of infravesical obstruction. Neurologic disorders have to be excluded. The aim of the operation is to decrease bladder capacity, and it is assumed that detrusor doubling will increase the contractility of the remaining bladder. The operation represents an alternative to intermittent self-catheterization and to long-term cystostomy. Better preconditions for spontaneous voiding are created; however, in most patients, a long learning phase is required until voiding without residual urine is achieved.

Indications

- Large bladder capacity after treatment of infravesical obstruction
- Large bladder capacity without neurologic disorders

Instruments

- Standard set for kidney surgery
- Hryntschak retractor
- Turner-Warwick electrical scissors

Suture materials

- Chromic catgut 5/0 for bladder mucosa
- Polyglycolic acid 4/0 for the detrusor muscle
- Plain catgut 4/0 for fixation of the cystostomy and for stay sutures

Operative technique step by step

- Insertion of an 18 Fr transurethral bladder catheter (Figure 2)

- Lower midline incision of Pfannenstiel incision (Figure 1)
- Division of the urachus
- Mobilization of the bladder (filled with 300–500 ml saline)
- Extraperitonealization of the bladder from the bladder dome down to the rectouterine fold (female) or the rectovesical fold (male) (extraperitonealization according to Völker) (Figure 3)
- Semicircular incision of the detrusor muscle using electrocautery and scissors; the mucosa remains intact (Figure 4)
- Elevation of the detrusor margins by Allis clamps and dissection of the detrusor from the bladder mucosa in lateral direction similar to the Lich–Grégoir technique for reflux repair (Figure 5)
- After preparation of two large detrusor flaps, the mucosa is incised and resected along the preparation line (Figure 6)
- Insertion of a 10 Fr cystostomy tube and fixation with plain 4/0 catgut
- Running suture of the bladder mucosa using 5/0 chromic catgut (Figure 7)
- Detrusor doubling with 4/0 polyglycolic acid U-shaped single stitches, thereby fixing the upper detrusor flap over the lower flap (Figure 8)
- Insertion of two paravesical drains (Figures 9 and 10)
- Wound closure

Surgical tricks

Turner-Warwick electrical scissors are helpful in dissecting the peritoneum from the bladder.

Postoperative care

The drains are removed after 4 days, the bladder catheter after 5 days. Voiding is initiated 1 week after the operation, first at intervals of 3 hours. The cystostomy tube stays until the patient is able to void without residual urine (<50 ml). Additional biofeedback training or relaxation of the pelvic floor by drugs may be helpful in achieving residual-free voiding.

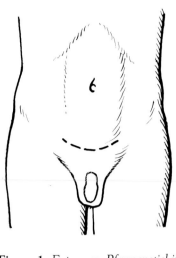

Figure 1. *Exposure: Pfannenstiel incision.*

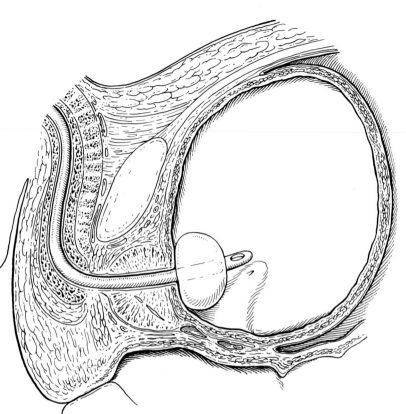

Figure 2. *Sagittal section for anatomic orientation. A bladder catheter is inserted before the operation. Note the course of the peritoneum down to the rectovesical space.*

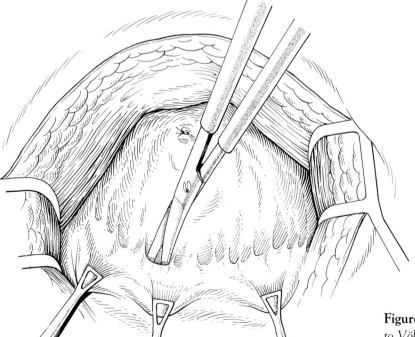

Figure 3. *Extraperitonealization of the bladder according to Völker (bladder filled with 300–500 ml saline). After division and ligature of the urachus, the peritoneum is dissected from ventral to dorsal with Turner-Warwick electrical scissors.*

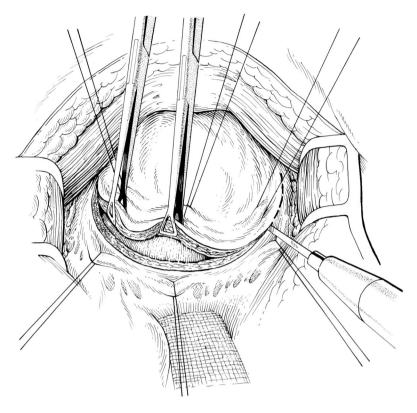

Figure 4. *Semicircular incision of the detrusor muscle between stay sutures, using electrocautery, without injuring the bladder mucosa. Allis clamps grasp the detrusor margins.*

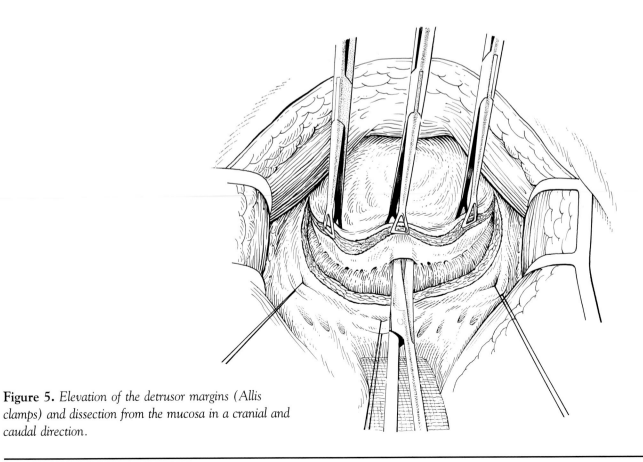

Figure 5. *Elevation of the detrusor margins (Allis clamps) and dissection from the mucosa in a cranial and caudal direction.*

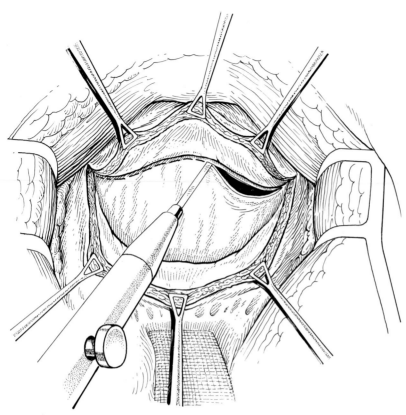

Figure 6. *Incision and resection of the mucosa using electrocautery. - - -, resection line.*

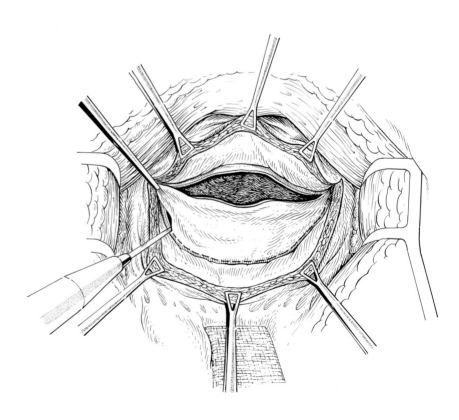

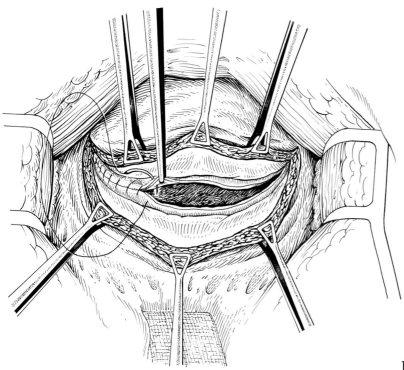

Figure 7. *Continuous suture of the mucosa (chromic catgut 5/0) for bladder closure, and insertion of a 10 Fr cystostomy tube before final closure.*

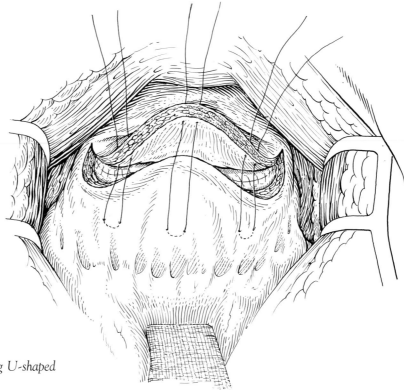

Figure 8. *Doubling of the detrusor using U-shaped sutures (polyglycolic acid 4/0).*

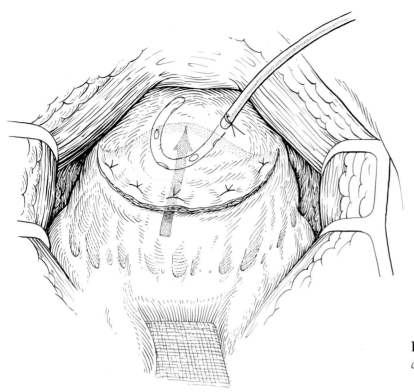

Figure 9. *Insertion of cystostomy with paravesical drainage.*

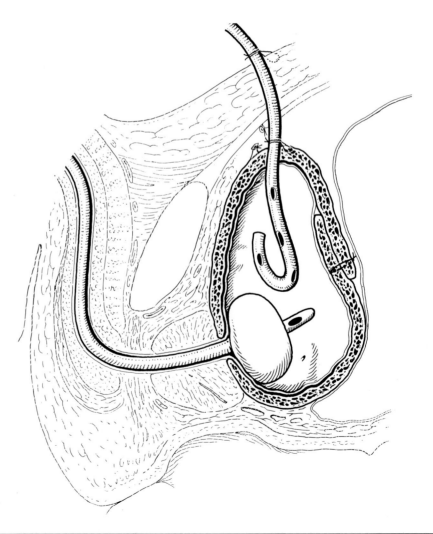

Figure 10. *Sagittal section: bladder catheter and cystostomy tube. Note the reduction in bladder volume by detrusor doubling in the area of the bladder dome.*

Sacral Neuromodulation for Treatment of Micturition Disorders and Fecal Incontinence

M. Hohenfellner, K.E. Matzel[a], D. Schultz-Lampel, S. Dahms,
R.A. Schmidt[b], E.A. Tanagho[c], J.W. Thüroff

Department of Urology,
University of Witten/Herdecke,
Wuppertal, Germany
[a]Department of Surgery,
University of Erlangen/Nürnberg,
Nürnberg, Germany
[b]Division of Urology,
University of Colorado,
Denver, Colorado, USA
[c]Department of Urology,
University of California San Francisco,
San Francisco, California, USA

Introduction

Actions of the detrusor, external sphincter and pelvic floor are coordinated by spinal and supraspinal reflex arcs (Figure 1). Pathologic hyperactivity or hypoactivity of these reflex arcs may result in functional disorders of the lower urinary tract. Sacral neuromodulation opens the possibility of correcting such pathologic neurologic interactions in selected patients. Its mechanism of action is twofold. During electrostimulation of the sacral spinal nerves (in most cases of the S3 segment) the parasympathetic lower motoneuron of the bladder is inhibited via activation of somatomotor afferents (Aα and Aγ neurons), while the sympathetics are stimulated, resulting in improved storage function of the lower urinary tract. Interruption of this kind of electrostimulation results in a rebound phenomenon in the sense that the parasympathetic lower motoneuron of the bladder is activated while the sympathetics are inhibited, thus inducing micturition. A precondition for implantation of a stimulation system for chronic sacral neuromodulation is a successful test stimulation demonstrating significant therapeutic efficacy.

In contrast to these indirect stimulation effects, sacral neuromodulation for treatment of fecal incontinence relies on direct stimulation of the somatic motoneurons of the sacral spinal nerves that innervate the striated anal sphincter.

Indications

- Functional or neurogenic micturition disorders resulting in detrusor hyperactivity or hypoactivity, bladder hypersensitivity or dyssynergia of the detrusor and the external anal sphincter. Experience to date shows that disorders due to nearly complete or complete spinal lesions are not likely to respond to sacral neuromodulation. Treatment of interstitial cystitis and/or pelvic pain draws unsatisfactory results in most cases, even if test stimulation was considered successful.

- Functional deficits of the striated anal sphincteric muscles without apparent gross defect.

Contraindications

General
- Skin disease(s) at the areas of implantation

- Pathologic anatomy of the sacrum, such as trauma sequelae or spina bifida

- Pregnancy

Micturition disorders
- Other relevant urologic pathologies that may contribute to the diagnosed micturition disorder (ureteral reflux, bladder diverticula, bladder stones, infravesical obstruction, carcinoma *in situ*)

- Anatomical bladder capacity <150 ml

- Stress incontinence

Special hazards of the procedure

- Dislocation of electrodes

- Infection of the implant

- Pain at the site of implantation

- Technical failure of the implant

- Iatrogenic intraoperative nervous lesions

- Exhaustion of the battery (usually after 5–8 years, requiring exchange of the stimulator)

- Activation or deactivation of the stimulator by powerful magnetic fields or microwaves

- Special care during high-frequency surgery following implantation of a stimulation system

Special instruments

Percutaneous and intraoperative test stimulation (Figure 2)
- Needle electrode (Medtronic 041828)

- Wire electrode (Medtronic 041830)

- Transparent skin adhesive dressing

- Test stimulator with leads and electrode (Medtronic Screener 3625)

Implant
- Antibiotic solution suitable for local irrigation

- Bipolar coagulation

- Neuropads

- Implants: electrode (Medtronic 3487A); extension lead (Medtronic 7495); neurostimulator Itrel II (Medtronic 7424) (Figure 3)

- Console programmer (Medtronic 7432)

- Magnet (Medtronic 7452)

Surgical technique step by step

Percutaneous stimulation
- Anesthesia can be general or local: the former has to avoid

muscle relaxation; the latter has to avoid electrical blockade of the sacral spinal nerves by inappropriate deep injection of the anesthetic.

- Prone position with support of the anterior superior iliac spine. The surgical drapes leave the anal sphincter, perineum and feet visible.

- The needle electrodes are inserted into one or both dorsal sacral foramina of the S3 segment (Figures 4 and 5). The needle is guided rectangular in relation to the surface of the sacrum, corresponding to a 60° angle in relation to the surface of the skin. Confirmation of the correct needle position (the needle is the cathode, the skin electrode the anode) by electrostimulation: S2 stimulation produces contraction of the superficial perineal muscles ('clamping') and outward rotation of the leg; S3 stimulation, contraction of levator ani ('bellow') and plantar flexion of the great toe or entire foot; and S4 stimulation, contraction of the levator ani ('bellow') without planar flexion of the great toe or entire foot (Figure 1).

- For subchronic sacral neuromodulation the needle electrodes are replaced by the stimulation wires, which are connected for 3–4 days to the external carry-on neurostimulator. During this time, the patient continues to record a micturition diary and cystometry is repeated. The test is regarded as successful if symptoms of storage failure are reduced by at least 50%; in detrusor areflexia, the test is considered a success if interruption of subchronic sacral neuromodulation results in micturition with less than 50 ml of residual urine.

Implant

- Delay between subchronic sacral neuromodulation and implant: ≥ 2 weeks.

- Preparation: marking of the desired subcutaneous position of the neurostimulator. Repeated total body skin disinfection. Prophylactic antibiotics.

- Prone position (as for percutaneous sacral neuromodulation) under general anesthesia without muscle relaxants (Figure 6).

- Median skin incision from S1 to S5. Exposure of the thoracolumbar fascia and identification of the appropriate foramen by probing and electrostimulation with the needle electrode (Figure 7). Exposure of the foramen by incision of the fascia and division of erector spinae muscle down to the bone without impairing the periosteum.

- Rinsing of the Quad electrode with antibiotic solution, application of friction collars and insertion of the electrode into the foramen. Repeated electrostimulation of all four con-

tact points to verify correct electrode position. Fixation of the electrode by suturing the friction collars to the periosteum and the sacroiliac ligaments (Figure 8). One of the friction collars has to be located as close to the foramen as possible to prevent movement of the electrode inside the foramen.

- The electrode lead is pulled subcutaneously through a small flank incision, which is then closed again temporarily (Figure 9). The sacral incision is rinsed with the antibiotic solution before being closed.

- The patient is brought into a lateral position for a hypogastric incision that exposes the external fascia and creates a pocket to take up the neurostimulator. From this incision the extension lead, which is plugged into the stimulator, is pulled through to the flank incision, where it is connected to the electrode lead (Figure 10). Redundant length of the extension lead is coiled and stored between the fascia and the stimulator. The stimulator is sutured to the fascia with its text-covered surface (the anode) facing the surgeon. The wounds are rinsed with antibiotic solution and closed (Figure 11).

Postoperative care

- The patient is mobilized as soon as possible

- On the first or second postoperative day, the functional parameters of the neurostimulator are programmed telemetrically by the physician; the patients themselves can activate or deactivate the neurostimulator using a hand-held (carry-on) magnet

- Initial setting of the active contact(s) and voltage (depending on the patient's perception of pain and muscular contraction): pulse width 210 μs; frequency 15 Hz; on/off ratio 5 : 1 s

- Superficial infections may be treated conservatively. Infections of the implant may require explantation of the stimulation system. In all cases of infection, the patient should be hospitalized to allow close observation, wound treatment and intravenous antibiotics if indicated

- Follow-up every 3–6 months

Surgical tricks

- Percutaneous and intraoperative localization of the sacral foramina with the needle electrode. The sacral foramen is covered with a small venous plexus, so correct needle position is often confirmed by a small bleed. When the needle is inserted correctly, leave it in position and use it as a landmark to localize the other foramina with a second needle

- Failure to achieve stimulation responses during the operation may be caused by application of muscle relaxants, a defect in the stimulation system (exchange the external stimulator wire and needle electrode), a dead battery, or wrong setting of the stimulation parameters of the external stimulator (check the range setting inside the case)

- After unpacking the various components of the implantable stimulation system, rinse them immediately with saline or antibiotic solution to prevent bacterial contamination by electrostatic charging. Do not wet the inside of the electrode ports of the stimulator

Special note

Evaluation of the efficacy, side-effects and risks of sacral neuromodulation is an ongoing process utilizing a prospective multinational multicenter protocol. As an evolution of the technique described here, a modification was developed in which both S3 spinal nerves are approached directly via a small laminectomy and equipped with tripolar cuff electrodes (Figure 12). This technique seems to improve efficacy in cases with dysfunction of the lower urinary tract while reducing the necessary voltage. If these preliminary results should be

confirmed in the long-term follow-up, this modification may evolve as the technique of choice in patients with voiding dysfunction. Until now, this technique has not been applied in patients with fecal incontinence.

Bibliography

1. Erlandson BE, Fall M. Intravaginal electrical stimulation in urinary incontinence. *Scand J Urol Nephrol* (Suppl. 44) (1977) 3–63.
2. Fall M. Electrical pelvic floor stimulation for the control of detrusor instability. *Neurourol Urodyn* **4** (1985) 329–35.
3. Schmidt RA. Advances in genitourinary neurostimulation. *Neurosurgery* **19** (1986) 1041–4.
4. Schmidt RA, Senn E, Tanagho EA. Functional evaluation of sacral nerve root integrity. *Urology* **35** (1990) 388–92.
5. Thon WF, Baskin LS, Jonas U, Tanagho EA, Schmidt RA. Surgical principles of sacral foramen electrode implantation. *World J Urol* **9** (1991) 133–7.
6. Matzel KE, Stadelmaier U, Hohenfellner M, Gall FP. Electrical stimulation of the sacral spinal nerves for treatment of fecal incontinence. *Lancet* **346** (1995) 1124–7.
7. Hohenfellner M, Schultz-Lampel D, Lampel A *et al.* Functional rehabilitation of the neurogenic bladder by chronic sacral neuromodulation. *Akt Urol* (in press).

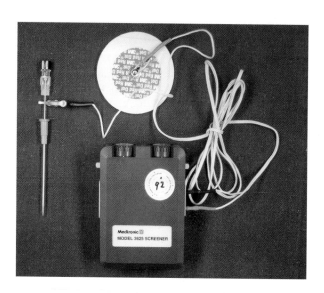

Figure 2. *System for percutaneous stimulation: needle electrode, external stimulator and skin electrode (anode).*

Figure 3. *Implantable stimulation system: stimulator, extension lead, Quad electrode and screwdriver.*

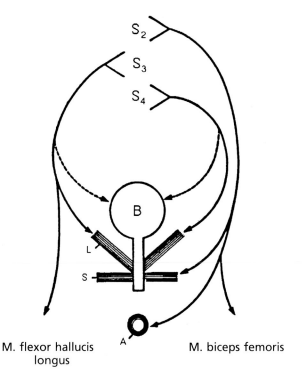

M. flexor hallucis longus   M. biceps femoris

Figure 1. *The bladder (B) is mainly innervated by neurons of the S3 segment. Somatic motoneurons of the same segment innervate the flexor hallucis longus muscle. The external anal sphincter (S) and pelvic floor (L) are innervated by somatic motoneurons of the S2, S3 and S4 segments. Motoneurons of the S2 segment approach the biceps femoris (outward rotator) muscle.*

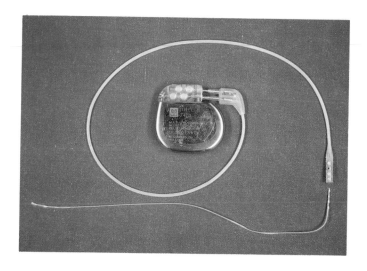

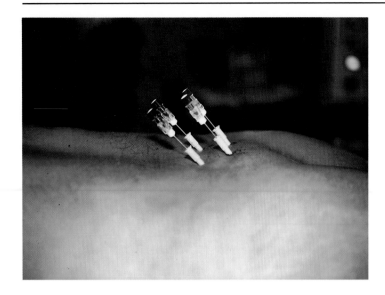

Figure 4. *The dorsal sacral foramina are located approximately 2 cm lateral to the sacral crest; their vertical separation is also approximately 2 cm. The S2 foramen is found 1 cm medial to and 1 cm below the posterior superior iliac spine; the S3 foramen is located at the level of the greater sciatic notch. The needle electrodes are inserted parallel to the axis of the foramina.*

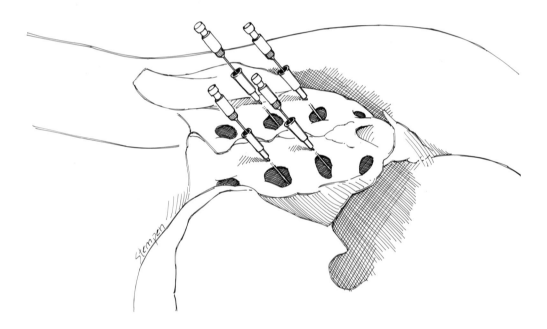

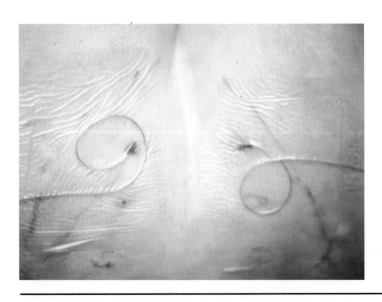

Figure 5. *Each S3 foramen is supplied with a wire electrode and covered with transparent dressing.*

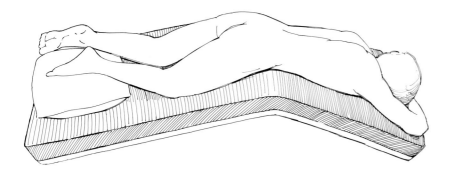

Figure 6. *Positioning of the patient.*

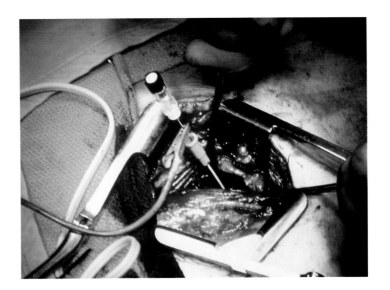

Figure 7. *Intraoperative stimulation with the needle electrode.*

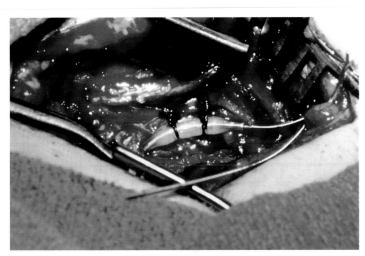

Figure 8. *The Quad electrode is implanted into the right S3 foramen and fixed by two friction collars.*

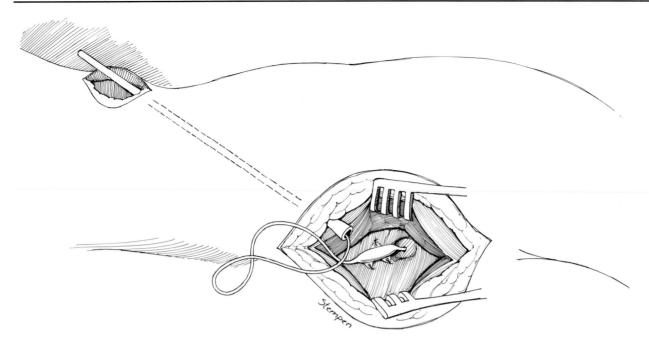

Figure 9. *Pull-through of the electrode lead from the sacral incision to the flank incision.*

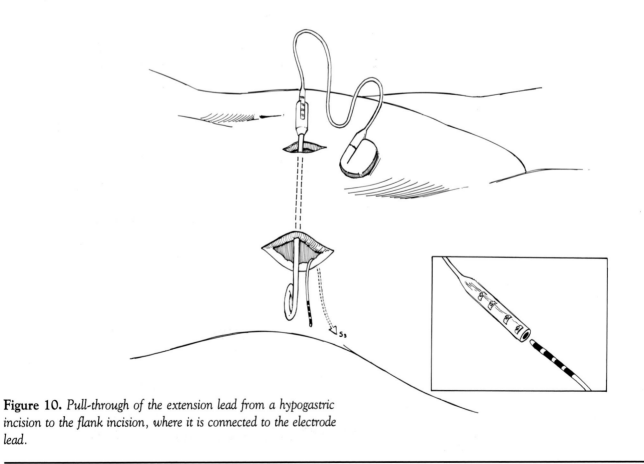

Figure 10. *Pull-through of the extension lead from a hypogastric incision to the flank incision, where it is connected to the electrode lead.*

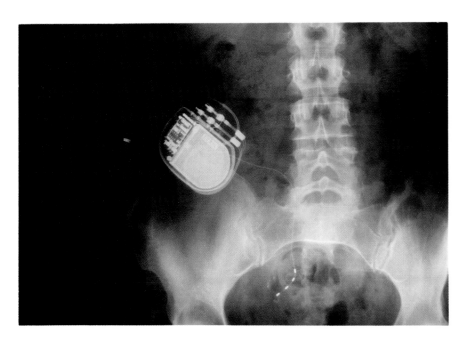

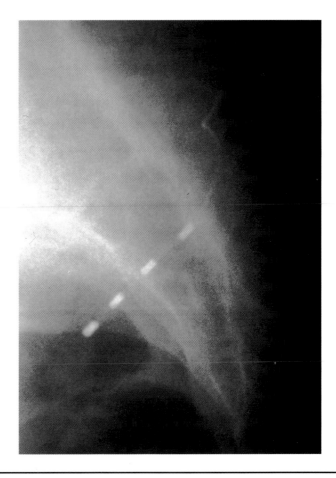

Figure 11. *(a) Implanted neurostimulator connected to a Quad electrode. (b) Quad electrode in the S3 foramen.*

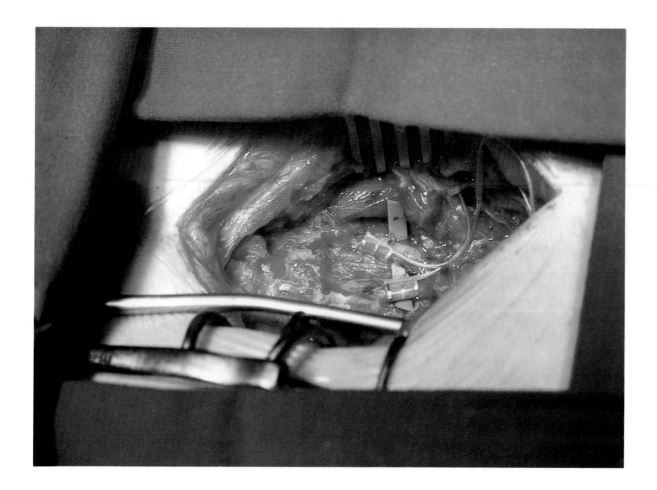

Figure 12. *Modified technique of sacral neuromodulation with two cuff electrodes fitted to each S3 spinal nerve.*

Sacral Rhizotomies for Continent Reconstruction of the Lower Urinary Tract

M. Hohenfellner, D. Schultz-Lampel, S. Dahms,
K. Schürmann[a], E.A. Tanagho[b], J.W. Thüroff
Department of Urology,
University of Witten/Herdecke,
Wuppertal, Germany
[a]Department of Neurosurgery,
Johannes Gutenberg University,
Mainz, Germany
[b]Department of Urology,
University of California San Francisco,
San Francisco, California, USA

Introduction

Paraplegic and tetraplegic patients experience dysfunctions of the lower urinary tract dependent on the level of the spinal lesion (Figure 1). Lesions above the sacral micturition center (S2–S4/5) may result – after a variable period of time – in pathologic activation or formation of spinal reflex arcs (Figure 2). The consecutive hyperreflexia of the detrusor and continence mechanism can be abolished by interruption of these reflex arcs by bisecting either the ventral or the dorsal roots of the sacral spinal nerves. In this way a hyperreflexic low-capacity high-pressure bladder can be changed into a high-capacity low-pressure reservoir with simultaneous reduction of infravesical resistance. (At present, we believe that not all of the ventral sacral roots should be bisected as a routine to avoid neurogenic lesions of the anal and urinary continence mechanism. However, there are no data available that would demonstrate that this assumption is of clinical significance. If implantation of a ventral sacral root stimulation system is intended, interruption of the sacral reflex arcs has to be limited strictly to dorsal sacral rhizotomies.)

The functionally reconstructed bladder may be emptied by different methods. The easiest way is clean intermittent catheterization. In urethral pathologies or other contraindications for urethral manipulations a continent vesicostomy may serve the same purpose. As a third possibility, a ventral sacral root stimulation system for restoration of voluntary telemetrically induced micturition can be implanted into selected patients.

Indications

Sacral rhizotomy is indicated in patients with near-complete or complete lesions of the spinal cord above the sacral micturition centre resulting in conservative refractory detrusor hyperreflexia. In extremely rare cases, sacral root surgery may also be eligible for patients with cerebral lesions. Autonomic dysreflexia is usually abolished by sacral deafferentation (exceptions may be seen in patients who swallow air while speaking and have therefore pneumatic overdistended bowels).

Contraindications

- Skin disease at the area of surgery
- Pathologic spinal anatomy such as trauma sequelae or spina bifida at the area of surgery
- History of meningitis or of intrathecal application of oily contrast media may be a contraindication for intradural procedures and enforce an extradural approach. A disadvantage of the latter is that ventral and dorsal roots are not as easily divided from each other extradurally as intradurally, and that the spinal nerves of the S4/5 segments are difficult to expose extradurally. Therefore, extradural deafferentation is more likely to be incomplete.
- Pregnancy.
- Low-compliance bladder due to fibrotic organization of the detrusor. Cystometric pressure waves usually indicate an intact and therefore relaxable detrusor. A steady increase of bladder pressure without pressure waves demonstrates in most cases detrusor fibrosis due to recurrent urinary tract infections, which has no or only minimal potential to be functionally corrected. Measurement of bladder capacity under spinal anesthesia is another helpful parameter to anticipate the ratio of functional and anatomic limitations of bladder capacity.
- In incomplete spinal lesions, the benefits of sacral root surgery have to be balanced against its side-effects.
- Reflex erections, as well as trigger mechanisms for induction of micturition and defecation, are eliminated by sacral root surgery.
- Relative incompetence of the continence mechanism may be abolished by improving the storage function of the bladder; however, significant lesions of the external sphincter (e.g. history of sphincterotomy) may require closure of the bladder neck in combination with a continent vesicostomy to take advantage of the sacral root surgery.

Special instruments

Laminectomy
- Ferguson suction tube with finger cut-off
- Bipolar electrocoagulation
- Liston–Key bone-cutting forceps (S-shaped)
- Double-action Stille–Leksell rongeur
- Echlin–Stookey rongeur
- Kerrison rongeurs
- Periosteal elevators
- Laminectomy retractor
- Absorbable sponge
- Bone wax
- Hydrogen peroxide solution

Dura and nerves
- Microscope or magnifier glasses ($2–4 \times$)
- Dura knife and scissor

- Nerve hooks
- Needle holder and scalpels for microsurgery
- External neurostimulator
- Urodynamic equipment for cystometry

Surgical technique

Intradural rhizotomies

- General anaesthesia without muscle relaxants
- Insertion of a bladder catheter to control the intravesical volume and measure the intravesical pressure
- Median skin incision from L4 to S4. Exposure and median incision of the thoracolumbar fascia (Figures 3 to 5). To expose the spinous processes and vertebral arches from the fascia and paravertebral muscles, the knife and periosteal elevators are kept in a cleavage plane between the bone and the periosteum (Figure 6) (otherwise severe bleeding may be encountered). Do not attempt localized hemostasis by electrocoagulation; insert gauze sponges into the wound and keep them in place by the valves of the laminectomy retractor
- When using the rongeurs (Figures 7 and 8) it is essential to bite the bone and not to tear it away. The ligamentum flavum may be dissected together with the bone or separately using toothed forceps and a knife
- Bleeding from the bone is controlled by local application of bone wax. Bleeding epidural blood vessels are controlled either with the bipolar coagulation forceps or by compression with hydrogen peroxide-soaked neuropaddies. Effective hemostasis is a prerequisite for successful completion of the following steps
- Opening of the dura and the arachnoid (Figure 9)
- Separation of the ventral and dorsal sacral roots with cotton pads and nerve hooks. The dorsal roots are located lateral to the ventral sacral roots and have a slightly larger diameter (Figure 10). Intraoperative electrostimulation (0.5–2 mA, 200 µs pulse width, 20 Hz) also confirms the motoric or sensoric nature and the level of the anatomic segment of the target root; additionally, the segment of the ventral sacral roots is identified, the stimulation of which elicits the most significant stimulation response (usually S3)
- Division and resection of 2–3 mm of length of the dorsal roots of S2–S4/5 bilaterally. If it is not intended to implant a ventral sacral root stimulator, the ventral roots of whichever segment has the most significant bladder contraction on electrostimulation may be bisected to increase the probability of interrupting all significant reflex arcs
- Closure of the dura (Figures 11 and 12)

Extradural rhizotomies

- Laminectomy from S1 to S4 to expose the sacral spinal nerves from S2–S4/5 (Figure 13). Electrostimulation of the sacral spinal nerves to confirm their segment levels and to identify the segment with the most prominent bladder response (Figure 14).
- Placement of a stay suture through the spinal ganglion and subepineural injection of saline (0.9%) or adrenaline (0.25 ml; 1 : 100 000).
- Slight traction of the stay suture exposes a groove between the ventral and dorsal sacral root. The dorsal root is located lateral to the ventral root and carries the bulge of the spinal ganglion.
- Microsurgical separation of the ventral and dorsal roots.
- Division of the dorsal roots by bisection of the spinal ganglion; bipolar coagulation of the stumps.

Complications

- Absence of intraoperative stimulation responses may be due to anesthetic application of muscle relaxants, a defective stimulation system (both electrodes held on a striated muscle in the area of the wound have to elicit a visible contraction), an empty bladder, or malfunctioning urodynamic equipment.
- Postoperative development of cerebrospinal fluid leakage should be encountered only very rarely. Usually conservative treatment by antibiotic prophylaxis, compressive dressings and a bed position that elevates the fistula on a level slightly higher than the rest of the liquor compartment will achieve spontaneous closure. Otherwise surgical closure of the fistula will be necessary.

Bibliography

1. Brindley GS, Polkey CE, Rushton DN. Sacral anterior root stimulators for bladder control in paraplegia: the first 50 cases. *J Neurol Neurosurg Psychiatr* **49** (1986) 1104–14.
2. Hohenfellner M, Paick J-S, Rocha TF *et al.* Site of de-afferentation and electrode placement: clinical implications. *J Urol* **147** (1992) 1665–70.
3. Hohenfellner M, Fahle H, Dahms S, Linn JF, Hutschenreiter G, Thüroff JW. Continent reconstruction of detrusor hyperreflexia by sacral bladder denervation combined with continent vesicostomy. *Urology* **47** (1996) 930–931.
4. Madersbacher H. Intradural spinal stimulation approach to selection/follow-up. *World J Urol* (1991) 122–5.
5. Sauerwein D. Die operative Behandlung der spastischen Blasenlähmung bei Querschnittslähmung. *Urologe* [A] **29** (1990) 196–203.

6. Schmidt RA, Bruschini H, Tanagho EA. Sacral root stimulation in controlled micturition: peripheral somatic neurotomy and stimulated voiding. *Invest Urol* **16** (1979) 130–4.

7. Schmidt RA, Bruschini H, van Gool J, Tanagho EA. Micturition and the male genitourinary response to sacral root stimulation. *Invest Urol* **17** (1979) 125–9.

8. Tanagho EA, Schmidt RA, Orvis BR. Neural stimulation for control of voiding dysfunction: a preliminary report in 22 patients with serious neuropathic voiding disorders. *J Urol* **142** (1989) 340–5.

9. Van Kerrebroeck PEV, Koldewijn E, Wijkstra H, Debruyne FMJ. Intradural sacral rhizotomies and implantation of an anterior sacral root stimulator in the treatment of neurogenic bladder dysfunction after spinal cord injury. *World J Urol* (1991) 126–32.

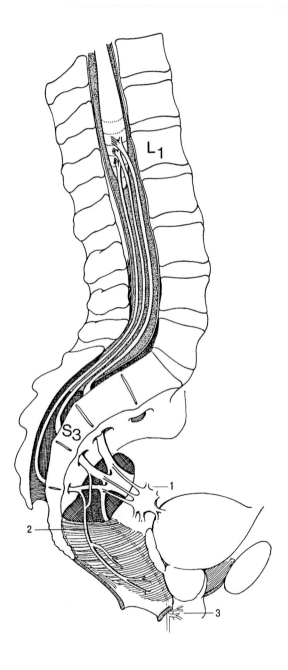

Figure 2. *Spinal lesions above the sacral micturition center may result in pathologic formation of sacral reflex arcs. Their sequelae (hyperreflexia of the lower urinary tract) may be corrected by dorsal sacral rhizotomies.*

◄ **Figure 1.** *Anatomy of the spinal column and the spinal micturition center. The detrusor is mainly innervated by parasympathetic neurons from the S3 segment and, to a lesser extent, from S2 and S4, which approach the bladder via the pelvic ganglion (1). The pelvic floor and external anal sphincter are innervated by somatomotor neurons running within the levator ani (2) and by the pudendal nerve (3) (S2–S4).*

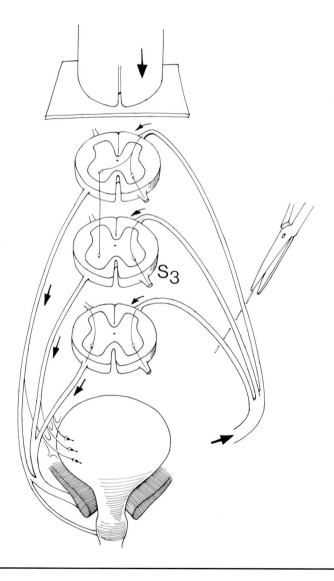

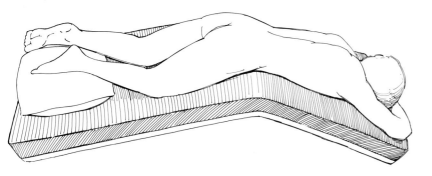

Figure 3. *Prone position with the table flexed about 45° to keep the caudal dural sac on a higher level than the head to minimize loss of liquor.*

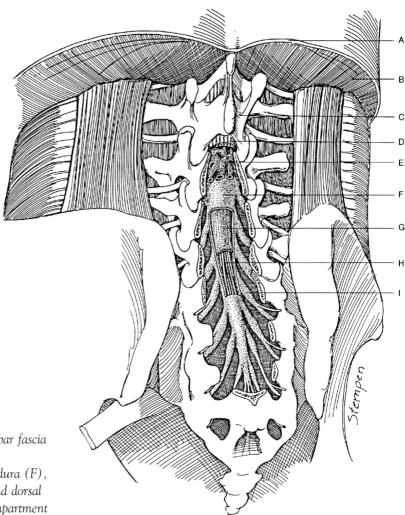

Figure 4. *Topography of the surgical field: thoracolumbar fascia (A), erector spinae muscle (B), sphenoidal spine (C), ligamentum flavum (D), vascular plexus and fat (E), dura (F), arachnoid (G), intradural compartment with ventral and dorsal sacral roots (H), spinal nerves within the extradural compartment (I).*

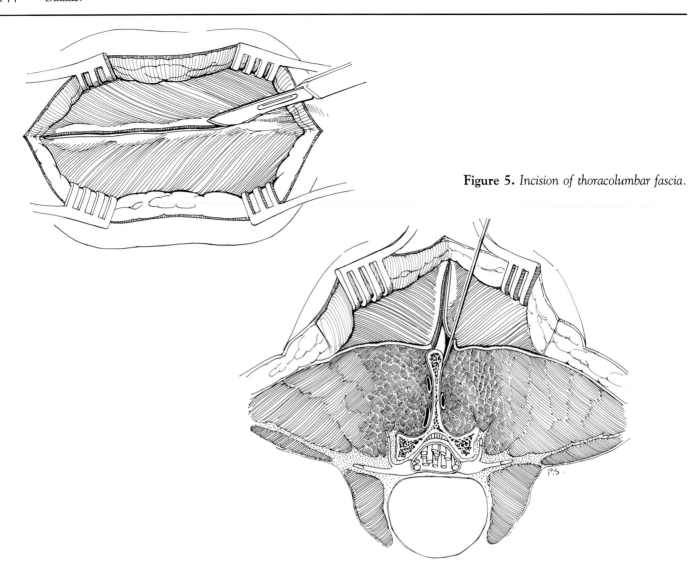

Figure 5. *Incision of thoracolumbar fascia.*

Figure 6. *Sharp dissection of thoracolumbar fascia and erector spinae muscle in a plane between the bone and periosteum.*

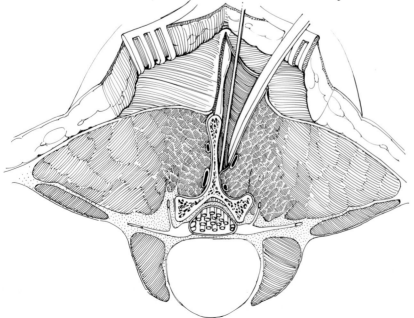

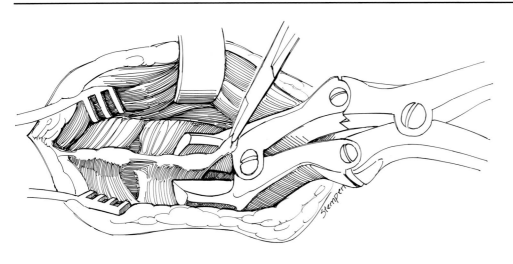

Figure 7. *Removal of spinous processes with (a) Liston–Key bone cutting forceps and (b) Stille–Leksell rongeur.*

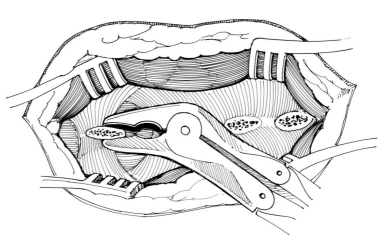

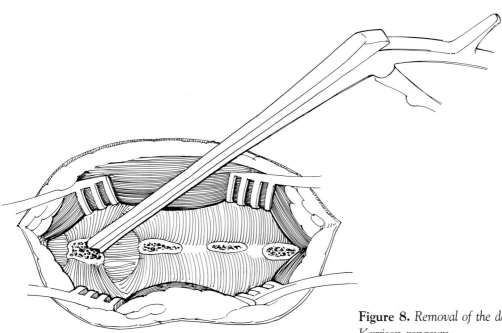

Figure 8. *Removal of the dorsal aspect of vertebral arches with Kerrison rongeurs.*

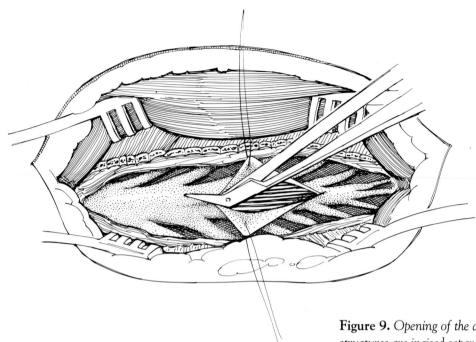

Figure 9. *Opening of the dura and arachnoidea. (If possible, both structures are incised separately.) Use monofile 5/0 stay sutures to keep the dura open.*

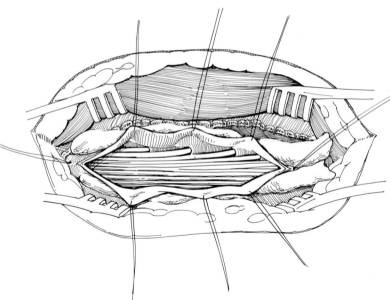

Figure 10. *Presentation of the intradural compartment. The cranial end of the dural incision is secured with a knotted stay suture to avoid uncontrolled ripping of the dura. Identification of the ventral and dorsal sacral roots via anatomic landmarks, and electrostimulation.*

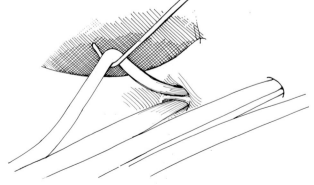

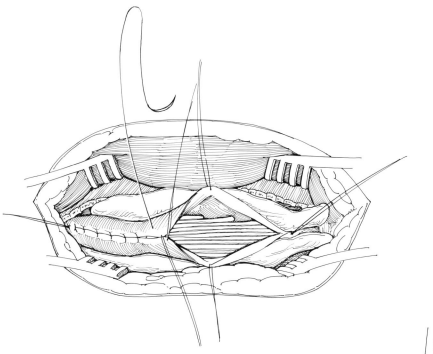

Figure 11. *Water-tight closure of the dura is accomplished by a running nonreabsorbable monofile suture. Take only a small rim of the dura and remove the stay sutures step by step.*

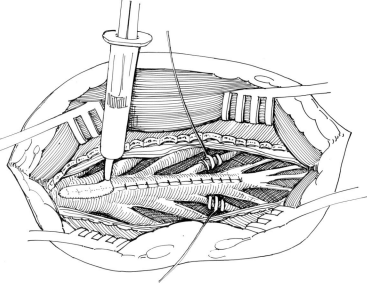

Figure 12. *Optionally, the suture can be sealed with fibrin glue. In this case, electrodes were positioned extradurally on the spinal nerve of the S3 segment for ventral sacral root stimulation.*

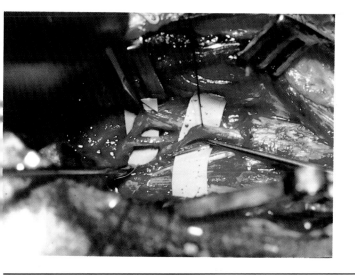

Figure 13. *Intraoperative view of the exposed sacral spinal nerves for extradural deafferentation. Stay suture in the spinal ganglion.*

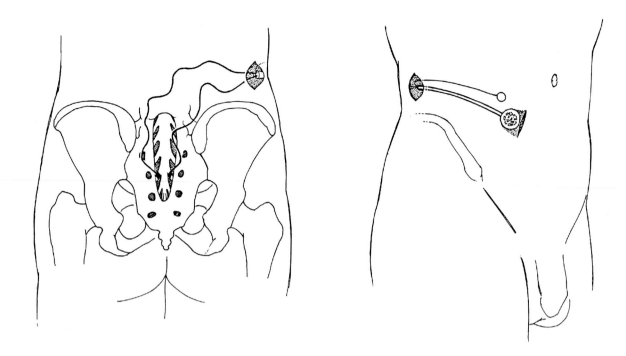

Figure 14. *Cable positioning and electrode placement.*

Fascial Sling Procedure in Men

J.W. Thüroff, M. Hohenfellner[a],
D. Schultz-Lampel
Department of Urology,
University of Witten/Herdecke, Wuppertal, Germany and
[a]Ruhr University, Herne, Germany

Introduction

Urinary incontinence in men still presents a therapeutic problem. Conservative therapy with drugs or physical treatment shows only limited effects, therefore reconstructive surgery is often necessary.

For surgical therapy, in most cases an artificial sphincter is implanted. This method is associated with the general problems of alloplastic implantation materials and artificial pressure around the whole circumference of the urethra, which could result in tissue atrophy, perforation of the sphincter cuff and infection of the alloplastic material.

In animal experiments a fascial sling procedure improves the urethral closure mechanism under stress conditions. Based on anatomic studies of the pelvic floor we have developed a modified fascial sling technique for therapy of urinary incontinence in men. Clinical trials have documented good or excellent postoperative results in 72.7% of cases.

Advantages

- Avoids the use of alloplastic materials
- Uses a pedicled fascial sling
- Standardizes the positioning of the sling
- Avoids cutting the sphincter or muscles of the pelvic floor
- Padding of the urethra with pubococcygeal muscle
- Suspends and elevates the pelvic floor without obstruction
- Allows unimpaired spontaneous micturition

Indications

- Incontinence after transurethral resection of the prostate (TURP)
- Incontinence after suprapubic enucleation of the prostate
- Incontinence after radical prostatectomy
- Neurogenic adynamic bladder with incontinence

Contraindications

- Neurogenic hyperactive bladder
- Reduced bladder capacity

Instruments

- Standard instruments
- Suture material: 3/0 Prolene (Ethicon, Edinburgh, UK)

Operative technique step by step

- Lower midline incision and semicircular incision above the anus
- Excision of a 1.5–2 cm × 20 cm pedunculated fascial sling out of the frontal rectus fascia with the base on the side of the symphysis (Figure 1)
- Opening of the retropubic space and preparation of the endopelvic fascia on both sides along the puboprostatic ligament
- Small longitudinal incision of the endopelvic fascia on both sides to provide an entrance and exit for the fascial sling (Figure 2)
- Preparation of the peritoneum around the anus, without cutting the central tendon, via the para-anal incision
- Preparation of the left ischiorectal fossa and blunt undermining of the urogenital diaphragm, with the transverse perineal muscle as the ventral, and the frontal rectal wall as the dorsal, border of the tunnel
- Perforation under digital control of the levator ani muscle coming from the perineum between the pubococcygeus (medial) and the ileococcygeus (lateral) muscles, clamping, and passage of the fascial sling on a stay suture
- Preparation of the right ischiorectal fossa and blunt undermining of the central tendon, creating a tunnel between the right and left fossa, with the prostate and urethra, the frontal rectal wall and the central tendon as borders of the tunnel.
- Passing the fascial sling from the left through the right fossa at right angles (Figure 3)
- Perforation to the right abdominal side, as described above, and passage of the sling through the right abdominal side
- Fixation of the free end of the sling under tension on the right Cooper's ligament with a 3/0 Prolene suture (Figure 4)

Postoperative care

Spontaneous micturition starts 6–8 days after the operation. The cystostomy tube is removed after confirmation of residual free emptying of the bladder.

Reference

1. Thüroff JW, Hohenfellner M, Schultz-Lampel D. Die Harninkontinenz des Mannes. *Akt Urol* **23** (1992) 149–57.

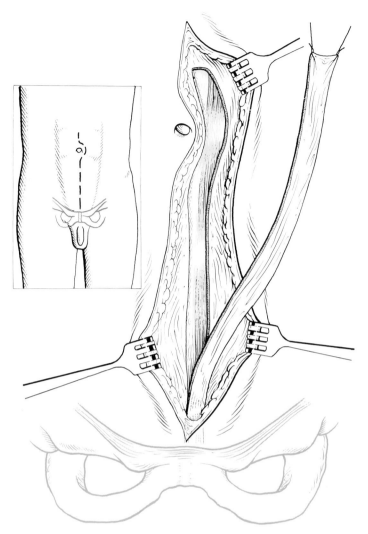

Figure 1. *Excision of a 1.5–2 cm × 20 cm pedicled fascial sling out of the frontal rectus fascia with the basis on the side of the symphysis.*

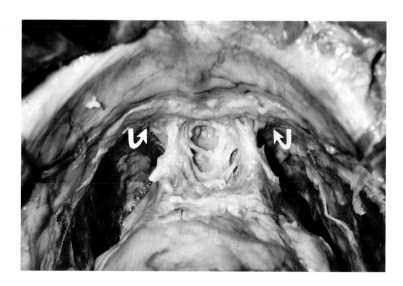

Figure 2. *Anatomic preparation: passing the fascial sling through the endopelvic fascia on both sides lateral to the puboprostatic ligament and between the origin of the pubococcygeus and ileococcygeus muscles.*

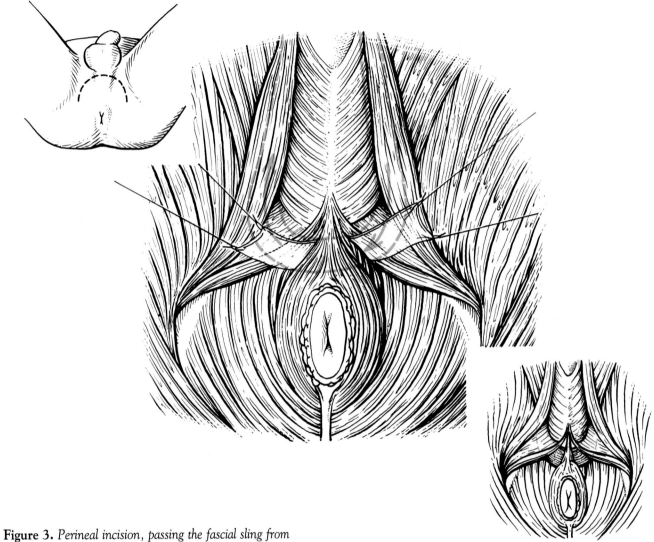

Figure 3. *Perineal incision, passing the fascial sling from the left abdominal side to the left ischiorectal fossa, then cranial to the central tendon between the membranes of the urethral/dorsal surface of the prostate and the frontal rectal wall to the right ischiorectal fossa, and to the right abdominal side.*

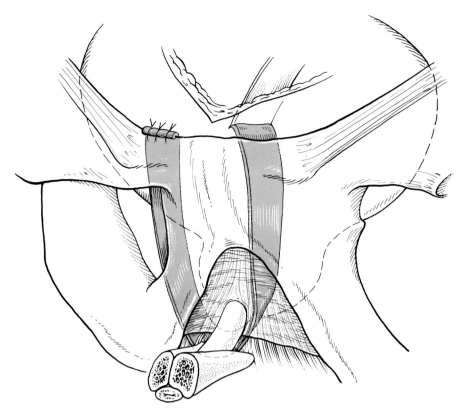

Figure 4. *Fixation of the fascial sling on Cooper's ligament.*

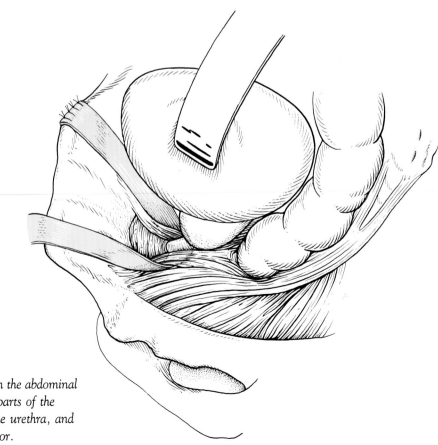

Figure 5. *Position of the fascial sling from the abdominal viewpoint. Medial approximation of the parts of the pubococcygeus muscle with padding of the urethra, and elevation and suspension of the pelvic floor.*

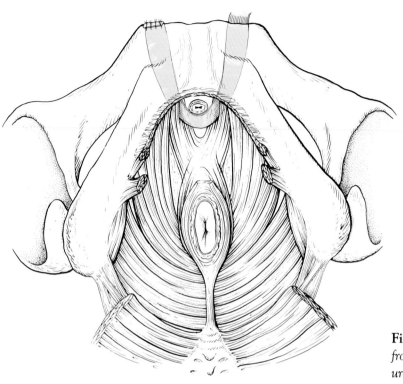

Figure 6. *View to the pelvic floor and the fascial sling from caudal (anatomical preparation after cutting of the urogenital diaphragm and the urethra): the fascial sling winds around parts of the pubococcygeus muscle on both sides.*

Figure 7. *View to the pelvic floor and the fascial sling from the abdomen.*

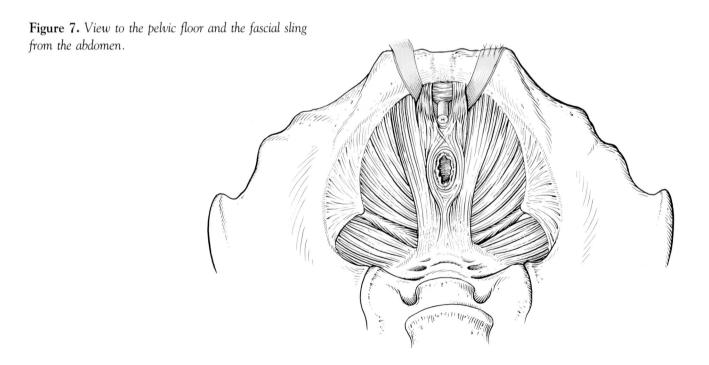

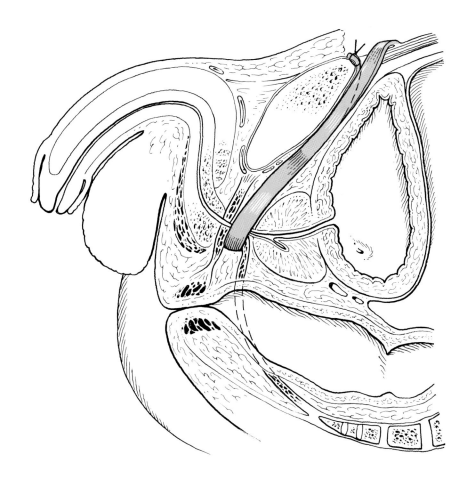

Figure 8. *Sagittal sectional image with presentation of the position of the fascial sling above the levator ani muscle (pubococcygeus muscle) and cranial to the central tendon and the urogenital diaphragm.*

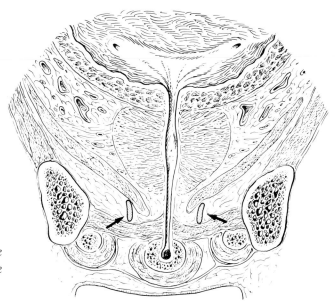

Figure 9. *Frontal sectional image with presentation of the position of the fascial sling between the levator ani muscle (pubococcygeus muscle) and the urogenital diaphragm (deep and superficial transverse perineal muscles).*

Vesicovaginal Fistula: Abdominal Approach

M. Stöckle[c], J. Leissner[a], F. Steinbach[b],
M. Fisch[a], M. Hohenfellner[a]
Department of Urology,
[a]*University of Mainz School of Medicine,*
Mainz, Germany
[b]*University of Magdeburg, Magdeburg, Germany*
[c]*University of Kiel, Kiel, Germany*

Comment

For a variety of reasons, the number of vesicovaginal fistulas treated by gynecologists has fallen. In developed countries, the most common cause of vesicovaginal fistula is gynecologic surgery in the small pelvis. Owing to a better and more sophisticated operative technique, the absolute number of postoperative fistulas has diminished. This is in contrast to underdeveloped nations, where most fistulas are caused by obstetric trauma. Interestingly, according to data from the Mayo Clinic (1800 fistulas over 30 years), the majority of fistulas (>50%) arose after uncomplicated vaginal or abdominal hysterectomy and not after extensive and complicated gynecologic surgery.

For many years, gynecologists favored the vaginal approach for fistula repair, which (especially in complicated fistulas) has a lower success and higher complication rate than the abdominal approach. Urologists, more orientated towards modern abdominal surgery, were more successful, so that recently younger gynecologists are very inexperienced in vesicovaginal fistula repair. However, the abdominal approach often results in overtreatment of small uncomplicated fistulas and therefore prevents quicker recovery of the patient.

Undoubtedly, the abdominal approach shows better results in complicated fistulas. However, in small (<2.5 cm) and nonradiation fistulas with a mobile vaginal stump, the vaginal approach for fistula repair (e.g. as described by Füth or Lazko) leads to success rates of up to 90%. Additionally, this technique avoids laparotomy and opening of the bladder, and provides quicker recovery with less morbidity. Therefore the surgeon, whether urologist or gynecologist, should be familiar with both routes of repair, and both departments should share their experience to gain the highest standard of treatment.

V. Friedberg, Denzlingen

Vesicovaginal fistula: abdominal approach

Introduction

The optimum approach for surgical repair of vesicovaginal fistulas remains a controversial issue. In our opinion, the vaginal approach should be reserved for uncomplicated and small fistulas. In contrast, indications for the abdominal approach are:

- Fistula close to the ureterovesical junction
- Fistula with a diameter of more than 2.5 cm
- Fistulas in which the bladder and ureter are prolapsed into the vagina
- History of multiple previous operations and suspected scarred paravesical tissue
- Vesicocervical fistula
- Complex vesicovaginal fistula after radiation

Decreased blood supply and scarred tissue in the fistula area often lead to recurrent fistula after operation. Therefore, interposition of healthy vascular tissue is mandatory. In our experience, an omental pedicle graft, with its abundant blood supply and lymphatic drainage, or a peritoneal flap gives the best chance of preventing recurrent fistula. Both tissue types may reabsorb urine extravasate and close small bladder leaks. Additionally, they prevent the formation of urine stones, which can occur when urine extravasate cannot be absorbed by the surrounding scarred tissue. Pechersdorfer *et al.* (1964) described first the placement of an omentum pedicle into the vesicovaginal septum.

Timing of surgery

Inflammatory and even destructive reactions of the surrounding tissue are characteristics of early fistula. Early fistula repair therefore often results in recurrent fistulas caused by dehiscent sutures or necrotized tissue. Thus, surgical fistula repair should not be attempted before the inflammatory reaction has subsided: we would wait at least 6 weeks after diagnosing the fistula. The subsiding inflammatory reaction can be confirmed by cystoscopy, and the fistula should be pale and noninflamed before repair is attempted.

Early surgical fistula repair is indicated only when the fistula has been diagnosed intraoperatively or in the early postoperative days, before the inflammatory reaction has started.

Preoperative care

Informed consent should be obtained for:

- Recurrent fistulas
- Ureteroneocystostomy in case of fistulas close to the ureterovesical junction
- Supravesical urinary diversion, especially after repair of complex fistulas due to radiation

Directly before the operation cystoscopy should be performed. Fistulas can be traced with 6 Fr or 7 Fr ureteral catheters. If necessary, lay the catheter into the fistula and clamp both ends of the catheter outside the body. Intraoperatively, after mobilization of the fistula, the catheter can be divided and pulled away.

Operative technique

- Exposure: lower midline incision, which can be lengthened cranially for mobilization of the omentum flap
- Mobilization and dissection of a 4 × 6 cm peritoneal flap (either a free flap or a pedicle from the attached bladder peritoneum)
- Opening the bladder and excision of the fistula with the surrounding tissue (at least 1 cm). If the fistula runs along one or two ureters, the ureter must be divided and ureteroneocystostomy performed
- Dissection of the vesicovaginal septum. Closure of the vagina with interrupted 3/0 absorbable sutures. The peritoneal flap or omental pedicle graft is brought into the pelvis and may be secured with a few absorbable sutures at the deepest point between the bladder and vagina. In heavily irradiated patients we favor the omentum pedicle graft, because often the peritoneum shows ischemic lesions and has a reduced blood supply

    It is important to fill the vesicovaginal space completely with peritoneal or omental tissue and drain it into the peritoneal cavity

- Closure of the bladder with interrupted 3/0 suture
- When the ureter has been divided from the bladder a ureteroneocystostomy using the psoas-hitch technique should be performed

- Paravesical drainage, suprapubic and transurethral catheter and wound closure

Special situations in radiation fistulas

In heavily irradiated patients the fistula must be excised until normal healthy tissue appears. The most important point to prevent recurrent fistulas is a tension-free closure of the fistula. When this is not possible, we recommend not closing the fistula but placing an omental pedicle graft into the vagina. Usually this closes the fistula, but prevents intercourse for a time. The patient should be informed of this possibility in advance and must agree with this condition. Before the catheter is removed, cystography should exclude any urinary extravasation.

If a ureteroneocystostomy must be performed, shorten the ureter until normal blood supply appears. It seems to be better to mobilize the bladder than the ureter; a tension-free anastomosis is mandatory. In cases of very short ureters the Boari-flap technique or bowel interposition becomes necessary.

Postoperative care

Mobilization of the patient on day 1; removal of splints and transurethral catheter between days 7 and 10. Cystography via the suprapubic tube on day 14: if no urinary extravasation is seen, the suprapubic catheter is removed.

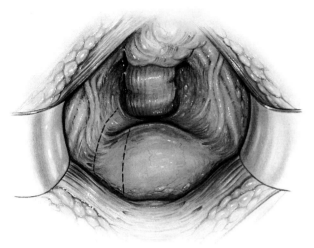

Figure 1. *Exposure of the bladder via median laparotomy. A peritoneal pedicle flap can be mobilized from the marked area.*

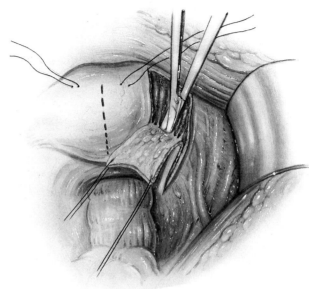

Figure 2. *Preparation of the pedicle flap and opening of the bladder between two stay sutures.*

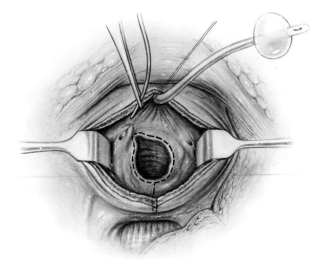

Figure 3. *Opening of the bladder, showing a transurethral catheter coming from the bladder, the ureteral orifices and a large vesicovaginal fistula. Open the bladder at the marked line for fistula excision.*

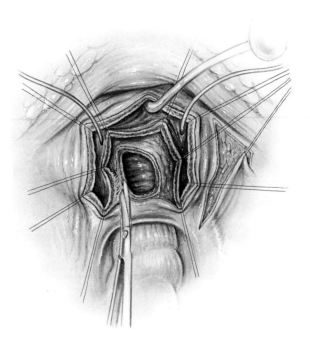

Figure 4. *Dissection of the vesicovaginal space.*

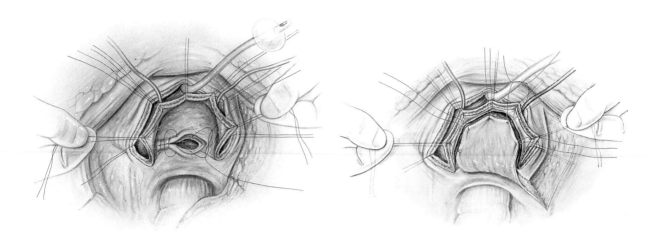

Figure 5. *Closure of the vagina with interrupted sutures. Knots should be placed inside the vagina to prevent any irritation of the bladder wall by suture material.*

Figure 6. *The peritoneal pedicle flap is brought into the vesicovaginal space and secured at the deepest point.*

Figure 7. *Closure of the bladder with interrupted sutures beginning at the bladder neck. Note that the ureters should not be irritated by the sutures.*

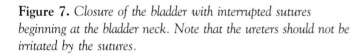

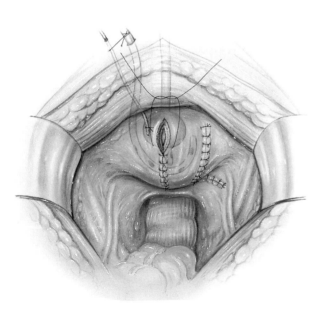

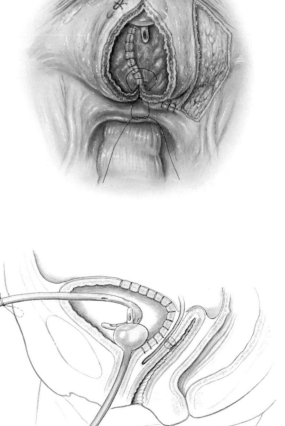

Figure 8. *The bladder closure is almost finished. The peritoneal defect in the paravesical area is already closed.*

Figure 9. *Cross-section after closure of the bladder and vagina.*

Figure 10. *In complex ureterovaginal and vesicovaginal fistulas a ureterocystoneostomy using the psoas-hitch technique is required. For tension-free anastomosis, a Boari flap may be necessary.*

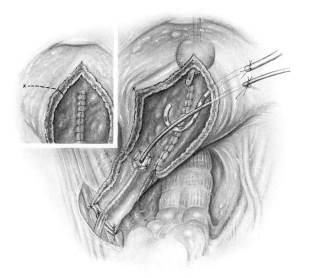

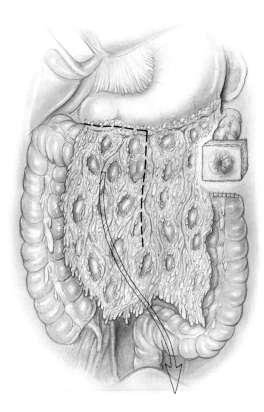

Figure 11. *In complicated fistulas an omental pedicle graft should be brought into the vagina to close the fistula (from either the right or the left colon). In vesicorectal or rectovaginal fistulas a colonic stoma is necessary.*

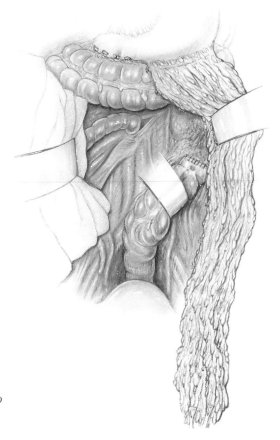

Figure 12. *Mobilization of an omental flap from the greater curvature of the stomach, which is brought lateral to the colon into the pelvis.*

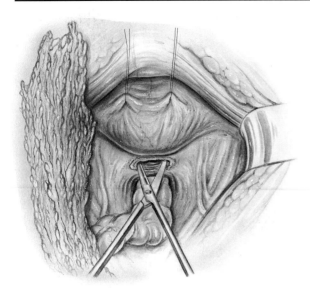

Figure 13. *In heavily irradiated patients the omental flap is placed inside the vagina without excision of the fistula.*

Figure 14. *Fixation of the omentum at the vulva. During the healing process, the omentum will be retracted into the vagina.*

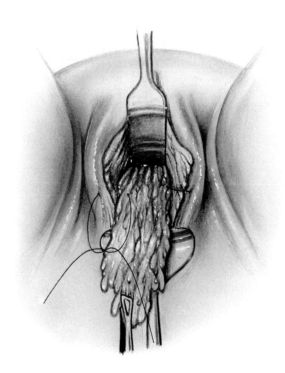

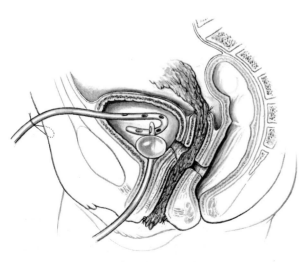

Figure 15. *Cross-section after interposition of an omental graft between the bladder and rectum.*

Bladder Diverticulectomy

S.W. Melchior, G.E. Voges, J. Fichtner,
R. Hohenfellner
*Department of Urology,
University of Mainz School of Medicine,
Mainz, Germany*

Acquired vesical diverticula usually occur in male adults, most often as a result of mechanical infravesical obstruction or neurogenic voiding disorders. The most frequent location is the ureterovesical junction.

Sequelae of diverticula include:

- Recurrent/persistent urinary tract infections
- Stone formation
- Obstruction of the ureter, large bowel or pelvic veins
- Vesicoureteral reflux (VUR)
- Malignant transformation

Treatment options

Asymptomatic diverticula should be endoscopically inspected once a year. Transurethral diverticulotomy with resection of the diverticular orifice and fulguration of the mucosa is adequate for small symptomatic diverticula. Open diverticulectomy is recommended for complicated diverticula exceeding 3 cm in diameter. Concurrent mechanical infravesical obstruction should be treated before diverticulectomy or in the same session. Also, coexisting VUR should be fixed by ureteroneocystostomy using the psoas-hitch technique. For open diverticulectomy, we usually prefer a combined extraintravesical approach.

Preoperative work-up

- History
- Physical examination
- Sonography of kidneys, bladder and prostate
- Intravenous urography and voiding cysturethrography in anterior–posterior, lateral and oblique views
- Chest radiography, ECG and blood work-up

Anesthesia

- Regional or general

Surgical technique (Figures 1–8)

- Perform urethrocystoscopy before surgery for inspection of the diverticulum (if not yet done)
- Place the patient in a supine extended position with the pelvis slightly elevated
- Make a midline suprapubic extraperitoneal incision of Pfannenstiel incision 3–4 cm above the symphysis (depending on the size of the diverticulum)

- Fill the bladder with 200–300 ml normal saline via a transurethral catheter
- After mobilizing the peritoneum upward and the perivesical tissue to the side, identify and retract the ipsilateral ureter
- Open the bladder between stay sutures
- Place a transurethral catheter into the diverticulum; insertion of an additional ureteral catheter may be helpful
- Filling the balloon of the catheter (depending on the diverticulum size) facilitates dissection of the diverticulum and the neck of the diverticulum *extra*vesically
- Pick up the diverticulum with a clamp and remove the catheter
- The diverticulum can now be removed by *intra*vesical circular excision around the diverticular entrance between stay sutures
- Close the bladder defect at the site of the former diverticulum in a two-layer technique by inverting the mucosa (using synthetic absorbable sutures)
- Close the bladder in a two-layer technique after inserting a suprapubic tube and a passive perivesical drain. The ureteral catheter should be in place for 6–7 days if the diverticulum was close to the ureteral orifice

Postoperative care

Remove the perivesical drainage on day 3, the transurethral catheter on day 3–5 and the suprapubic tube on day 7 if voiding occurs without problems.

Bibliography

1. Das S, Amar AD. Vesical diverticulum associated with bladder carcinoma: therapeutic implications. *J Urol* **136** (1986) 1013–14.
2. Fellows GJ. The association between vesical carcinoma and diverticulum of the bladder. *Eur Urol* **4** (1978) 185–6.
3. Kelalis PP, Mclean P. The treatment of diverticulum of the bladder. *J Urol* **98** (1967) 349–52.
4. Mclean P, Kelalis PP. Bladder diverticulum in the male. *Br J Urol* **40** (1968) 321–4.
5. Melchior SW, Voges GE, Stöckle M, Müller SC. Divertikeltumoren der Harnblase. *Urol A Suppl* (1992) A61.
6. Montague DK, Boltuch RL. Primary neoplasms in vesical diverticula: report of ten cases. *J Urol* **116** (1976) 41–2.
7. Smith MS. Vesical diverticulectomy: In: Glenn JF (ed.) *Urologic Surgery*. Philadelphia: J.B. Lippincott (1983).

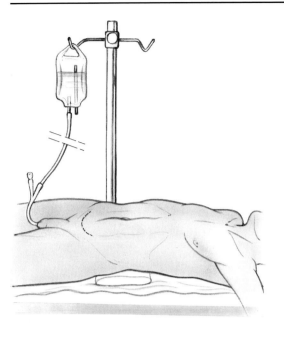

Figure 1. *Pfannenstiel incision 3–4 cm above the symphysis.*

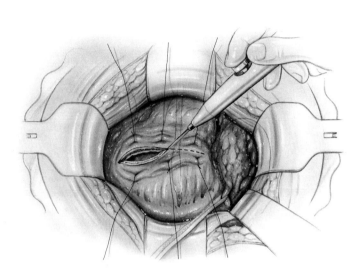

Figure 2. *Transverse incision of the bladder between stay sutures after dissection of the ureter.*

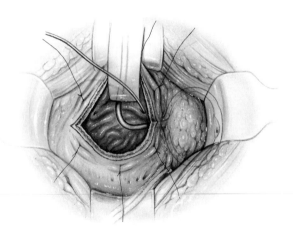

Figure 3. *Insertion of a ureteral catheter and placing of the transurethral catheter in the diverticulum.*

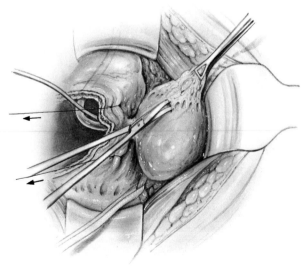

Figure 4. *Dissection of the diverticulum.*

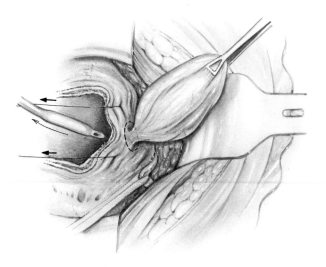

Figure 5. *Grasping of the diverticulum with a clamp and removal of the catheter (ureteral catheter not shown).*

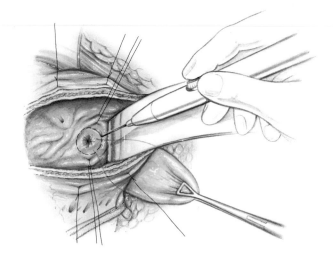

Figure 6. *Circular excision of the diverticular orifice (ureteral catheter not shown).*

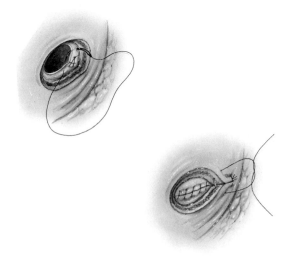

Figure 7. *Closure of the bladder in a two-layer technique.*

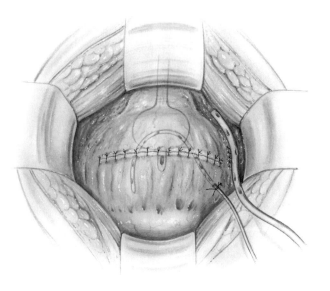

Figure 8. *Operative site after bladder closure.*

Continent Vesicostomy

J. Fichtner, R. Hohenfellner
Department of Urology,
University of Mainz School of Medicine,
Mainz, Germany

Introduction

The incorporation of the efferent segment in the pouch during continent urinary diversion results in a higher leakage-point pressure and a larger functional capacity than the use of extraluminar efferent segments.[1] Accordingly, the concept of a submucosally embedded seromuscular tube (Boari tube) as the efferent segment for a Mainz pouch (developed by Lampel and Thüroff[2]) can be transferred to the bladder. This procedure, which was originally planned as a simplification of the continence mechanism in cases where the appendix was not available, has been successfully used in 34 cases. Similarly, a submucosally embedded Boari tube may be used for creation of a continent vesicostomy. This procedure offers advantages and alternatives to repeated implantations of artificial sphincters in cases of urethral lesions, in the Mitrofanoff procedure, cecal augmentation with appendicocecal or ileal stoma, transureteroureterostomy with catheterization through a ureteral stump, and other forms of continent urinary diversion.

Indications

- Irreversible loss of the urethra or the continence mechanism, with normal bladder capacity and a normal upper urinary tract
- Neurogenic adynamic bladder with incontinence
- Congenital anomalies, e.g. urogenital sinus

Contraindications

- Reduced bladder capacity
- Dilated upper urinary tract
- Neurogenic hyperactive bladder

Instruments

- Standard instruments for urethral operations
- Ring retractor
- Suture material: polyglycolic acid 4/0, chromic catgut 5/0

Operative technique step by step (Figures 1–13)

- Lower midline incision with butterfly-flap plasty at the limit of the pubic hair growth for later construction of the pseudoumbilical stoma

- Extraperitoneal mobilization of the bladder (filled with 300 ml saline)
- Extraperitonealization of the bladder dome after division of the urachus. In cases with attached peritoneum (e.g. secondary operations) this part remains with the bladder and the peritoneal reflection is closed by a running suture after mobilization
- Parallel incision of the detrusor muscle after placement of stay sutures for demarcation of the tube over a length of 8 cm and 3 cm width
- Lateral blunt and sharp dissection of the intact mucosal layer (2 cm on each side) for creation of the submucosal trough
- Placement of mucosal stay sutures, parallel opening of the bladder along the marked Boari flap and inspection of the ureteral orifices
- Two-layer closure of the tube with running 5/0 chromic catgut mucosal suture and interrupted 4/0 polyglycolic acid sutures of the detrusor muscle over an 18 Fr balloon catheter (30% tissue shrinkage). Placement of a lateral cystostomy tube
- Running 4/0 chromic catgut suturing of the vesical mucosa for creation of the submucosal trough with interrupted sutures at the insertion of the tube
- Embedding of the tube and closure of the overlying detrusor muscle with interrupted 4/0 Vicryl sutures (Ethicon, Edinburgh, UK)
- Fixation of the tube after incision of the fascial layer, and semicircular anastomosis of both cutaneous flaps with the tube – a pseudoumbilical stoma is thus created
- Paravesical drainage and wound closure

Surgical tricks

The lateral mobilization of the vesical mucosa at both edges of the marked flap is especially important for later successful embedding of the created tube and should encompass at least 3 cm to each side.

Postoperative care

The balloon catheter is removed 3 weeks after surgery, and clean intermittent catheterization is then started. The cystostomy tube is removed after confirmation of residual-free emptying of the bladder.

Special situations

In incontinent patients the bladder has to be completely separated from the urethra at the bladder neck and is then closed by two-layer suturing with interposition of omentum or a free peritoneal flap.[3] (Division of the bladder neck at least 2 cm distal to the base of the tube is necessary for preservation of the blood supply.)

References

1. Stenzl A, Klutke CG, Golomb J, Raz S. Tapered intraluminal versus imbricated extraluminal valve: comparison of two continence mechanisms for urinary diversion. *J Urol* **143** (1990) 607–11.
2. Lampel A, Hohenfellner M, Schultz-Lampel D, Wienold D, Thüroff JW. Submuköser Seromuskularis-Conduit: Eine neue Technik des kontinenten Stomas beim Mainz-Pouch. *Akt Urol Operative Techniken* **24** (1993) 6.16: I–VII.
3. Voges GE, Müller SC, Stöckle M, Hohenfellner R. Antegrade (deszendierende) radikale retropubische Prostatektomie. *Akt Urol* **22** (1991) I–XIV.

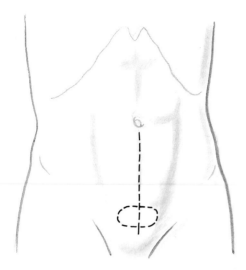

Figure 1. *Lower midline incision with semicircular distal butterfly plasty.*

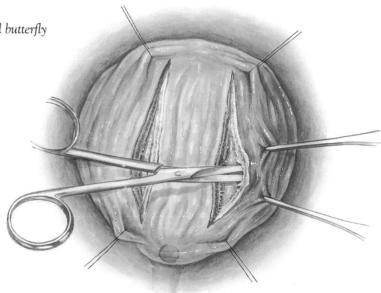

Figure 2. A 3 × 8 cm Boari flap is formed and the mucosa mobilized laterally.

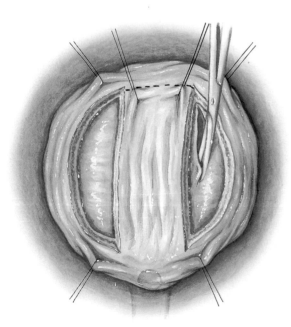

Figure 3. *Incision of the bladder along the flap.*

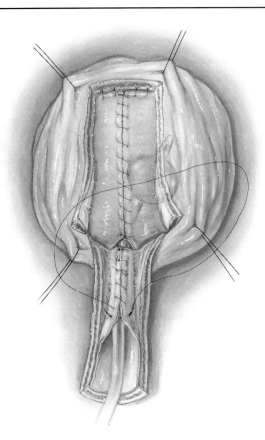

Figure 4. *Running readaptation of the lateral mucosal edges and closure of the tube with running suture over an 18 Fr balloon catheter.*

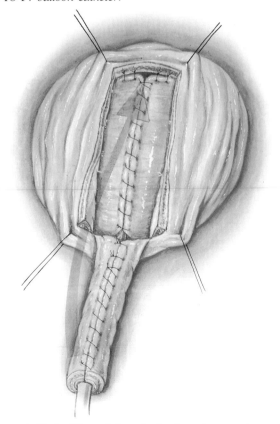

Figure 6. *Embedding of the tube in the submucosal trough.*

Figure 5. *The detrusor muscle of the tube is sutured.*

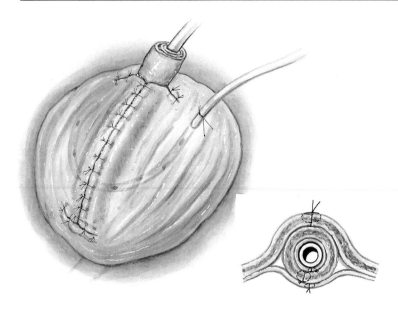

Figure 7. *Interrupted sutures of the detrusor muscle over the embedded tube.*

Figure 8. *Star-shaped incision of the fascial layer for pull-through of the tube.*

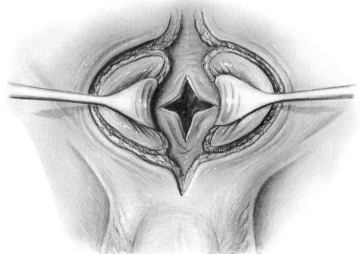

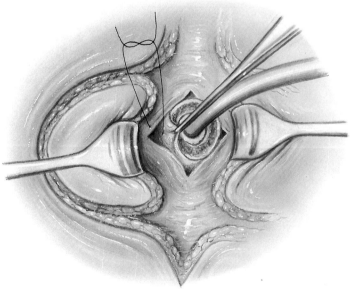

Figure 9. *Anchoring of the tube to the rectus fascia.*

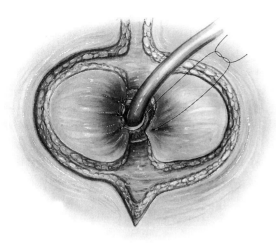

Figure 10. *Semicircular anastomosis of both cutaneous flaps with the tip of the tube.*

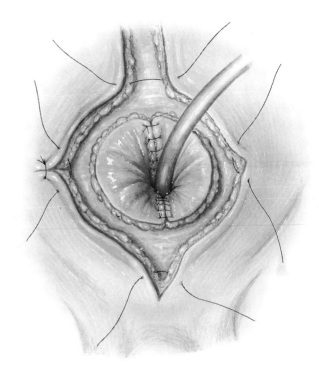

Figure 11. *Skin closure with suturing of the lateral wound edges to the funnel.*

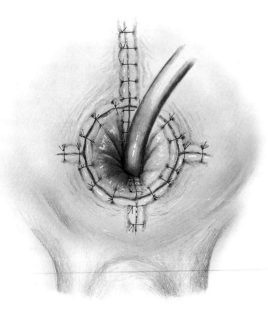

Figure 12. *A pseudoumbilical stoma in the area of pubic hair growth is created.*

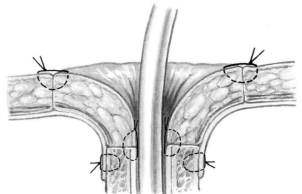

Figure 13. *Cross-section of the stoma with indwelling catheter.*

Modified Boari Hitch Technique (Übelhör Procedure) for Ureteral Neoimplantation

R. Wammack, M. Fisch, R. Hohenfellner
Department of Urology,
University of Mainz School of Medicine,
Mainz, Germany

Introduction

The original technique described by Boari (Casati and Boari 1894, Ockerblad 1947) of replacing a ureter by a vesical flap is not often performed. Cases treatable with the Boari-flap procedure represent borderline indications in the sense that ureteral defects are present which cannot be treated by a psoas-hitch technique so that ureteral replacement by bowel or renal autotransplantation would have to be carried out. Both are elaborate procedures.

The parallel bladder incision originally recommended by Boari can compromise the blood supply of the distal part of the flap, which is the area where ureteral implantation is to be performed. Subsequent fibrosis and stenosis at the site of ureteral implantation is often the result. These disadvantages are obviated by implementation of Übelhör's modification of the Boari procedure.

Indications

- Ureteral injuries, stenosis and fistulas which cannot be breached using the psoas hitch technique and which extend beyond the ureter's crossing with the major iliac vessels

Contraindications

- Reduced bladder capacity

Instruments

- Standard instruments for bladder surgery
- Ring retractor
- Suture material: polyglycolic acid 3/0 and 4/0, and chromic catgut 4/0 and 5/0

Operative approach

The optimal operative approach depends on the primary disease. Generally, access can be gained transperitoneally or extraperitoneally. In cases with extensive adhesions and scar tissue formation, a transperitoneal approach by a midline lower abdominal incision is more beneficial than an extraperitoneal approach.

Preoperative treatment

Before ureteral neoimplantation, adequate bladder capacity should be present and there should be no evidence of mucosal inflammation.

Operative technique step by step (Figures 1–14)

- The generous primary incision towards the bladder outlet is followed by a vertical incision. This incision can be extended in the direction of the contralateral ureteral orifice until the desired length of flap is obtained
- The broad basis of the flap guarantees a good vascular supply up to the equally broad distal portion of the flap, enabling safe ureteral implantation
- Ureteral implantation is performed in an open-ended technique analogous to the procedure described for the psoas-hitch technique (see Chapter 3.8)

Postoperative care

The indwelling catheter is removed around day 8 while the bladder remains drained by the suprapubic cystostomy. The ureteral stent is removed on day 10 and after documentation of residual-free voiding; the cystostomy tube can be removed thereafter. The drain in the vicinity of the anastomosis site is progressively retracted starting on day 3. During the first 5–6 days, an antibiotic is routinely administered, and infection prophylaxis with a furantoin derivative is continued for 1 week thereafter.

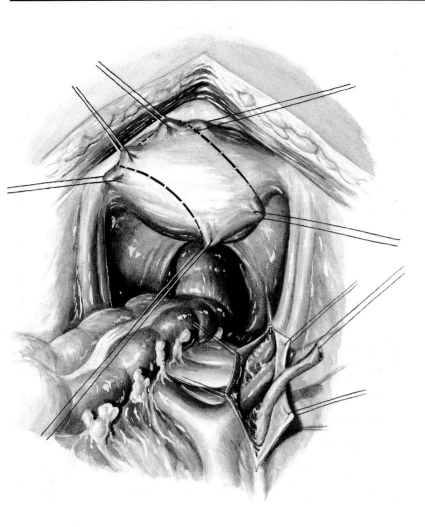

Figure 1. *Classic incision for creating a Boari flap.*

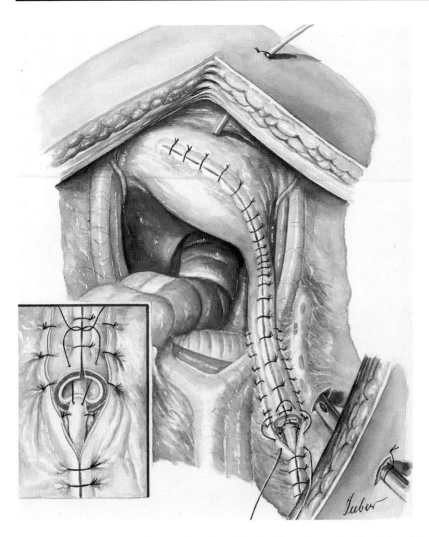

Figure 2. *Classic Boari flap with unfavorable blood supply to the distal flap (danger of stricture at the ureteral implantation site).*

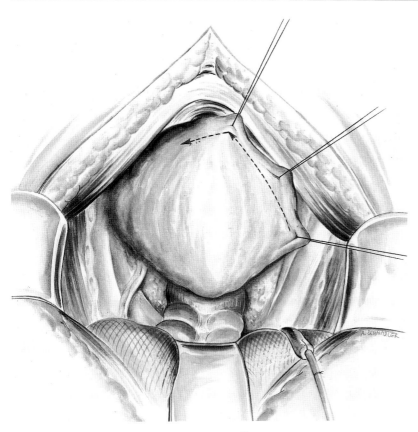

Figure 3. *Modified incision as described by Übelhör: placement of three stay sutures in the lateral bladder wall.*

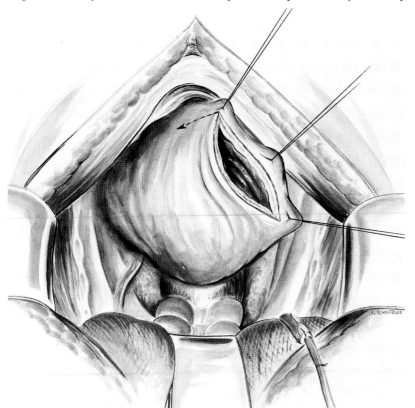

Figure 4. *Upper and lower stay sutures mark the borders of the incision in the direction of the bladder outlet.*

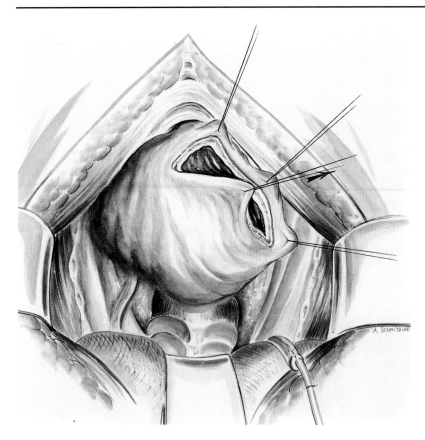

Figure 5. *An additional stay suture placed at a corner of the newly created flap pulls the flap to the side.*

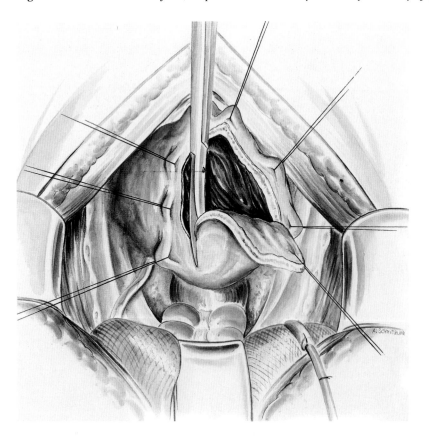

Figure 6. *Change in the direction of incision (vertical). The incision can be extended in the direction of the bladder base. Creation of a triangular flap.*

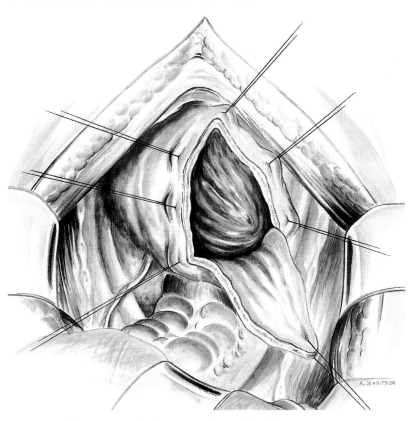

Figure 7. *Traction on the flap causes longitudinal deformation.*

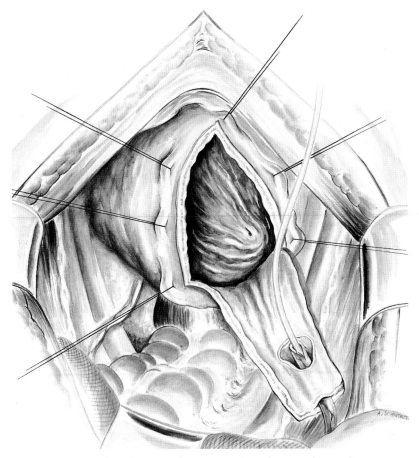

Figure 8. *Ureteral implantation by means of a submucosal tunnel using an Übelhör-ended technique.*

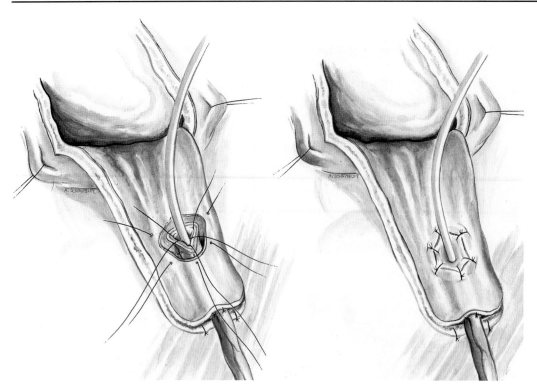

Figure 9. Ureteral anastomosis by ureteromucous single-stitch sutures (5/0 chromic catgut). Fixation of the cranial end of the flap to the psoas muscle produces the rectangular shape of the flap.

Figure 10. Completed ureterovesical anastomosis. Placement of a ureteral stent (6 Fr).

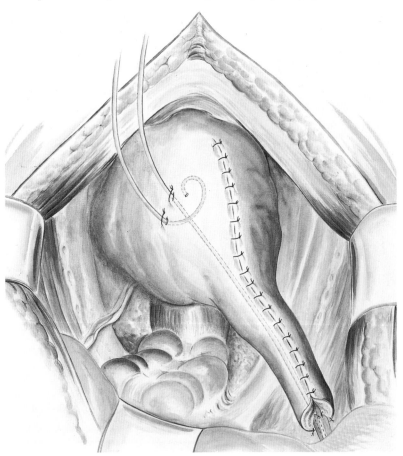

Figure 11. Closure of the bladder with a 5/0 chromic catgut running suture for the mucosa, 4/0 polydioxanone single-stitch detrusor sutures. A ureteral stent and cystostomy (12 Fr) have been led out by means of separate incisions.

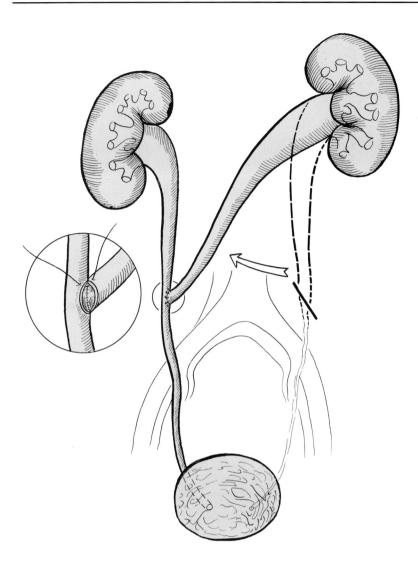

Figure 12. *Transureteroureterostomy: end-to-side ureteral anastomosis.*

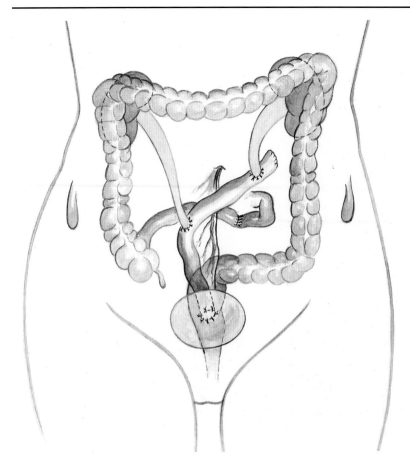

Figure 13. *Bilateral ureteral replacement by means of an isolated ileal segment.*

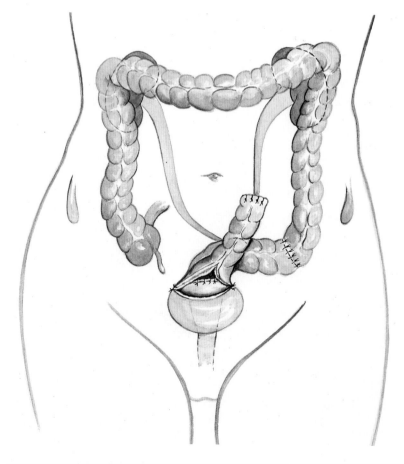

Figure 14. *Bilateral ureteral replacement and augmentation of the subtotally resected bladder by an isolated segment of sigmoid colon (ureterocolocystoplasty).*

Psoas Hitch Technique for Ureteral Neoimplantation

R. Wammack, M. Fisch, R. Hohenfellner
Department of Urology,
University of Mainz School of Medicine,
Mainz, Germany

Introduction

Open antirefluxing ureteral implantation by means of a submucosal tunnel is far superior to all other forms of ureteral neoimplantation. Experience has shown that it is of the utmost importance to approximate the ureter and bladder maximally and fix the bladder to the psoas muscle. These aims are accomplished by extensive vesical mobilization, transection of the lateral umbilical cord, transection of the ureter far away from the site of an infected fistula at a level demonstrating healthy and viable tissue, and the establishment of an absolutely tension-free anastomosis between the ureter and bladder.

Indications

- Reflux (not treatable by the Grégoir technique)
- Primary obstructive megaureter
- Distal ureteral injuries
- Distal ureteral stenosis
- Ureterovaginal fistula

A defect of the terminal 6–7 cm of the ureter can usually be treated using this technique.

Contraindications

- Reduced bladder capacity
- Lesions above the ureter's crossing with the major iliac vessels

Instruments

- Standard instruments for bladder surgery
- Ring retractor
- Suture material: polyglycolic acid 3/0 and 4/0, chromic catgut 4/0 and 5/0

Operative approach

The optimal operative approach depends on the primary disease. Generally, access can be gained transperitoneally or extraperitoneally. In cases with extensive adhesions and scar tissue formation, a transperitoneal approach by a midline lower abdominal incision is more beneficial than an extraperitoneal approach.

Preoperative treatment

Before ureteral neoimplantation is performed, adequate bladder capacity should be present and there should be no evidence of mucosal inflammation. The absence of inflammation is one of the most crucial prerequisites for a successful outcome.

Operative technique step by step

- Extraperitoneal approach by means of a parainguinal incision
- Exposure of the ureter at the level of its crossing with the major iliac vessels
- Following of the ureter distally is not possible without further preparation because of extensive scar tissue formation
- Transection of the ureter (Figure 1), ligation of the distal end and placement of a stay suture at the proximal end (Figure 2). The difference between well-vascularized healthy ureteral tissue and damaged whitish anemic ureteral tissue can generally be recognized easily
- Filling of the bladder with saline solution via an indwelling catheter and determination of the distance to the proximal ureteral stump
- Dissection of the peritoneum off the bladder and mobilization of the bladder using both blunt and sharp preparation techniques
- Ligation and transection of the lateral umbilical cord
- Placement of several stay sutures in the bladder, which is subsequently drained
- Reassessment of the distance between the ureter and bladder. To achieve reliable antirefluxing ureteral implantation, the ureter must not only reach the site of planned implantation in the total absence of tension, but extend over this site by 1.5 cm. Generally, a distance of 4–5 cm can be bridged easily by preparation and mobilization of the contralateral bladder wall
- Fixation of the bladder to the psoas muscle fascia (Figure 3) by two 3/0 Dexon sutures (Davis and Geck, Gosport, UK)
- Opening of the bladder between stay sutures to the point of the proposed ureteral entrance into the bladder (Figure 3)
- Tunnelling of the bladder mucosa in the direction of the old ureteral orifice using scissors
- The ureter is pulled through the submucosal tunnel by its stay suture with the aid of a slightly curved dissection clamp (Figure 4)

- Spatulation of the distal 0.5 cm and establishment of ureteral anastomosis to the bladder mucosa using 4/0 chromic catgut sutures (Figure 4)

- A ureteral stent is advanced into the renal pelvis for protection of the anastomosis. It is led out along with the cystostomy tube through separate incisions (Figure 4)

- Bladder closure in two layers (Figure 5) using running chromic catgut suture (5/0) for the mucosa and interrupted single-stitch polyglycolic acid sutures (4/0) for the muscular layer

- Drainage of the perivesical space

Surgical tricks

With a transperitoneal approach, the entire implantation site can be completely extraperitonealized by a peritoneal flap, having previously been dissected from the bladder. After radiation therapy, the peritoneum occasionally adheres rigidly to the bladder, tears easily and makes the creation of such a flap very difficult. In such cases, the implantation site can remain intraperitoneal without disadvantage. Intraperitoneal drainage is, however, advisable.

A 16 Fr silicone catheter inserted as a suprapubic cystostomy guarantees reliable bladder drainage in the unfortunate event of the transurethral catheter being clogged (e.g. by blood clots). Such a safety valve can compensate for shortcomings in postoperative care or nonspecifically trained nursing staff.

Postoperative care

The indwelling catheter is removed around day 8, while the bladder remains drained by the suprapubic cystostomy. The ureteral stent is removed on day 10 and after documentation of residual-free voiding; the cystostomy tube can be removed thereafter. The drainage tube in the vicinity of the anastomosis site is progressively retracted starting on day 3. During the first 5–6 days, an antibiotic is routinely administered, and infection prophylaxis with a furantoin derivative continues for 1 week thereafter.

Special situations

Irradiated patients

In complicated cases and after radiotherapy, the stent can remain in place for up to 3 weeks.

Bilateral fistulas

Whether fistulas can be repaired in a one-stage procedure depends on the level of the lesion and the bladder capacity. If sufficient bladder capacity is present and the lesions are located below the ureters' point of crossing the major iliac vessels, direct ureteroneocystostomy of the longer ureter and ureteral neoimplantation by means of the psoas-hitch technique for the shorter ureter is possible during a single operation. Lesions above the ureters' crossing with the iliac vessels, have required a two-stage procedure until recently. Reconstruction of the worst affected ureter would have been attempted first. After 6–8 weeks, the bladder capacity would usually have reached normal levels again and reconstruction of the contralateral ureter would be performed. This procedure has been replaced by a single-stage bilateral implantation of both ureters into the cecal segment used to augment the bladder.

Common errors and complications

One of the most serious surgical errors is establishment of the ureterovesical anastomosis under tension. Obstruction and failure of the operation are then almost certain.

If upper urinary tract dilatation does not subside within a period of 6–9 months, revisional surgery must be planned. Statistics on late results should not only judge the condition of the upper urinary tract but also document whether the operation was successful in preventing urinary tract infections and vesicoureteral reflux. Only if all three of these criteria are met can the operation be termed a success. The need to avoid urinary tract infection is especially important for patients who have had radical gynecologic tumor surgery and subsequent neurogenic voiding dysfunction.

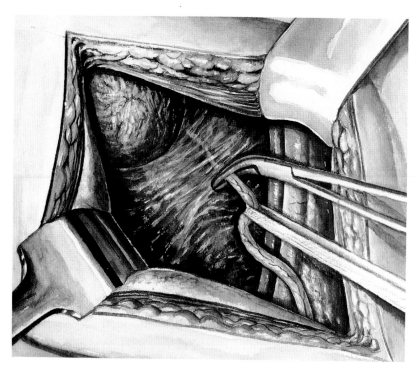

Figure 1. *Extraperitoneal approach. Division of the ureter.*

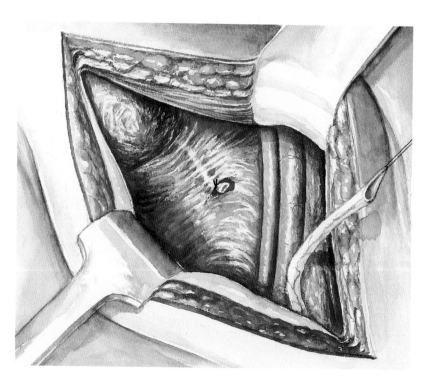

Figure 2. *Ligation of the distal ureter and placement of a stay suture in the proximal ureter.*

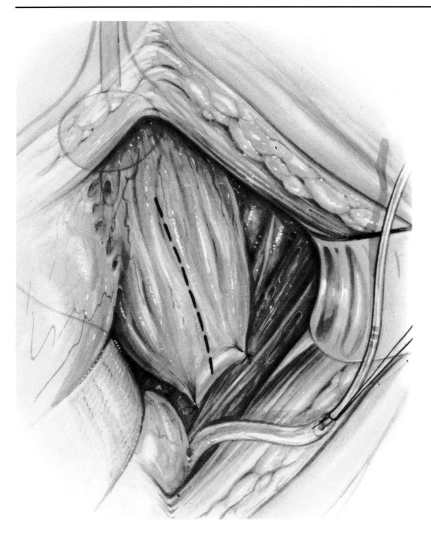

Figure 3. *Fixation of the bladder to the psoas muscle fascia and longitudinal opening of the bladder.*

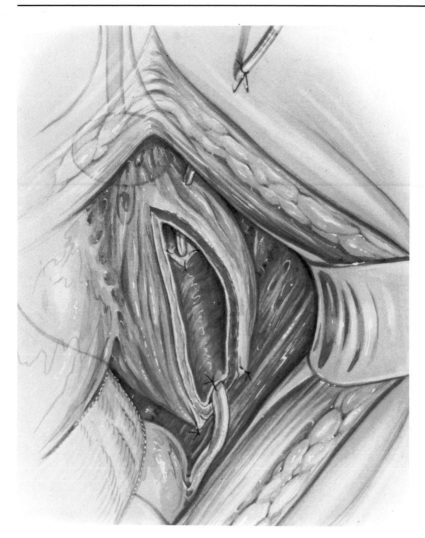

Figure 4. *Ureteral implantation by means of a submucosal tunnel. Ureteromucous adaptation. A ureteral stent is led out through bladder wall and skin.*

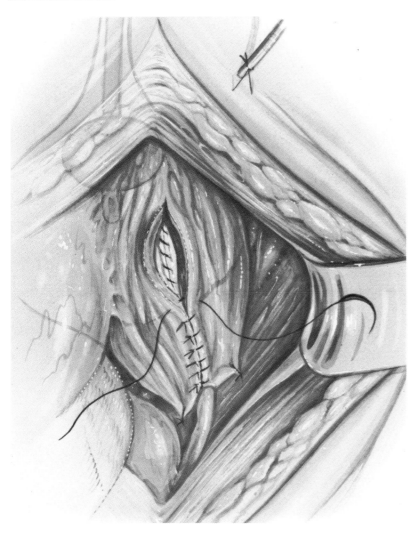

Figure 5. *Two-layer closure of the bladder.*

Retropubic Prostatectomy using a Modified Millin Technique without a Postoperative Transurethral Catheter

H. Baur, W. Schneider
Department of Urology,
Krankenhaus der Barmherzigen Brüder,
München-Nymphenburg, Germany

Comment

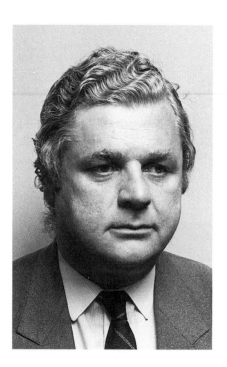

Transurethral resection of the prostate (TURP) is the therapy of first choice for the treatment of benign prostatic hyperplasia (BPH). In most clinics, the decision of which kind of treatment should be chosen is made by transrectal palpation and endoscopic inspection of the prostate; nevertheless, determination of the volume of the prostate is more exact by transrectal ultrasonography. The risk of underestimating the volume of the prostate is high, unless transrectal ultrasonography is used, and so BPH with a prostate weight of more than 60 g is often treated by TURP. Adenomas of up to 90 g can also be resected transurethrally within 60 minutes without any problems.

The authors of this well-illustrated paper describe the technique of open surgery for adenomas more than 60 g in weight. Of the techniques for open surgery of the prostate, I prefer the retropubic adenomectomy first described by Millin. This easy technique is combined with a low morbidity and excellent results. The most important fact, as described by the authors, is to pay careful attention to every step of the operation. After preparation of the frontal plane of the prostate it is incised transversally 2 cm distal to the bladder neck. During this step careful hemostasis is very important. Then the adenoma is enucleated under visual control and the urethra cut in the region of the apex of the prostate. To preserve the biggest part of the urethra, the adenoma is split at the midline and the urothelium detached. Usually this is not necessary because, in most cases, especially when the adenoma has a large middle lobe, it is possible to fix the lower part of the trigone deep onto the back wall of the capsule of the prostate. The completeness of enucleation is checked, especially in the region of the middle lobe. Ligation of the vesicoprostatic vessels and insertion of a cystectomy tube into the bladder are interesting modifications but are usually not used in our institution. As noted by the authors, it is important to start the stitches of the capsule sutures at the lateral end of incision on both sides. The single sutures should close the capsule of the prostate in a figure-of-eight suture.

I agree with the authors that it is very important for all urologists to be able to perform an open prostatectomy. As they do, I prefer the retropubic technique to the transvesical one because it gives a better chance of controlling hemorrhages.

John M. Fitzpatrick, Dublin

Retropubic adenectomy of the prostate

Introduction

Open prostate adenomectomy has undergone a renaissance. In extensive studies conducted by Roos *et al.*[1] in 1989, transurethral prostate resection was associated with a four to six times higher rate of reoperation, as well as a higher postoperative mortality rate than open adenomectomy. The technique used for adenomectomy should take into account the typical side-effects, such as catheter-induced infection with polyresistant hospital microorganisms or postoperative urethral strictures, especially in view of the severe irritation of the urethra caused by the resectoscope (which is moved as many as 2000 times during the transurethral resection of large adenomas). On the other hand, although digital enucleation does less damage to the urethra, the method requires a Foley catheter to tamponade the prostatic cavity. Millin introduced retropubic adenomectomy in 1945. This chapter describes a further development of the original Millin technique, which obviates the need for a postoperative transurethral catheter.

Indication

- Benign prostatic hyperplasia with a prostate weight of >50 g

Instruments

- Standard instruments for operations in the pelvis
- Millin retractor
- Suture material: chromic catgut 1/0, 2/0; plain catgut 2/0

Exposure

The patient is positioned for surgery in an extended frog-leg position with his legs slightly abducted and lowered. The retropubic gap is exposed through a Pfannenstiel incision by spreading apart the abdominal rectus muscles and through the gaps of the prevesical fascia.

Operative technique

- Intrapelvic vasectomy at the junction between the external iliac vein and the peritoneum to prevent inflammation of the epididymis
- Preventive hemostasis by ligating the vesicoprostatic vascular bundle (Grégoir suture with chromic catgut 1/0) on both sides after the three-blade Millin retractor is inserted (Figure 1)
- Exposure of the exact point of transition from the bladder outlet to the ventral capsule by crossed Kader retractors (Figure 2)
- Generous partial excision of the ventral prostatic capsule, and oval-shaped excision of the bladder outlet. Excision of the adenoma distal to the interureteric bar. Indigo carmine is given intravenously to mark the position of the ureteral orifices and to permit inspection for proper functioning (Figures 3 and 4)
- After digital enucleation the adenoma is cut away from the urethra at the level of the apex under direct vision (Figure 5). The prostatic cavity is inspected (Figure 6) and residual parts of the tumor can be detected and removed under visual control
- Reducing the prostatic cavity and final hemostasis by gathering up sutures (chromic catgut 1/0)
- Deep retrigonization to create a continuous transition from the prostatic cavity to the bladder (plain catgut 2/0) (Figure 7). The ventral prostatic cavity is closed with interrupted 1/0 chromic catgut sutures after an 18 Fr cystostomy has been placed (Figure 8)
- Drainage by an 18 Fr silicone tube placed over the row of sutures

Postoperative care

Following the retropubic adenomectomy it is routine to maintain continuous urine drainage for 5 days. On day 6 the cystostomy is closed and, when spontaneous micturition without residual urine is achieved, the drainage tube is removed.

References

1. Roos NP, Wenneberg JE, Malenka DF *et al.* Mortality and reoperation after open and transurethral resection of the prostate for benign prostatic hyperplasia. *N Engl J Med* **320** (1989) 1120–4.
2. Baur H, Altwein JE, Schneider W. Retropubische Adenomektomie der Prostrata. *Akt Urol* **21** (Suppl Operative Techniken) (1990) I–VIII.

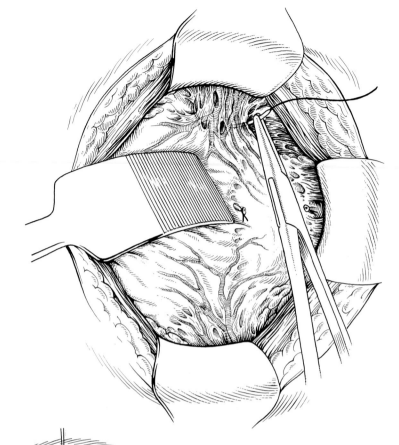

Figure 1. *The retropubic region is exposed, the ventral prostate capsule freed of fat tissue, and the dorsal veins of the penis ligated and transected. The vesicoprostatic bundle is ligated by a 1/0 chromic catgut mass suture.*

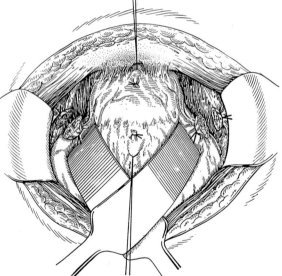

Figure 2. *Exposure of the bladder outlet with Kader retractors. The distal capsule suture in the region of the puboprostatic ligaments and the proximal suture of the bladder outlet are tied. The vesicoprostatic bundles are ligated and transected on both sides.*

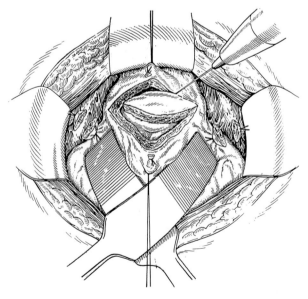

Figure 3. *Circumcision of the adenoma distal to the ureteral orifices. Situation immediately before the digital enucleation of the adenoma. Marking of the position and function of the ureteral orifices by intravenous indigo carmine.*

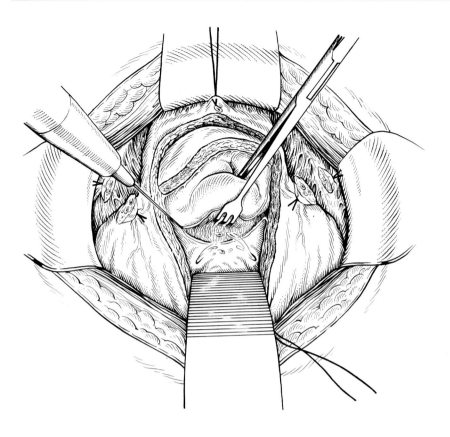

Figure 4. *Broad partial excision of the ventral prostate capsule and oval circumcision of the bladder outlet with electrocautery between the preliminary sutures.*

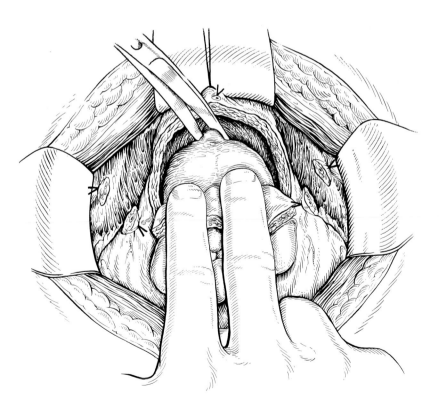

Figure 5. *Sharp separation of the adenoma from the distal urethra made possible by prior broad excision of the ventral prostate capsule.*

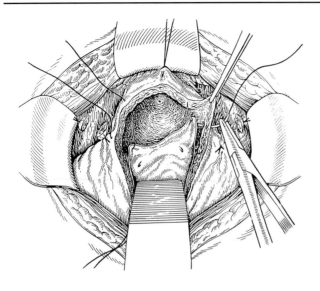

Figure 6. *Situation after enucleation. The 1/0 chromic catgut gathering sutures are brought into position on both sides to reduce the volume of the fossa and transpose the trigone.*

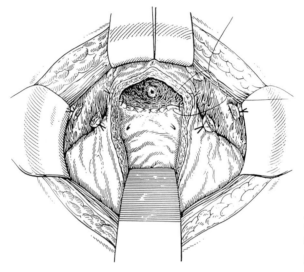

Figure 7. *Deep retrigonization to create a wide nonobstructive junction from the fossa to the bladder.*

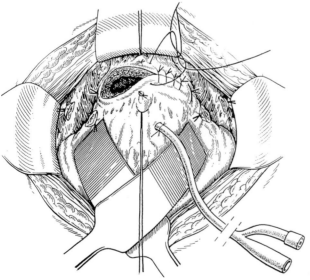

Figure 8. *Closure of the ventral prostate capsule with 1/0 chromic catgut interrupted sutures. Cystostomy (18 Fr) in position.*

Suprapubic Prostatectomy

K. Weingärtner, R. Hohenfellner[a]
Department of Urology,
Philipps University Medical School,
Marburg, Germany
[a]Department of Urology,
University of Mainz School of Medicine,
Mainz, Germany

Comment

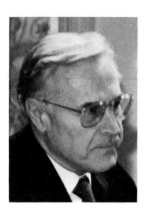

Today, transurethral resection of the prostate (TURP) is preferred to open surgery for adenoma of prostate in 90% of cases. The reasons for this are that modern instruments are much more efficient, and that the diagnosis of benign prostatic hyperplasia (BPH) is made early so that the average weight of the adenomas is about 30 g (much lower than 30 years ago).

I agree with the authors of this article about the indications and preoperative work-up. We also do not perform preoperative cystoscopy, and have not seen any disadvantage in this in the last couple of years. Urethral strictures can be diagnosed by urine flow measurements; larger bladder stones, tumors or diverticula should be seen on intravenous pyelography in most cases.

I see no advantage to the use of an electric knife for cutting the endovesical part of the adenoma: bimanual enucleation has been our preferred technique for decades and has the advantage that small knots of adenoma can be felt between the palpating fingers. The incidence of recurrences is low using this technique. The danger of contaminating the area is minimal. Minor bleeding can be managed very well by inserting a balloon catheter and closing the Z-sutures at the ureter angles above the catheter. We rarely see postoperative hemorrhage if we drain the catheter balloon step by step in the first postoperative days. The danger of postoperative stricture can be decreased by excising the fossa and bladder at the 6 o'clock position. We use triple-lumen catheters, never bigger than 20 Fr, so that a suprapubic cystostomy is not necessary. This helps to decrease postoperative wound leakage.

Postoperative irrigation with normal saline for the first four days has proved useful. Blood clots can be washed out with a bladder syringe. We no longer give prophylactic antibiotics, and start therapy only when fever rises above 38 °C.

Bibliography

1. Haschek H, Plum H. Einzeitig suprapubische Prostatektomie mit primärem Blasenverschluss. *Urol Int* **15** (1963) 52–64.
2. Haschek H, Schumann F. Operationsvorbereitung und Nachbehandlung des kreislaufgefährdeten Prostatikers. *Urologe* **2** (1963) 153–5.
3. Haschek H. Zur Technik der Blutstillung bei suprapubischer Prostatektomie. *Urologe* **2** (1963) 156–9.
4. Haschek H, Schumann F. Todesfälle nach suprapubischer Prostatektomie. *Wien Klin Wochenschr* **113** (1963) 782–7.
5. Haschek H, Reuter HJ. Vergleich der Spätergebnisse nach suprapubischer Prostatektomie und transurethraler Elektroresektion (je 1000 Fälle). *Urol Int* **23** (1968) 454–69.
6. Haschek H. Die operative Behandlung des Prostataadenoms. *Wien Klin Wochenschr* **90** (1978) 181–4.
7. Haschek H, Porpaczy P, Schmidbauer CP. Bakterieller Hospitalismus ist abhängig von Antibiotikapolitik und Krankenhaushygiene. *Med Klin* **77** (1982) 15–17.
8. Schmidbauer CP, Haschek H. Effektive Massnahmen zur positiven Kosten–Nutzenrelation am Beispiel der Diagnose und therapie des Prostataadenoms und der Steinerkrankung des oberen Harntraktes. Kongressbericht 19. Kongress d. Ges f. Urologie, San Francisco, 1982.
9. Schramek P, Schmidbauer CP. Sekundäreingriffe nach Prostataadenomchirurgie. *Acta Chir Austr* Suppl. **43** (1982) 142–3.
10. Schramek P. Spätergebnisse und Rezidivoperationen nach Adenomchirurgie. *Akt Urol* 11 (1980) 103–6.

H. Haschek, Vienna

Suprapubic prostatectomy

Introduction

Transurethral resection of the prostate (TURP) is the operative treatment of choice for more than 90% of patients presenting with obstructive voiding symptoms due to benign prostatic hyperplasia. For the remaining subset of patients a variety of open surgical procedures can be offered, including:

- Suprapubic or transvesical prostatectomy
- Retropubic or transcapsular prostatectomy
- Perineal prostatectomy

None of these procedures involves total removal of the prostate because a tissue plane exists between the adenoma and the compressed true prostate, which is left intact. Suprapubic prostatectomy, first described by Fuller[1] and popularized by Freyer and Harris,[2,3] is an open surgical procedure for enucleation of the prostatic adenoma via an extraperitoneal approach.

Indications

- Adenomas with an estimated weight of more than 60 g
- Association with large bladder calculi
- Sizable diverticula of the bladder justifying removal
- Ankylosis of the hip preventing proper positioning of the patient for TURP

Preoperative diagnostic procedures

- Check for diabetes, cardiovascular disease, chronic obstructive pulmonary disease, hypertension, cerebral insult, neurogenic bladder, especially associated with Parkinson's disease
- Transrectal ultrasonography of the upper urinary tract, bladder and prostate
- Retrograde urethrography of the kidney, ureter and bladder
- Urinalysis and urine culture
- Check indication for autologous blood

Instruments

- Suture material: plain catgut 0, polyglycolic acid 2/0

- Jackson–Pratt drain (10 Fr)
- Catheters: 18 Fr three-way Foley catheter, 10 Fr suprapubic cystostomy

Patient position

- Supine position with the table slightly hyperextended and the legs stretched

Operative technique step by step

- Vertical midline incision from below the umbilicus to the symphysis
- Catheterization and filling of the bladder with 200–300 ml water or normal saline
- Extaperitoneal exposure of the bladder; blunt or sharp dissection of the peritoneum superiorly
- Transverse opening of the bladder wall between two stay sutures (Figure 1)
- Identification of both ureteral orifices and exposure of the bladder neck
- Incision of the mucosa around the bladder neck to prevent uncontrolled rupture during enucleation (Figure 2)
- Insertion of the index finger in the prostatic urethra and fracturing the anterior commisure (Figure 3)
- Enucleation of the prostatic adenoma sweeping circumferentially posterior using simultaneous counterpressure by the index finger of the opposite hand inserted in the rectum (Figure 4)
- Sharp or blunt dissection of the urethra at the apex without displacement of the urethra cephalad, thus preventing damage of the external urethral sphincter (Figure 5)
- Digital control of the prostatic fossa for complete enucleation of the adenoma
- Tamponade of the fossa for approximately 5 minutes
- Figure-of-eight suture ligatures of 0 plain catgut (Figure 6), starting in the middle of the trigone and at the 3–4 and 8–9 o'clock positions at a safe distance from the ureteral orifices (Figure 7)
- Insertion of a transurethral catheter (18 Fr three-way Foley) and closure of the ventral portion of the prostatic fossa with two or three full-thickness suture ligatures of 0 plain catgut (Figure 8)

- Filling of the balloon of the catheter with 40–60 ml (in the bladder, not the prostatic fossa)

- Water-tight single-layer interrupted closure of the bladder with 2/0 polyglycolic acid suture after placement of a suprapubic cystostomy (Figure 9)

- Drainage of the retropubic space and wound closure

Postoperative care

- Intravenous fluids only on the day of surgery; oral nutrition is started on day 1 after surgery

- Prophylactic intravenous antibiotic coverage for 2–3 days, e.g. with a cephalosporin. This can be changed to oral therapy, which is maintained until 3–5 days after removal of the transurethral catheter

- Removal of the transurethral catheter on day 3–5. Removal of the suprapubic tube on day 6 or 7, provided the patient has no residual urine

Surgical tricks

- Ureteral orifices very close to the margin of resection should be stented for 4–6 days to avoid problems from the upper tract

References

1. Fuller E. Six successful and successive cases of prostatectomy. *J Cutan Genitourin Dis* **13** (1895) 229.
2. Freyer PJ. A new method of performing prostatectomy. *Lancet* **i** (1900) 774.
3. Harris SH. Suprapubic prostatectomy with closure. *Br J Urol* **1** (1929) 285.

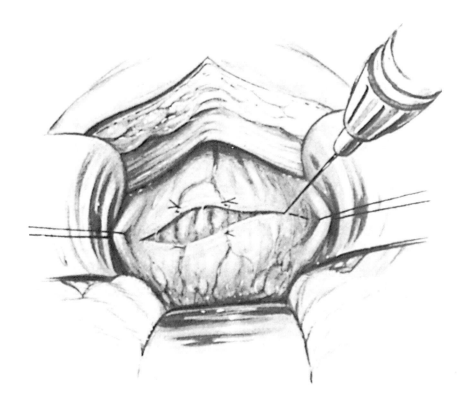

Figure 1. *Transverse opening of the bladder wall with electrocautery.*

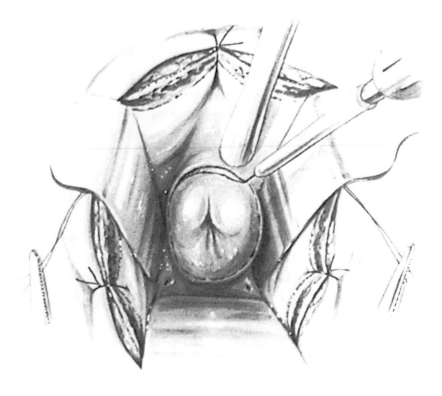

Figure 2. *Incision of the bladder mucosa around the bladder neck using electrocautery.*

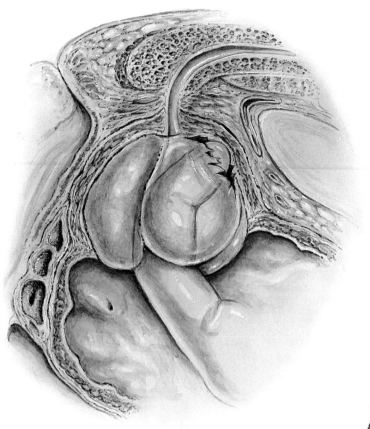

Figure 3. *Fracture of the anterior commissure with the index finger.*

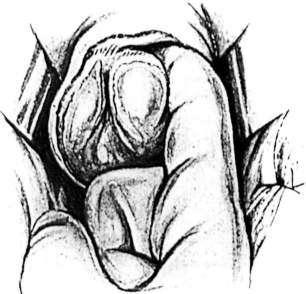

Figure 4. *Blunt enucleation of the prostatic adenoma with the index finger under simultaneous digital rectal control.*

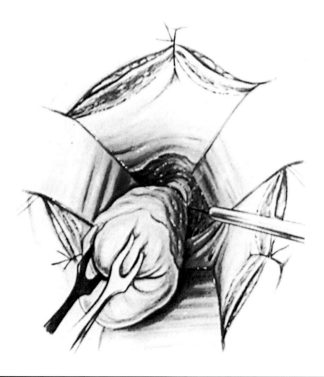

Figure 5. *Sharp dissection of the prostatic urethra from the apex.*

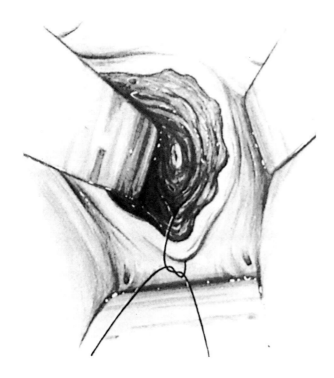

Figure 6. *Hemostasis is achieved by figure-of-eight suture ligations (0 plain catgut) beginning in the middle of the trigone.*

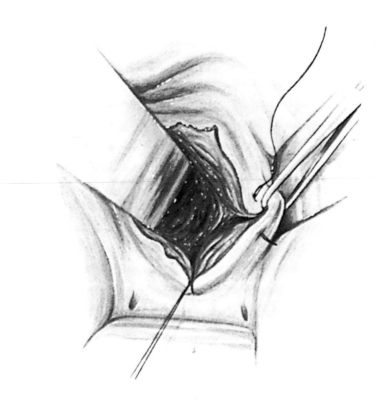

Figure 7. *Suture ligations at the 3–4 and 8–9 o'clock positions at a safe distance from the ureteral orifices for hemostasis.*

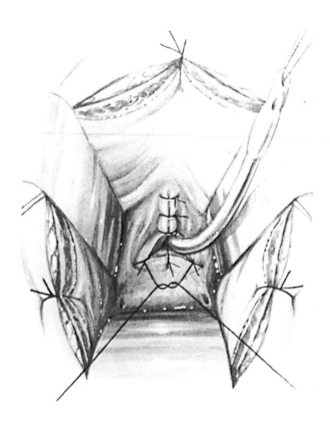

Figure 8. *After placement of a transurethral catheter, the anterior portion of the prostatic fossa is closed by full-thickness suture ligations with 0 plain catgut.*

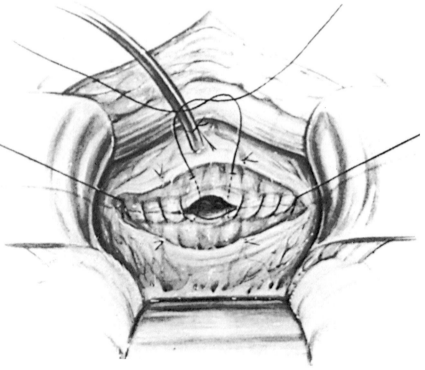

Figure 9. *Water-tight single-layer closure of the bladder with 2/0 polyglycolic acid interrupted sutures.*

Retropubic Ascending Radical Prostatectomy

F. Schreiter
Urologische Abteilung,
Allgemeines Krankenhaus Hamburg,
Hamburg, Germany

Comment

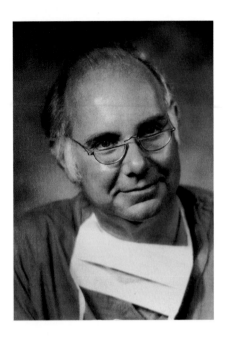

Radical retropubic prostatectomy is not an easy operation. Professor Schreiter has beautifully outlined in this chapter his technique of the ascending (Walsh) procedure.

We at Stanford have extensively investigated how cancer 'escapes' from the prostate, and based on these findings I want to stress and re-emphasize some important points of the operation.

Almost 50% of all positive margins occur over the apical surface of the prostate, not only posteriorly but also anteriorly to the urethra. Efforts to preserve Walsh's periurethral pillars (the prostatoischial ligaments of Müller) and efforts to dissect the dorsal vein complex from the underlying anterior fibromuscular stroma of the prostate can easily expose cancer at the anterior apex. We suggest that the dorsal vein complex should be cut 3–4 mm distal to the urethra including all the fascial investments. After cutting the proximal membranous urethra, this incision finally exposes the thick triangular termination of Denonvilliers' plate immediately beneath the urethra as it proceeds inferiorly to the perineal membrane. This terminal plate of Denonvilliers' fascia can be several millimeters thick. It is important to separate this fascia cleanly and cut it as far distally as possible, because it is sometimes invaded with cancer. On reaching the longitudinal muscle of the anterior wall of the rectum the surgeon is in the correct plane and Denonvilliers' fascia, with its firmly attached prostatic capsule, will remain intact. The rectourethralis muscle inserts quite distally into the posterior side of Denonvilliers' terminal plate and is not seen in the retropubic approach to

the prostate unless the surgeon is too far down the membranous urethra. This approach to the apex of the prostate has reduced the frequency of positive apical margins in our series remarkably and has not had any adverse affect on continence.

Positive posterolateral and rectal margins can be avoided by understanding the histologic components of the lateral pelvic fascia in relation to Denonvilliers' fascia and by recognizing that perineural space invasion by intraprostatic cancer is the most common method of spread into the periprostatic fat. Because of the latter observation, a safe policy is never to perform the nerve-sparing radical prostatectomy on the side of the palpable nodule in clinical stage B disease. However, even when a bilateral nerve-sparing radical prostatectomy is done for clinical stage A cancer, or on the contralateral side to a palpable stage B cancer, or bilaterally in cystoprostatectomy for bladder cancer, it is easy to separate Denonvilliers' fascia from an unsuspected peripheral zone cancer. Indeed, it is surprisingly easy to leave all of Denonvilliers' fascia behind and fail to recognize it. Part of the solution is to recognize that the anterior leaf of the periprostatic fascia (a part of the lateral pelvic fascia) sweeps from the lateral surface of the prostate and around the lateral edge of the neurovascular bundle, forming the posterior leaf of the periprostatic fascia before flushing with Denonvilliers' fascia. When the anterior leaf is incised immediately above the neurovascular bundle to push the neurovascular bundle laterally from the prostate capsule, it is important not to bluntly separate the neurovascular bundle posteriorly from the prostate. After the apex of the prostate has been turned cephalad, the posterior leaf of the periprostatic fascia just lateral to the base of the prostate can be cut sharply under direct vision.

Approaching the junction of the distal and middle thirds of the prostate at approximately the level of the verumontanum, the surgeon should be aware that about 12% of ejaculatory ducts penetrate the prostate on the posterior surface of the gland rather than at its base. Because, with rare exceptions, clinical stage B cancers reach the seminal vesicles by following the ejaculatory ducts, the surgeon must be very careful to avoid damaging Denonvilliers' fascia at any time. This is important because two-thirds of patients with seminal vesicle invasion have invasion of Denonvilliers' fascia near the midline near the base of the prostate. Moreover, Denonvilliers' fascia is only about 0.2 mm thick in the midline and must not be breached.

Margins at the superior pedicle are caused by perineural space invasion where extracapsular cancer has travelled several centimetres within the perineural spaces. These pedicles should be taken as far posteriorly toward the hypogastric vessels as possible on the side of the palpable nodule in clinical stage B disease. They have to be shortened on the side of the nerve-sparing dissection as emphasized by Walsh[3], but the neurovascular bundles can usually be seen as they proceed from the posterolateral edge of the prostate toward the hypogastric complex.

Malizia, in a brilliant dissection of the vesical neck that followed the longitudinal muscle fibers of the vesical neck into the base of the prostate, has shown us how to preserve every muscle bundle of the vesical neck. Because there is no true capsule between the vesical neck smooth muscle bundles and prostatic acini and ducts, this dissection will leave positive margins in a small percentage (2–5%) of patients otherwise curable by radical prostatectomy. More important, however, is Malizia and Wein's observation that these completely preserved vesical necks are incompetent: in the standing position urine is held at the distal striated sphincter – not at the preserved vesical neck. This is an important observation because it means that every surgeon should take a wide margin at the vesical neck as illustrated in this chapter.

Thus with a better understanding of how cancer escapes from the prostate, the urologic surgeon can:

- Avoid leaving a positive margin by inadvertently cutting into the incorrect plane owing to a misunderstanding of the periprostatic fascias

- Sharply reduce the high incidence of positive margins at the apex of the prostate

- Achieve an even wider surgical margin and a better chance of cure by avoiding a nerve-sparing operation

The transfer of this knowledge to the surgical procedure may improve the long-term results in patients who have extracapsular extension of their prostatic cancer – which includes, unfortunately, about half of clinical stage B radical prostatectomies.

T.A. Stamey, Stanford, California

Retropubic ascending radical prostatectomy

Introduction

Before the 1960s, radical prostatectomy was a recommended treatment for organ-confined prostate cancer. Because of insufficient clinical staging and therefore poor comparability of results, the opinion that external or interstitial radiotherapy gives better results became more and more accepted.

In the 1980s, Paulson[1,2] showed that radical prostatectomy at a comparable stage is superior to radiotherapy. Improvements in surgical technique[3] led to lower morbidity, and especially to less incontinence and impotence; for example, the rate of postoperative incontinence decreased below 10%. Incontinent patients could be treated by the use of an artificial sphincter prosthesis.

In Europe the retropubic approach is the favorite for radical prostatectomy. The major advantage compared with the perineal procedure has to be seen in the concurrent realization of a pelvic lymphadenectomy. The ascending technique from the apex to the bladder is the usual procedure because of the possibility of ligating the dorsal venules of the penis early and sparing the neurovascular bundles under visual control.

Indications

- Clinical stage T2 tumors of the prostate

Contraindications

- Cancer not confined to the prostate on clinical staging

Instruments

- Standard instruments for abdominal operations
- Balfour retractor
- Special right-angle clamp for ligation of the dorsal vein of the penis
- Vessel loops

Operative technique step by step (Figures 1–25)

- Place the patient in a 20° Trendelenburg position
- Midline incision between the navel and the pubic bone
- Extraperitoneal lymphadenectomy of the lymph node packages of the external and internal iliac arteries, the obturator fossa and the deep paravesical lymph nodes; if there are suspicious nodes, additional removal of the lymph nodes of the common iliac artery
- Preparation of the retropubic space and incision of the endopelvic fascia beside the prostate on both sides
- Sharp cutting of the prostatic ligaments near the symphysis with preservation of the veins of the Santorini plexus and the dorsal vein of the penis

- Blunt removal of the prostate from the levator muscle and the urogenital diaphragm

- Palpation of the 18 Fr transurethral catheter, tunneling under the dorsal vein of the penis above the urethra with a right-angled clamp, placement of a free suture and ligation of the vein. Additional ligation with stitches on the left and right side and positioning of three stitch ligatures, proximally in the periprostatic fascia

- Sharp penetration with scissors to the apex of the prostate and opening of the periprostatic fascia on both sides

- Tunneling under the urethra at the apex with preservation of the borders of the periprostatic fascia within the neurovascular bundles and passing a vessel loop through

- Incision of the frontal wall of the urethra and positioning of the first two anastomosis sutures with 2/0 Maxon (Davis and Geck, Gosport, UK)

- Partial withdrawal of the catheter and cutting of the back wall of the urethra with preservation of the seminal colliculus

- Cutting of Denonvilliers' fascia at the origin of the rectourethral muscle

- Blunt preparation of the prostatic back wall to the seminal vesicles

- In a nerve-sparing operation, cutting of the periprostatic fascia near the apex of the prostate with preservation of the neurovascular bundles

- Sharp preparation of the prostate at the frontal wall of the bladder, blunt removal at the trigone and sharp cutting of the bladder mucosa at the trigone

- Preparation of the seminal vesicles and ligation of the ductus deferents. Cutting of the prostate pillars after ligation and removal of the whole package

- Reconstruction of the bladder neck with 5/0 noninterrupted Maxon suture so that the opening measures 18 Fr; eversion of the bladder mucosa and single-stitch suturing with 3/0 Maxon

- Positioning of the back anastomosis sutures at 5 and 7

o'clock under retraction of the frontal anastomosis sutures at 1 and 11 o'clock

- Tying of the anastomosis sutures after placing of a 16 Fr balloon catheter

- Placing of one suction drainage tube at the anastomosis and two lateral Easyflow drainage tubes

- If the tumor is found not to be confined to the prostate, large-scale excision of the periprostatic fascia including the neurovascular bundles

Postoperative care

- Removal of the suction drainage after a week

- Removal of the Easyflow drainage tubes after lymph secretion stops

- Removal of the transurethral catheter after 2 weeks if the anastomosis is dense on cystography; if cystography shows any extravasation remaining, the catheter is left in place for another week or until the anastomosis becomes dense

Special situations

A nerve-sparing operation should be performed only on small tumors confined to the prostate, with sufficient safety margins confirmed by frozen sections.

References

1. Paulson DF, Lin GH et al. Radical surgery vs. radiotherapy for adenocarcinoma of the prostate. J Urol **128** (1982) 502–4.
2. Paulson DG, Robertson JE, Daubert LM et al. Radical prostatectomy in stage A prostatic adenocarcinoma. J Urol **140** (1988) 535–9.
3. Walsh PC. Radical prostatectomy for treatment of localized prostatic carcinoma. Urol Clin **7** (1980) 583–91.

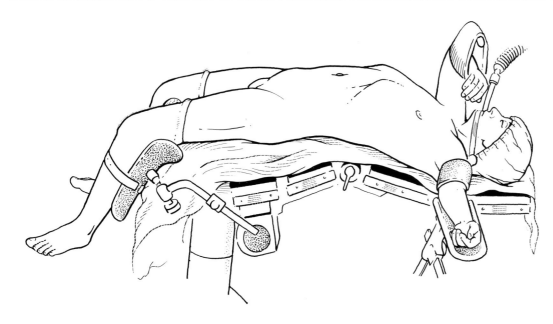

Figure 1. *Position of the patient in a 20° Trendelenburg position with the upper part of the body lowered.*

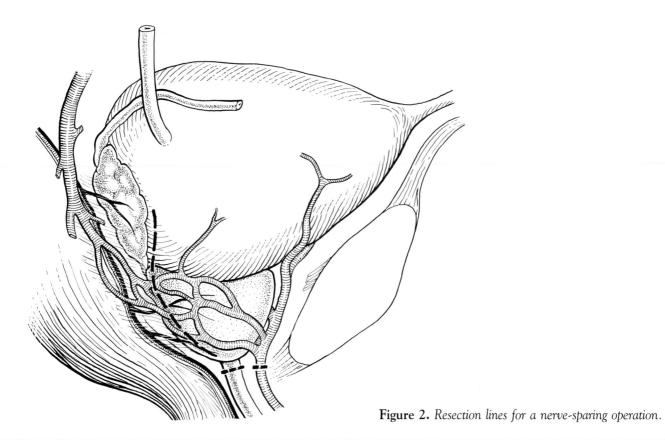

Figure 2. *Resection lines for a nerve-sparing operation.*

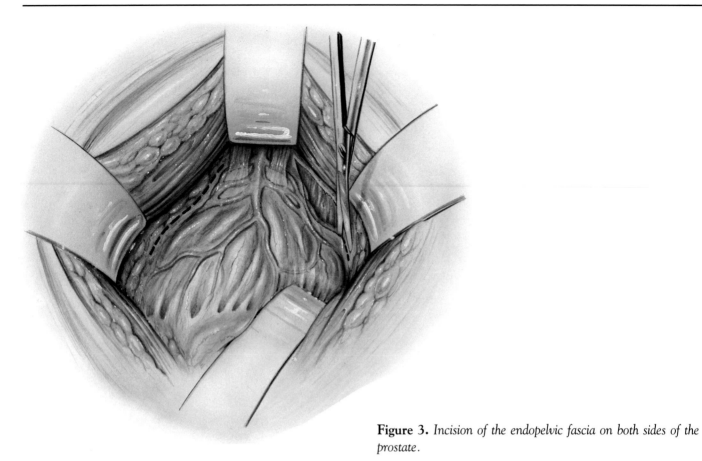

Figure 3. *Incision of the endopelvic fascia on both sides of the prostate.*

Figure 4. *Cutting of the puboprostatic ligaments near the pubic bone.*

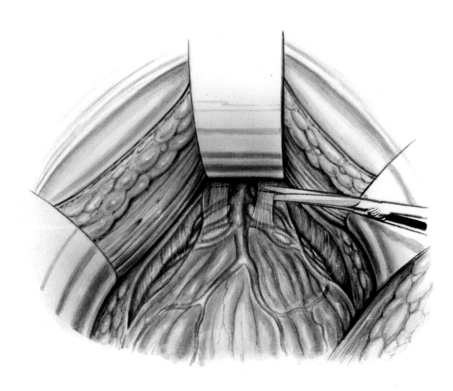

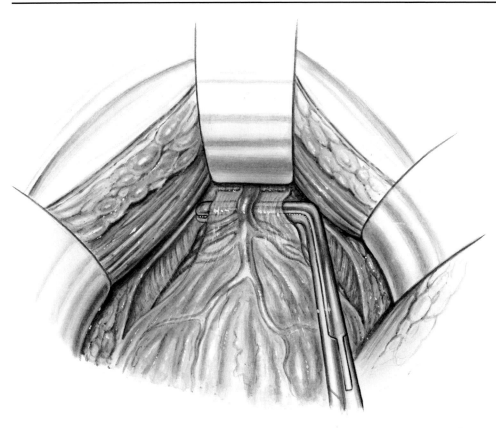

Figure 5. *Tunneling under the dorsal vein of the penis with a special right-angled clamp. The vein is embedded in the endopelvic fascia.*

Figure 6. *Cutting of the dorsal vein of the penis and the endopelvic fascia above the right-angled clamp.*

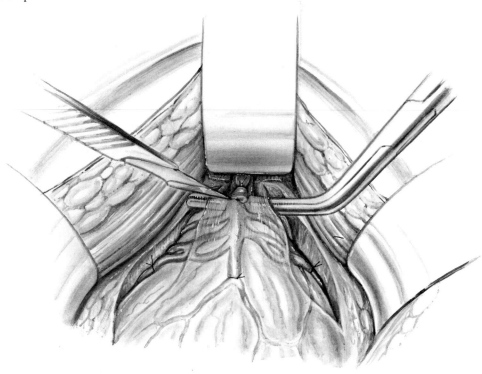

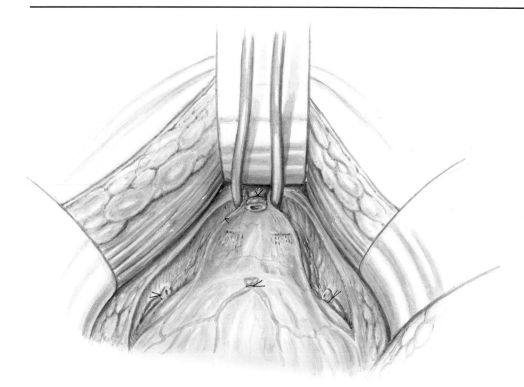

Figure 7. *After preparation of the frontal wall of the prostate, tunneling under the urethra within the endopelvic fascia and positioning of a vessel loop.*

Figure 8. *Cutting of the frontal wall of the urethra and positioning of the anastomosis sutures at 11 and 1 o'clock.*

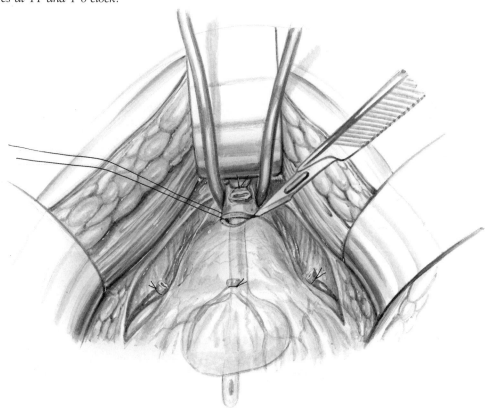

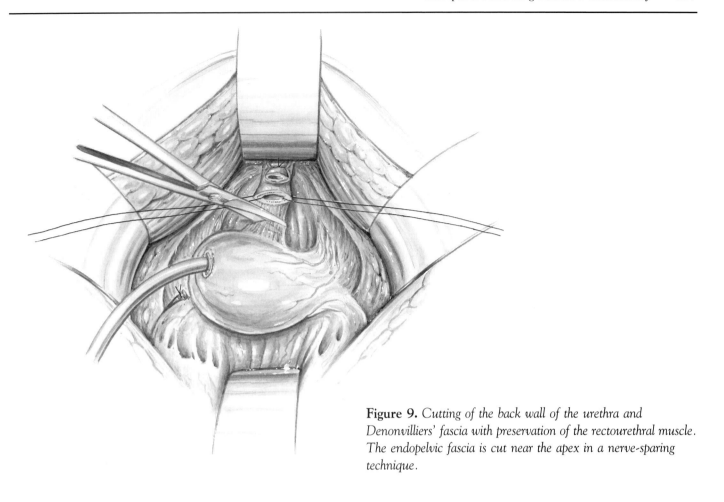

Figure 9. *Cutting of the back wall of the urethra and Denonvilliers' fascia with preservation of the rectourethral muscle. The endopelvic fascia is cut near the apex in a nerve-sparing technique.*

Figure 10. *Cutting of Denonvilliers' fascia (lateral view).*

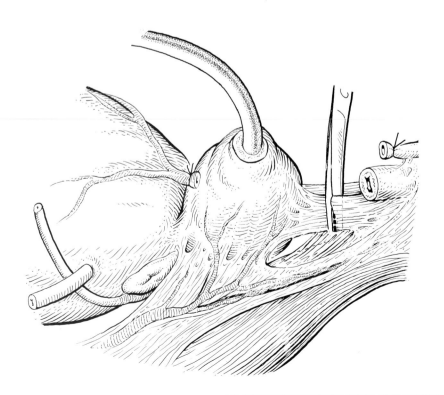

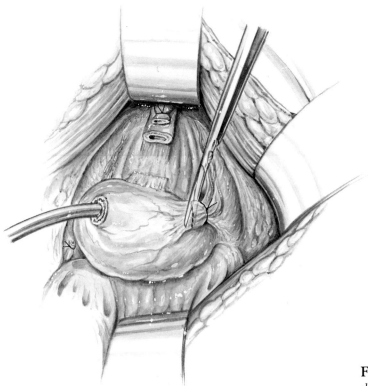

Figure 11. *Cutting of the lateral prostate pillars after ligation of the lateral prostatic arteries.*

Figure 12. *Incision of Denonvilliers' fascia near the base for preparation of the seminal vesicles.*

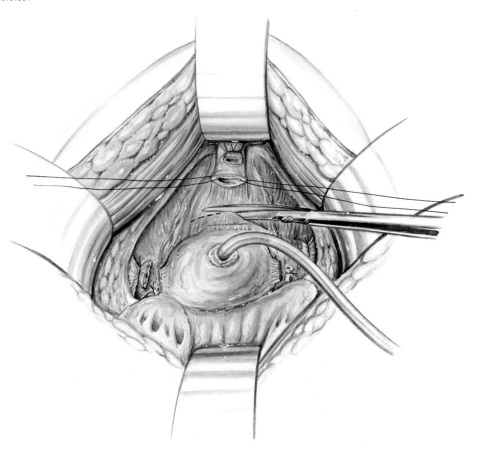

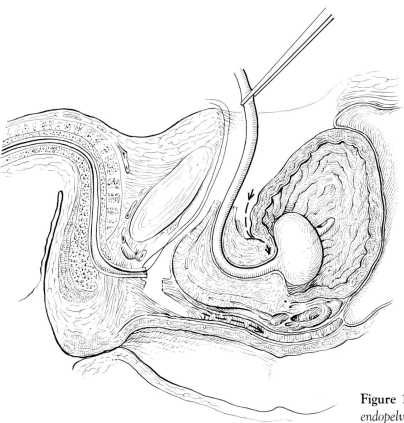

Figure 13. *Resection line between Denonvilliers' fascia and the endopelvic fascia and method of cutting at the front wall of the bladder neck.*

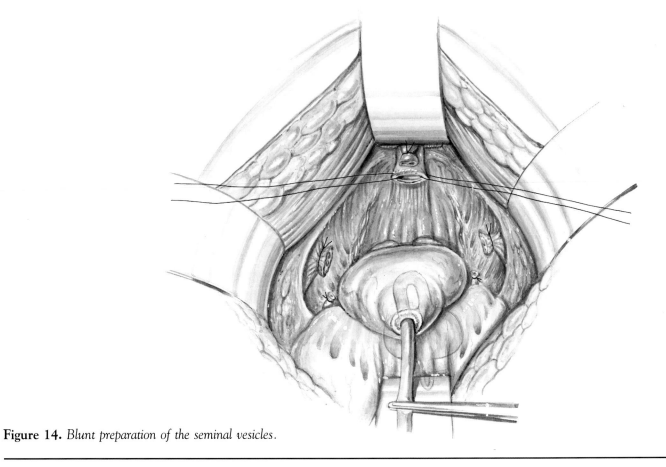

Figure 14. *Blunt preparation of the seminal vesicles.*

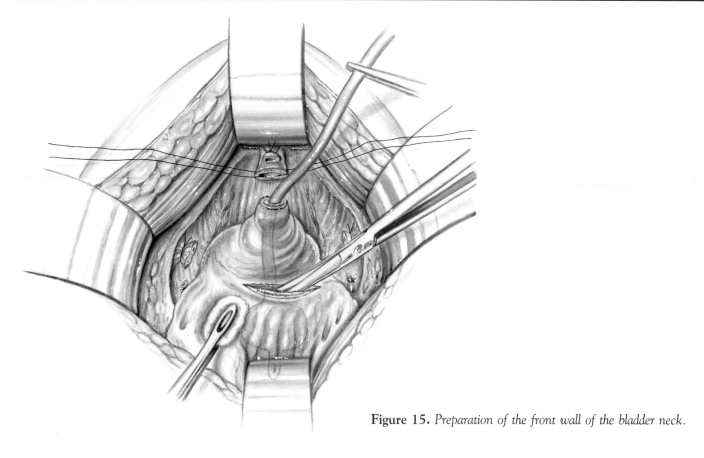

Figure 15. *Preparation of the front wall of the bladder neck.*

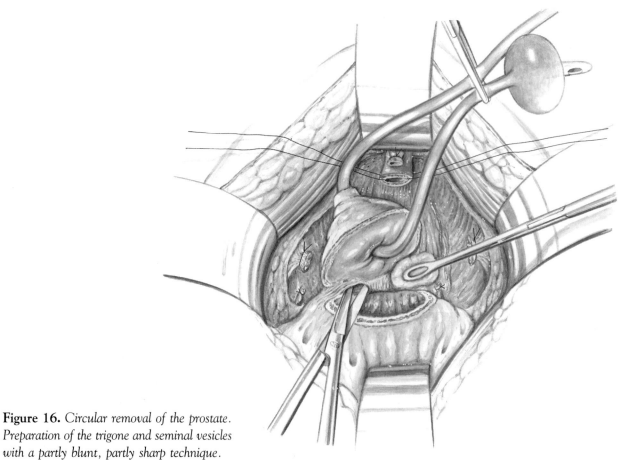

Figure 16. *Circular removal of the prostate. Preparation of the trigone and seminal vesicles with a partly blunt, partly sharp technique.*

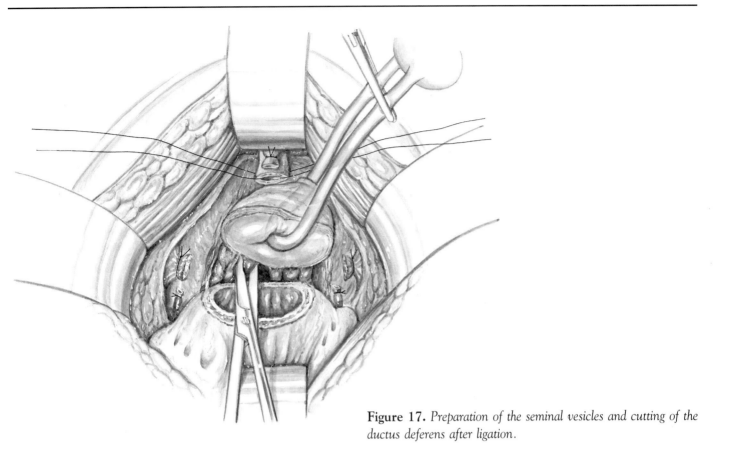

Figure 17. *Preparation of the seminal vesicles and cutting of the ductus deferens after ligation.*

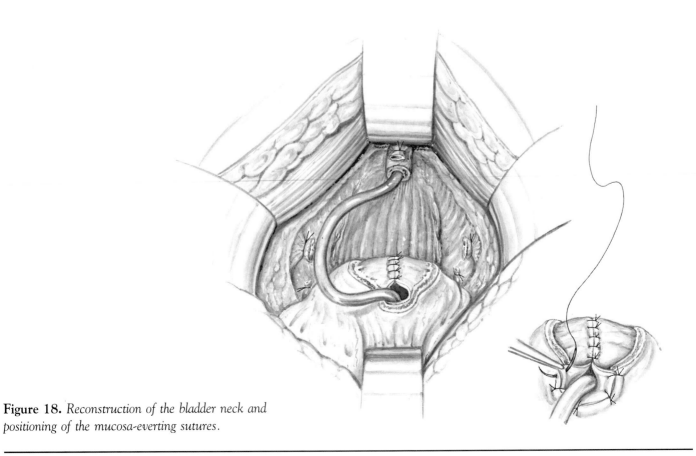

Figure 18. *Reconstruction of the bladder neck and positioning of the mucosa-everting sutures.*

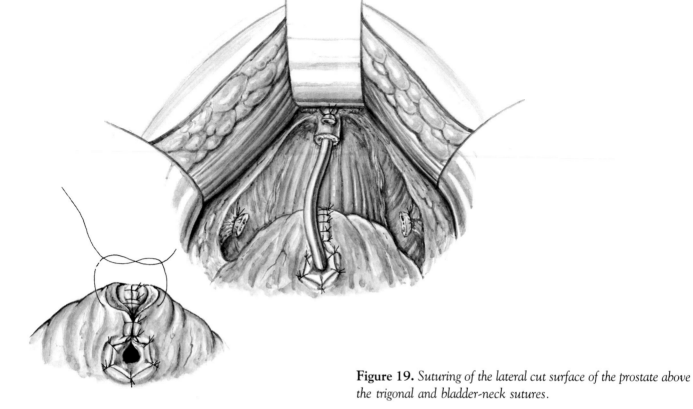

Figure 19. *Suturing of the lateral cut surface of the prostate above the trigonal and bladder-neck sutures.*

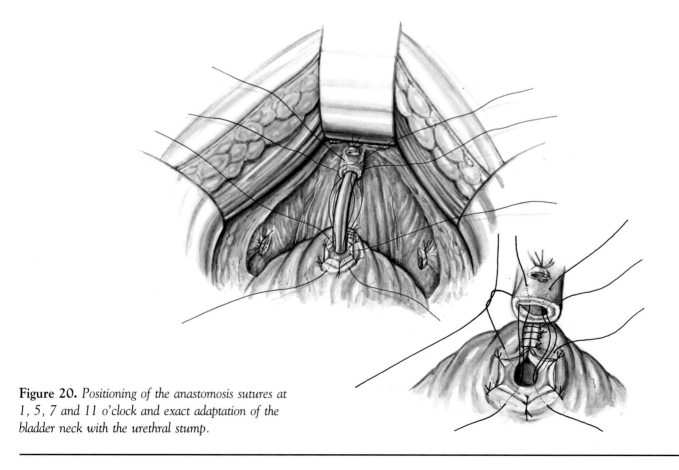

Figure 20. *Positioning of the anastomosis sutures at 1, 5, 7 and 11 o'clock and exact adaptation of the bladder neck with the urethral stump.*

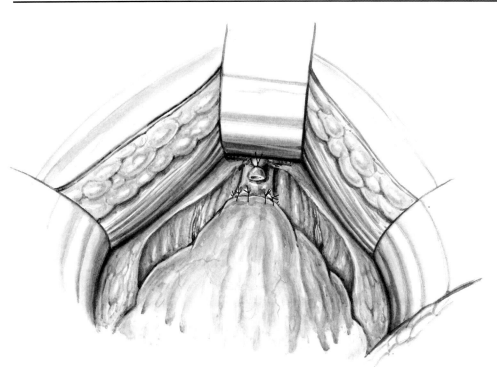

Figure 21. *Tension-free waterproof anastomosis of the bladder neck to the urethral stump.*

Figure 22. *Operation without nerve sparing: resection of the endopelvic fascia within the neurovascular bundles.*

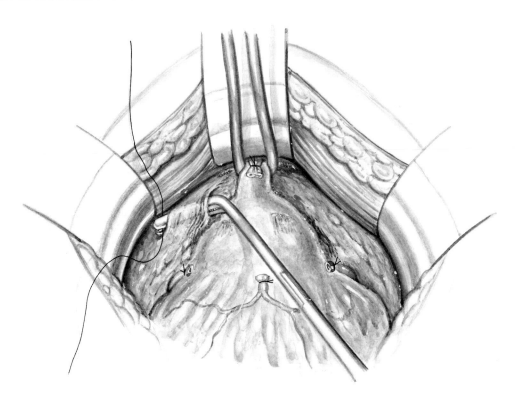

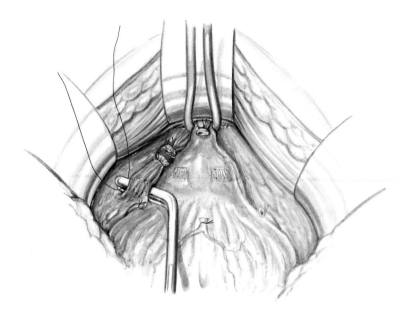

Figure 23. *Removal of the neurovascular bundles.*

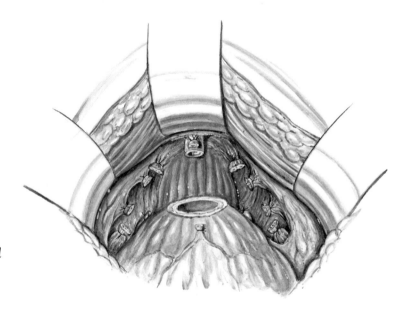

Figure 24. *Appearance after extended resection of the prostrate and the endopelvic fascia including the neurovascular bundles.*

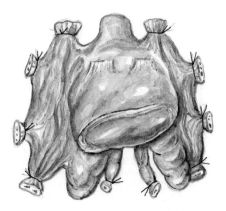

Figure 25. *The whole prostate package, including seminal vesicles and endopelvic fascia with neurovascular bundles, after removal.*

The Antegrade (Descending) Approach for Radical Retropubic Prostatectomy

G.E. Voges, S. Schumacher, M. Stöckle[a], J. Fichtner,
S.C. Müller[b], R. Hohenfellner

Department of Urology,
University of Mainz School of Medicine,
Mainz, Germany
[a]University of Kiel, Kiel, Germany
[b]University of Bonn, Bonn, Germany

Comment

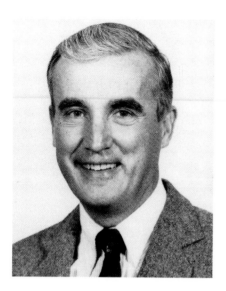

The antegrade approach is a very sound anatomic approach with several advantages. One of the weakest points in total prostatectomy beginning at the apex is the seminal vesiculectomy portion of the dissection. As described here, it is done first under conditions of primary exposure and vascular control. There is no need for haste. A hidden bonus of this technique, with the bladder neck still intact, is that it is applicable to nerve-sparing cystectomy procedures. Another advantage is the planned avoidance of dissection against the apex itself, with opening of the apical areolar tissue and peeling and preservation of the apical neurovascular bundles, which is another weak point of the nerve-sparing technique as described by Walsh. By definition, the Walsh technique invites positive apical margins of dissection.

Third, closure of the bladder neck as done here follows anatomic and functional principles. If the detrusor is dissected carefully and reapproximated well, as shown, a functional equivalent of a baseplate is restored.

My education in total prostatectomy began with the perineal approach under Wyland Leadbetter. Later the Campbell technique, also a descending approach with division of the bladder neck first, was used successfully in conjunction with pelvic lymph node dissection for pathologic staging. In recent years, the nerve-sparing technique of Walsh has been used here, but we have misgivings about the incidence of positive margins (40–70%) and possible inadequacy of local tumor control. Time will tell, but increasing evidence of clinical local recurrence (i.e. residual unresected tumor) in the USA is rapidly accumulating. This may demand a reassessment of nerve-sparing techniques or at least of selection procedures for nerve-sparing operations. In the meantime, a significant prostatectomy series without nerve sparing is necessary. Hopefully this technique will find wide acceptance and will serve for comparison with nerve-sparing prostatectomy.

John P. Donohue, Indianapolis

The antegrade (descending) approach for radical retropubic prostatectomy

Introduction

Radical prostatectomy is presently the preferred therapy for patients with clinically localized prostate cancer. Excellent long-term disease-free and cancer-specific survival, with low treatment-related morbidity, have been observed when an aggressive surgical approach to this disease is implemented. The retropubic approach to the prostate in combination with a modified pelvic lymph node dissection was revolutionized in the early 1980s by Walsh *et al.* Their studies of the pelvic anatomy and neuroanatomy has allowed the urologic surgeon to perform a nerve-sparing radical retropubic prostatectomy in appropriately selected patients.[1,2]

We prefer the antegrade (descending) approach for radical retropubic prostatectomy – a modification of the Campbell procedure. This technique offers several advantages over techniques starting with the mobilization of the apex:

- The antegrade approach allows an earlier decision on local operability

- The early dissection of the lymphovascular pedicles minimizes blood loss and prevents possible iatrogenic dissemination of tumor cells during mobilization of the prostate

- The mobile prostate allows better visualization of the apex of the gland during ligation of the dorsal vein complex and during transection of the membranous urethra

We have modified the antegrade approach for radical retropubic prostatectomy based on the detailed analysis of positive surgical margins of Stamey *et al.*[3,4] and their recognition of the sites of cancer penetration into the periprostatic fat and knowledge of the precise areas where Denonvilliers' fascia is commonly invaded and the mechanisms by which cancer spreads into the seminal vesicle. This technique allows wider surgical margins, especially during apical dissection.

Patient selection

Patients selected for radical prostatectomy should have clinically localized disease and should be in good general health with at least a 10-year life expectancy.[5]

Preoperative evaluation

Patients should have documented adenocarcinoma of the prostate (at least quadrant biopsies should be available before surgery is scheduled).

- Digital rectal examination in the knee-elbow position
- Prostate specific antigen (PSA) determination
- Ultrasonography of the upper urinary tract
- Chest radiography
- Bone scan (may be omitted in patients with PSA <5 ng/ml and a well-differentiated tumor)
- Optional transrectal ultrasonography and intravenous urography

Preoperative preparation

- Donation of autologous blood before operation
- Cleansing enema the night before surgery
- Antibiotic prophylaxis administered when the patient is called to the operating room
- Minidose heparin (subcutaneous injection into the upper arm)
- Optional sequential compression stockings

Special instruments

- Special Overholt clamp
- Turner-Warwick needle holder
- Ring retractor (e.g. Bookwalter retractor)
- Vascular instruments
- Satinsky scissors

Operative technique step by step (Figures 1–13)

- Supine hyperextended posture, with the table in the Trendelenburg position (10–20° angle)
- Rectal tube (22 Fr); after skin preparation, placement of an indwelling 20 Fr Foley catheter with 10 ml balloon
- Midline lower extraperitoneal abdominal incision from the symphysis to the umbilicus
- Blunt mobilization of the peritoneum off the posterior rectus fascia, transversus abdominis muscle and iliac vessels
- The vasa deferentia are divided. The proximal end is left on traction and is the guide for the retrovesical dissection. Placement of the ring retractor
- Modified bilateral pelvic lymph node dissection: all lymphatic tissue bordered by Cooper's ligament (inferiorly), the obturator nerve (posteriorly), the external iliac vein (laterally) and the bifurcation of the iliac vessels (proximally).

Transection of the lateral umbilical ligament facilitates pelvic lymphadenectomy and retrovesical dissection

- Fatty tissue is bluntly swept off the anterior surface of the prostate to expose the endopelvic fascia and the puboprostatic ligaments

- Incision of the endopelvic fascia (Metzenbaum scissors or long scalpel) away from the surface of the prostate to reduce the risk of bleeding from the medially located veins of Santorini. The incision is extended towards the puboprostatic ligaments; all levator ani muscle bundles are displaced laterally from the lateral periprostatic fascia. This allows palpation of the lateral surface of the prostate and the membranous urethra. The insertion of a wet compress makes dissection easier and stops bleeding in this area

- Dissection continues immediately along the vas deferens to the tip of the seminal vesicles. Small vessels have to be carefully coagulated. The 'ureter bundle' is retracted laterally with a vessel retractor

- Using the index and third finger along the vas deferens, the space behind Denonvilliers' fascia at the base of the prostate is opened. This space is developed further by bluntly sweeping the rectum off Denonvilliers' fascia down to the apex of the prostate. The rectal tube is the guide on the dorsum of the fingers. During this maneuver the prostate is continuously palpated between the second and third finger dorsally and the thumb, which is placed on the anterior surface of the prostate

- The operation continues with the dissection of the vesicle neck. Careful traction on the Foley catheter aids in the localization of the vesicle neck. Additionally, the crossing smooth muscle fibers in the area of the bladder neck show the preferred area of dissection. Two rows of 2/0 polyglyconate sutures (Maxon; Davis and Geck, Gosport, UK) are placed distally and proximally to the bladder neck to reduce bleeding from the dorsal vein plexus. The sutures remain long and tagged during the entire preparation. Traction on these sutures is extremely important during the further dissection of the vesicle neck

- Incision of the bladder neck starts between the suture lines, first with electrocautery then with scissors, and proceeds to the Foley catheter. Even though there is no anatomic capsule between the prostate and bladder, it is possible to preserve longitudinal muscle fibers of the vesicle neck into the base of the prostate. On the other hand, reconstruction of the widely opened bladder neck is so reliable that positive surgical margins in this area in a small percentage of patient otherwise curable by radical prostatectomy should not be accepted

- The catheter is pulled out of the bladder and retracted caudally and upwards. A vessel hook is inserted into the ventral opening of the bladder neck, allowing localization of both orifices

- The trigone is cut about 1 cm in front of the interureteric rim using electrocautery

- Using scissors and electrocautery, dissection continues in the midline until the ampulla of the vas and the anterior surface of the seminal vesicle are just visible

- With the index and third fingers, the bladder can now be bluntly swept off the anterior surface off the seminal vesicles

- Simultaneous digital elevation of the prostate retrovesically can be helpful in some cases

- The right and left vas are pulled through and retracted caudally to aid in the complete mobilization of the seminal vesicles

- The bladder is retracted cephalad and the seminal vesicles are completely mobilized. Both seminal vesicles can now be pulled through

- At the base of the prostate Denonvilliers' fascia is now clearly visible. This fascia is frequently invaded by tumor and must be removed with the prostate

- Traction on the vas and seminal vesicles exposes the superior pedicles and neurovascular bundles. Division of the superior pedicles deep in the pelvis

- Removal of the periprostatic wet compresses and division of the lateral pedicles of the prostate deep in the pelvis. (In selected cases a nerve-sparing procedure can easily be performed. In the descending technique, separation of the neurovascular bundle starts at the base of the prostate with a sharp separation of the superior pedicle and the neurovascular bundle off the dorsolateral base of the prostate.)

- The prostate is now completely mobile dorsolaterally

- Residual fibers of the endopelvic fascia laterally and the puboprostatic ligaments are divided close to the symphysis pubis. The prostate is now completely mobile

- A fine right-angled clamp (Overholt) is inserted superficially below the dorsal vein complex about 2–3 mm distal to the apex of the prostate. The clamp is only minimally opened, not to injure the external sphincter. The dorsal vein complex is then ligated with a 2/0 polyglycolic suture (e.g. Dexon; Davis and Geck) as distally as possible. Alternatively, a partially straightened 26 G needle on a polyglycolic suture can be placed through the dorsal vein complex near the inferior edge of the symphysis pubis as far distally as possible

- Transection of the dorsal vein complex immediately proximal to the suture (no. 10 scalpel or electrocautery) onto the membranous urethra and the Foley catheter.

Opening of the membranous urethra in a semicircular manner with the Satinsky scissors

- Placement of the 11 and 1 o'clock sutures (two of a total of four anastomotic sutures) to the vesicle neck

- The Foley catheter is pulled back into the membranous urethra and then pulled out of the wound. Very careful cephalad traction on the Foley catheter (not to injure the external sphincter) is helpful during dissection of the posterior lip of the membranous urethra

- Transection of the posterior membranous urethra and the thick triangular termination of Denonvilliers' fascia and removal of the surgical specimen. The 5 and 7 o'clock sutures are fully anchored into the distal Denonvilliers' plate before passing the sutures into the wall of the membranous urethra. At all times the dissection stays in front of the apical surface of the prostate. (The surgical specimen is carefully linked before formal fixation. This allows a reliable assessment of positive surgical margins.)

- Continuous bleeding from the dorsal vein complex is now controlled

- Placement of a cystostomy and fixation with 3/0 catgut

- Reconstruction of the bladder neck starting laterally with resorbable suture material (2/0 or 3/0 Maxon) until a 20 Fr Foley catheter is just passable into the bladder. The mucosa is carefully everted using interrupted 3/0 catgut

- The 5 and 7 o'clock anastomotic sutures are placed at their appropriate position in the vesicle neck

- A 20 Fr 20 ml silicone catheter is passed through the penis into the bladder, but is not inflated

- Sutures are now placed in the vesicle neck at the 1 and 11 o'clock positions

- The catheter is now inflated with 20 ml sterile water

- Approximation of the bladder to the membranous urethra with slight traction on the catheter. The 5 and 7 o'clock sutures are tied, followed by the 11 and 1 o'clock sutures

- Two silicone drains are placed perivesically

- The rectus muscles are loosely approximated and the rectus fascia is securely closed

Postoperative management

- Appropriate analgesia

- The patient is mobilized on day 1; pelvic floor training is started on the same day

- Drains are progressively removed, starting on day 2

- The silicone catheter is clamped on day 4; the cystostomy stays open

- Patient is usually discharged on day 7 with appropriate antibiotic therapy

- On day 14, cystography is performed and the catheter is removed. At the same time a first postoperative prostate specific antigen (PSA) level is obtained

Complications

Intraoperative
- Bleeding from the dorsal vein complex

- Dissection of the obturator nerve (primary suture)

- Rectal lesion (double-layer closure, free peritoneal patch optionally)

- Ureteral lesion (ureteral neocystotomy, e.g. psoas hitch, Boari hitch)

Early postoperative
- Loss of the silicone catheter with urinary extravasation (careful attempt to reposition the catheter, probably under cystoscopic guidance)

- Thromboembolic complications (early mobilization, modified pelvic lymphadenectomy, low-dose heparinization,[6] sequential compression stockings)

- Lymphocele (ultrasound-guided percutaneous puncture or drainage)

References

1. Reiner WC, Walsh PC. An anatomical approach to the surgical management of the dorsal vein and Santorini's plexus during radical retropubic surgery. *J Urol* **121** (1979) 198–200.
2. Walsh PC, Lepor H, Eggleston JC. Radical prostatectomy with preservation of sexual function: anatomical and pathological considerations. *Prostate* **4** (1983) 473–85.
3. Stamey TA, Villers AA, McNeal JE, Link PC, Freiha FS. Positive surgical margins at radical prostatectomy: importance of the apical dissection. *J Urol* **143** (1990) 1166–73.
4. Voges GE, McNeal JE, Redwine EA, Freiha FS, Stamey TA. Morphologic analysis of surgical margins with positive findings in prostatectomy for adenocarcinoma of the prostate. *Cancer* **69** (1992) 520–6.
5. Voges GE, Hohenfellner R. Prostatakarzinom: keine Behandlung – eine Option bei klinisch lokalisiertem Tumor? *Akt Urol* **21** (1990) 232–3.
6. Kröpfl D, Krause R, Hartung R. A method to avoid lymphoceles in heparinised patients. *J Urol* **139** (1988) 168A.

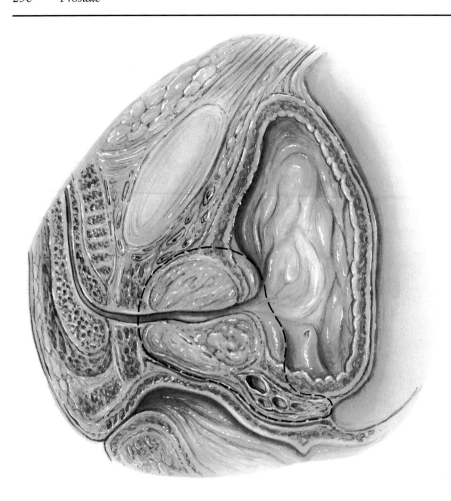

Figure 1. *Resection margins during radical prostatectomy. Because of a close approximation of the prostate to the other pelvic organs (bladder, rectum, membranous urethra with the external sphincter and pelvic side wall) dissection with a wide surgical margin is not possible.*

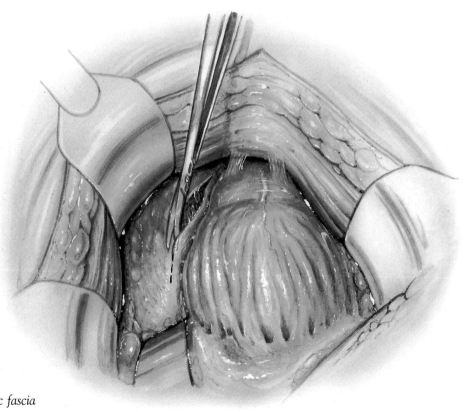

Figure 2. *Incision of the endopelvic fascia away from the surface of the prostate.*

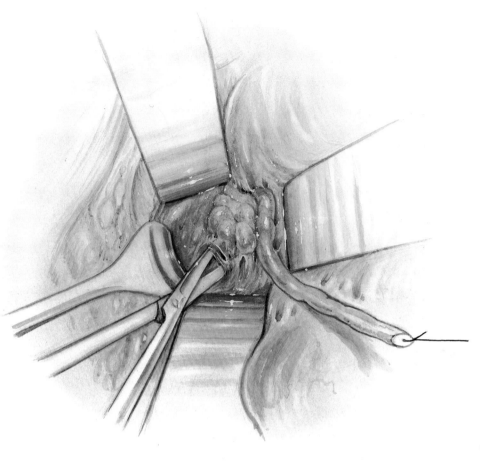

Figure 3. *Sharp dissection immediately along the vas deferens to the seminal vesicles. Careful mobilization of the left seminal vesicle (on the right the bladder is retracted medially; the head of the patient is to the bottom of the picture). Small vessels are carefully coagulated, especially at the tip of the seminal vesicles. The vessel retractor on the left side retracts the ureter bundle laterally. During the complete maneuver, careful exposure of the surgical field with long narrow retractors is extremely important.*

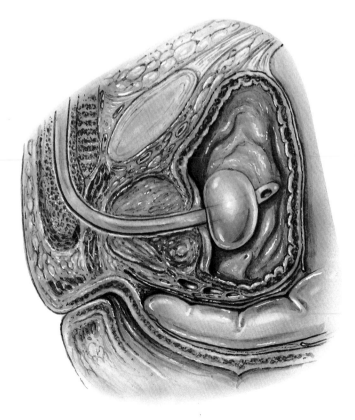

Figure 4. *After removing all retractors the index and third finger follow the vas deferens and open the space behind Denonvilliers' fascia. Blunt dissection to the apex of the prostate with preservation of Denonvilliers' fascia on the dorsal surface of the prostate.*

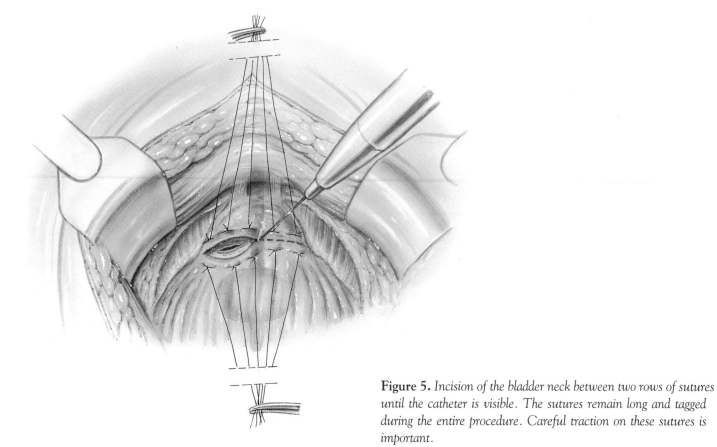

Figure 5. *Incision of the bladder neck between two rows of sutures until the catheter is visible. The sutures remain long and tagged during the entire procedure. Careful traction on these sutures is important.*

Figure 6. *(a) After localization of both orifices the trigone is cut about 1 cm in front of the interior track rim until the ampulla of the vas and the anterior surface of the seminal vesicles are visible.*

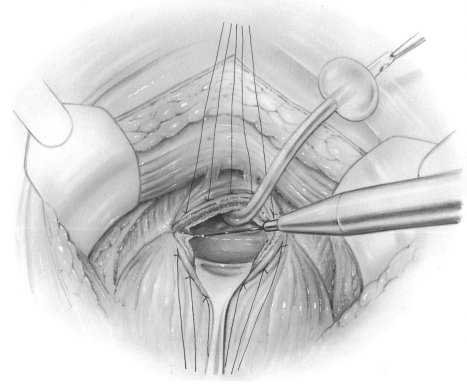

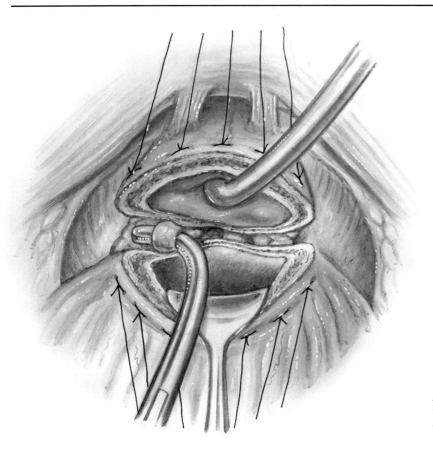

Figure 6. *(b) Both vasa are pulled through, followed by complete mobilization of the seminal vesicles.*

Figure 7. *Cephalad retraction of the bladder, and ligature and division of the superior pedicles deep in the pelvis. During a nerve-sparing procedure in carefully selected cases, the superior pedicle neurovascular bundles can easily be dissected off the dorsolateral base on the prostate at this point.*

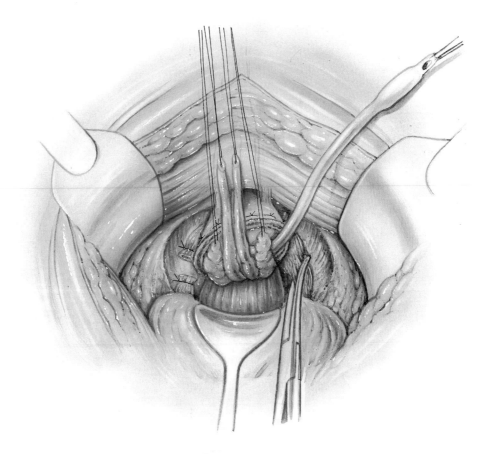

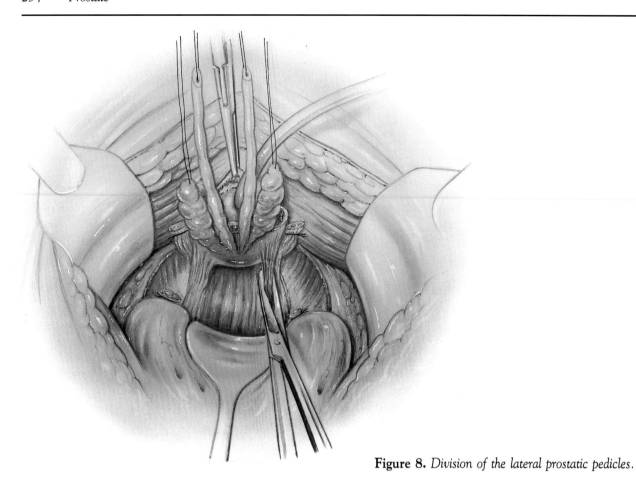

Figure 8. *Division of the lateral prostatic pedicles.*

Figure 9. *Division of the puboprostatic ligaments using the Satinsky scissors.*

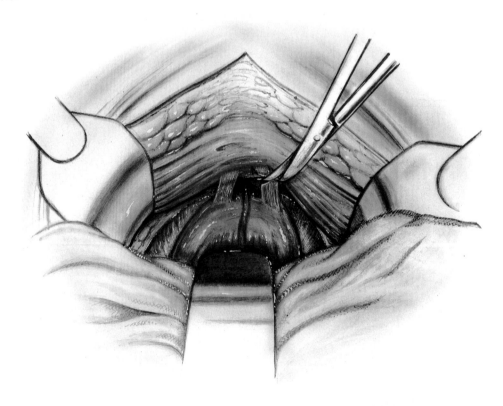

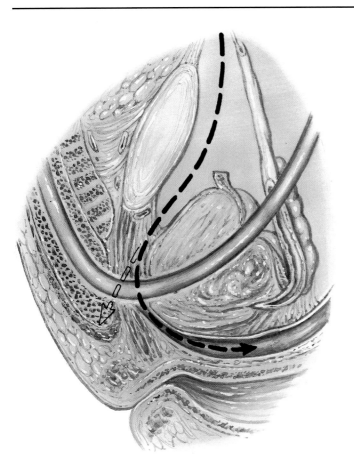

Figure 10. *Optimal plane of dissection at the apex (solid arrow). Erroneous preparation along the wrong plane (open arrow) leads to loss of a functional urethra and increases the risk of bleeding.*

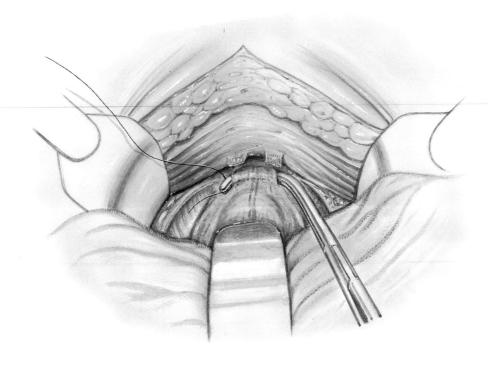

Figure 11. *(a) A fine right-angled clamp is passed below the dorsal vein complex. A 0 Dexon suture is pulled through and tied. The dorsal vein complex is transected immediately proximal to the suture (scalpel or electrocautery) onto the catheter.*

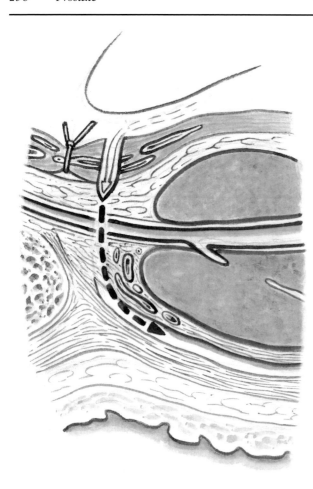

Figure 11. *(b) At all times the dissection stays in front of the apical surface of the prostate. This decreases the rate of positive apical resection margins.*

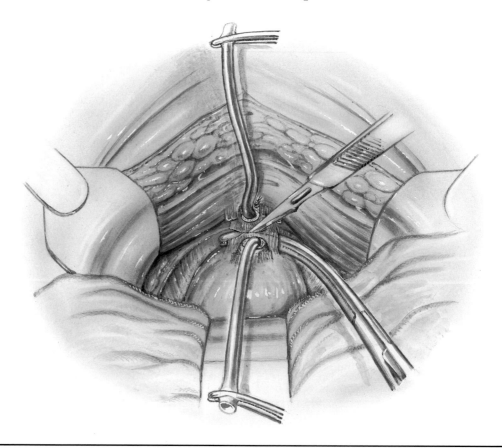

Figure 12. *Elevation and transection of the distal end of Denonvilliers' fascia. The 5 and 7 o'clock anastomotic sutures should be fully anchored into the distal end of this fascia.*

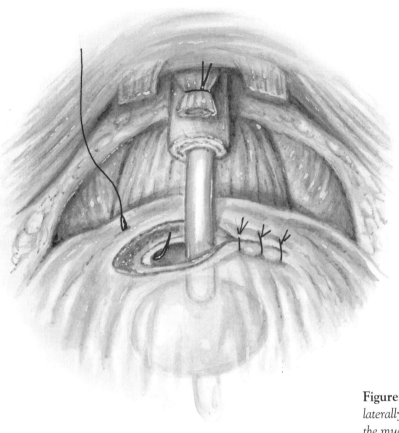

Figure 13. (a) Reconstruction of the bladder neck starting laterally after inspection of both orifices. (b) Careful eversion of the mucosa at the bladder neck for a water-tight mucosa-to-mucosa anastomosis between the urethral stump and the bladder neck.

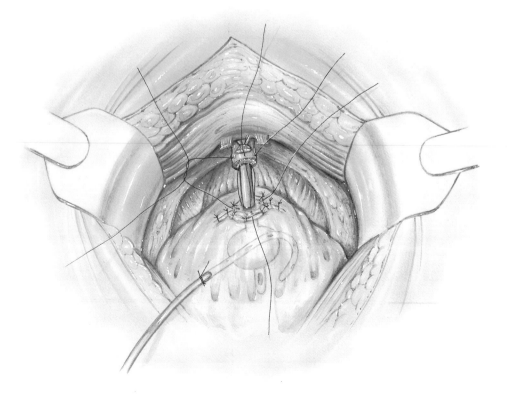

MINT: Minimally Invasive Nonexpensive TURP

J. Fichtner, A. Macedo, M. Wöhr,
M. Yoshioka, R. Hohenfellner
Department of Urology,
University of Mainz School of Medicine,
Mainz, Germany

Introduction

The variety of new and different technologies (Table 1) for surgical treatment of benign prostatic hyperplasia (BPH) as alternatives to the gold standard transurethral resection of the prostate (TURP) implies both medical and economic problems for the treating physician. A stepwise therapy from the less invasive procedure to finally TURP seems to be restricted to few fully equipped centers. However, in a small and selected group of patients at high medical and anesthesiologic risk or who request prograde ejaculation, the need for a minimally invasive alternative to conventional TURP may arise.

Table 1.

	Cost of purchase (US$)	Cost of single-use material (US$)
TURP (transurethral resection)	16000	35
TULAP/VLAP (transurethral laser ablation)	53000	340
TUNA (transurethral needle ablation)	26500	1100
TUMT (transurethral microwave)	400000	540
ILK (interstitial laser coagulation)	46500	200

MINT (minimal-invasive nonexpensive TURP) allows use of the routine TURP equipment with a conventional high-frequency energy source to perform a minimally invasive procedure of short duration (10 min). In a modification of the original Nesbit technique,[1] the resection is restricted to creation of a channel beginning at the 12 o'clock position and widening to 11 and 1 o'clock without involvement of the lateral and median lobes. The bladder neck can be preserved and thus theoretically antegrade ejaculation is preserved in patients who request this particularly. In contrast to the resection technique of Flocks,[2] beginning resection at 12 o'clock avoids the risk of falling lateral lobes, and a sufficient micturition channel is created even with removal of only minor amounts of tissue. In addition, there is very low risk of bleeding owing to the poor blood supply of the prostate anteriorly.

So far MINT has been performed at our institution in 56 patients, the majority being in complete retention. They were not eligible for a standard TURP because of high medical risk. At an average follow-up of 9 months, residual-free micturition resulted in 81%.

Indications

Symptomatic obstructive adenoma in patients with:

- High medical or anesthesiologic risk
- Limited life expectancy
- The wish for prograde ejaculation

Contraindications

- Associated bladder diverticulum and stones
- Extensive strictures not manageable by endoscopy
- Severe cerebral sclerosis, Parkinson's disease

Instruments

- 24 Fr resectoscope with angled loop, 0° optic and sufficient lubricant
- Energy source: Erbotom ICC 350 high-frequency cautery with automatically induced sparkling release (650 V effectively with 200 W) and high coagulation effect vene with cutting cautery
- 20 Fr irrigation catheter
- Optional trocar cystostomy for low-pressure resection

Anesthesia

Spinal

Surgical technique step by step (Figures 1–6)

- Insertion of the 24 Fr resectoscope with optional trocar cystostomy. Fixation of the shaft with the left hand at the level of the verumontanum, and rotation of the loop to the 12 o'clock position
- Eversion of the loop until just distal to the bladder neck and slow resection of a first channel
- Hemostasis by slowly gliding the loop back over the exposed tissue
- Creation of a tunnel by adding resection channels at 11 and 1 o'clock and of a resulting plateau due to the underlying lateral lobes
- Landmarks are the bladder neck, the prostatic capsule (laterally) and the verumontanum (distally)
- Optionally a bladder neck incision at 12 o'clock can be added at the end of the procedure (Turner-Warwick)

Surgical tricks

Extremely careful resection with slow movement of the loop is mandatory for achievement of a good coagulation effect. Use of the surgeon's left hand is of great importance both for fixation of the shaft at the level of the verumontanum and for control of the resectoscope movements.

Follow-up

- Constant irrigation for 12 hours
- Antibiotics for 3 days
- Removal of the transurethral catheter after 24 hours
- Assessment of residual urine volume with the suprapubic catheter; removal of the catheter when the residual volume is below 50 ml

References

1. Nesbit RM. *Transurethral Prostatectomy*. Springfield, IL: Charles C. Thomas (1943).
2. Flocks RH. The arterial distribution within the prostate: its role in transurethral prostatic resection. *J Urol* **37** (1937) 524.

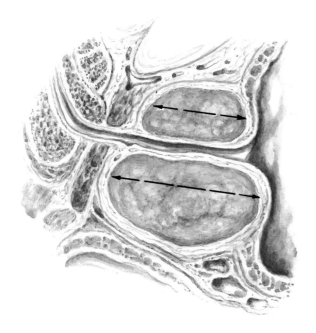

Figure 1. *Extent of the anterior prostatic tissue.*

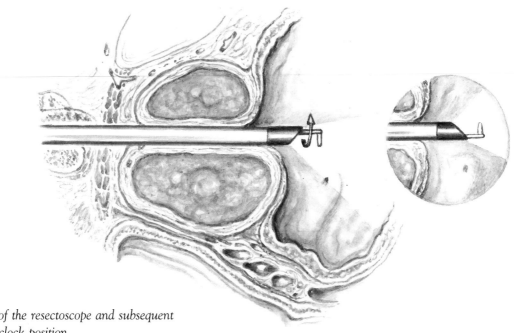

Figure 2. *Insertion of the resectoscope and subsequent rotation to the 12 o'clock position.*

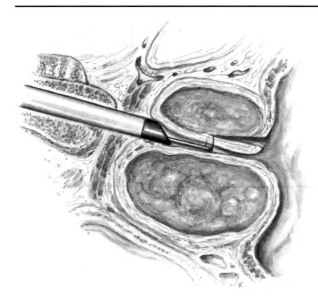

Figure 3. *The first cut at 12 o'clock with slow movement of the loop.*

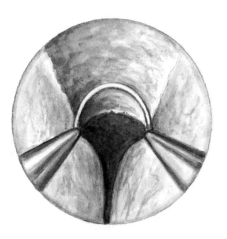

Figure 4. *Resulting channel at 12 o'clock.*

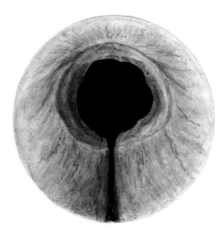

Figure 5. *Completion of the micturition channel after resection from 11 to 1 o'clock with resulting plateau due to the underlying lateral lobes.*

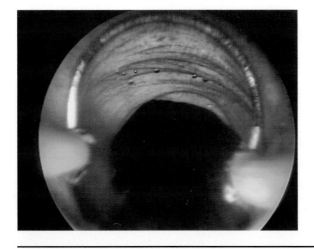

Figure 6. *Final endoscopic appearance.*

Radical Perineal Prostatectomy

D.F. Paulson
Professor and Chief,
Division of Urology,
Department of Surgery,
Duke University Medical Center,
Durham, North Carolina, USA

Introduction

Radical perineal prostatectomy can be accomplished via a radical retropubic or perineal route. Since PSA has allowed us to exclude many patients from node dissection, perineal prostatectomy has increased in popularity due to decreased morbidity, decreased blood loss, and shortened hospital stay.

Indications

Perineal prostatectomy is appropriate for any patient with clinically localized adenocarcinoma of the prostate.

Preoperative preparation

Preoperative osmotic mechanical bowel cleansing combined with non-absorbable oral antibiotics the day before surgery and a neomycin enema on the morning of surgery.

Instruments

- Lowsley retractor
- Young tractor
- Baby Deaver retractors
- Weighted vaginal speculum
- Standard instruments for surgery
- Suture material: 0, 2–0, 4–0 monofilament absorbable sutures

Exposure

Anterior rectal curvilinear incision.

Operative technique step-by-step (Figures 1–8)

- In the exaggerated lithotomy position, the weight of the patient is borne across the upper back and positioning maintained by towels or pillows placed beneath the sacrum and small of the back
- The incision is a generous inverted 'U' which encircles the anus, with the arms carried posterior to the anus
- The anus is excluded from the field by the use of drapes and Allis clamps. Fibrofatty tissue on either side of the midline is incised with cutting cautery, giving access to ischio-rectal fossa

- The central tendon is isolated by placing a finger beneath the central tendon anterior to the rectum and the central tendon is divided at the skin margin
- Muscular fibers overlapping the anterior rectal fascia are elevated and, using the anterior rectal fascia as a guide, a plane is established on either side of the rectourethralis to the base of the prostate
- The urethra is exposed in the midline at the apex of the prostate and the neurovascular fascia may be separated from the urethra. This fascial layer which is adherent to prostatic substance may be preserved or sacrificed in accordance with extent of disease
- The urethra is sharply divided and, using a Young tractor to bring the prostate into the operative field, the prostate is bluntly dissected from beneath the dorsal venous complex and liberated from the detrusor musculature
- The urethra is divided at the bladder neck and the bladder allowed to retract into the pelvis. The fascia overlying the vas deferens and seminal vesicles is incised to expose the vas deferens. The vas deferens and seminal vesicles may be used to identify the plane between the vasculature and seminal vesicles, these vessels being controlled either with electrocautery or surgical clips
- Following division of the vasculature, the seminal vesicles may be mobilized to their tips and the vascular supply to the seminal vesicles controlled with surgical clips
- Following removal of the specimen, the bladder is closed from 6 to 12 o'clock with interrupted 0 absorbable sutures and the anastomies between the urethra and bladder neck is accomplished by 4 quadrant sutures of 00 absorbable monofilament. This direct anastomosis is supported by Dee's modification of Vest sutures in which 0 absorbable sutures at each quadrant of the vesicle neck are brought through the perineal body and secured beneath the skin

Surgical tricks

- Dissection of the prostate from beneath the dorsal venous complex prior to division of the urethra allows for mobilization of a long length of membraneous urethra
- Identification of the seminal vesicles and vas deferens allows identification of the proper plane to mobilize and secure the vascular supply of the prostate

Postoperative care

The perineal drain is removed on the second day and the catheter is usually removed on the 14th to 18th postoperative day. The patient is discharged on the morning of the second to third postoperative day.

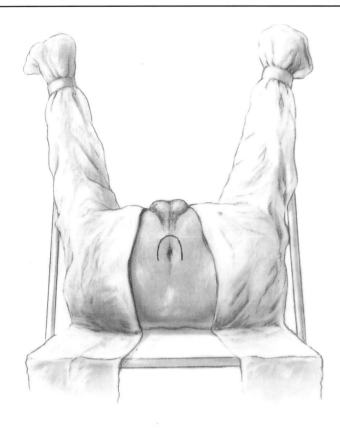

Figure 1. *In the exaggerated lithotomy position, the weight of the patient is borne across the upper back and positioning maintained by towels or pillows placed beneath the sacrum or small of the back.*

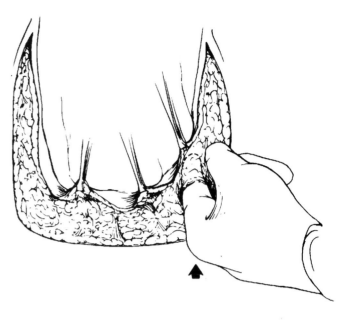

Figure 3. *The anus is excluded from the field by the use of drapes and Allis clamps. The fibrofatty tissue to either side of the midline is incised with cautery to permit access to the ischial rectal fossa.*

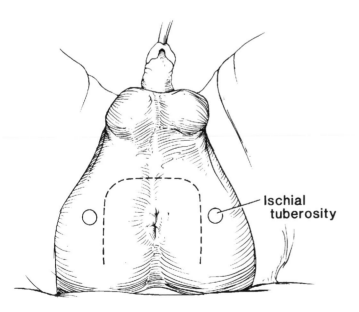

Figure 2. *The incision is a generous inverted 'U' and is carried posteriorly to the anus.*

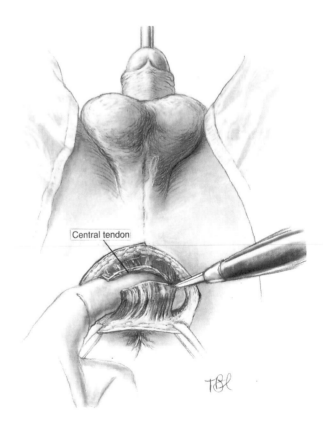

Figure 4. *The central tendon is isolated by placing a finger anterior to the rectum and is divided at the skin margin.*

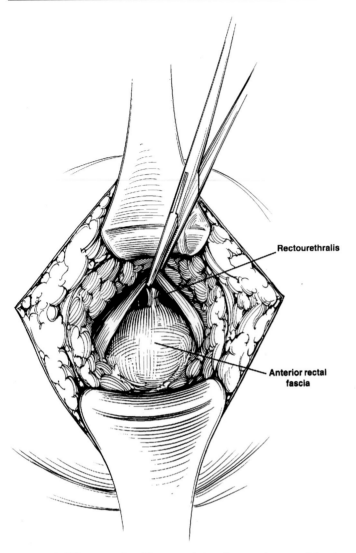

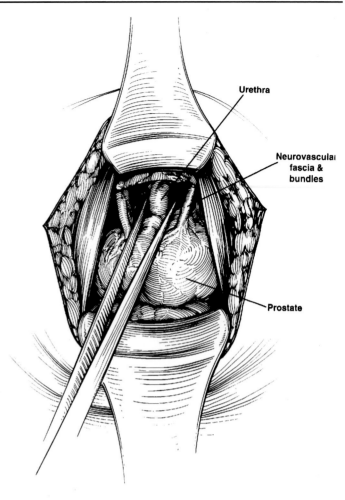

Figure 5. *The muscular fibers overlying the anterior rectal fascia are elevated and, using the anterior rectal fascia as a guide, a plane established on either side of the rectourethralis to the base of the prostate.*

Figure 6. *The urethra may be exposed in the midline at the apex of the prostate and the neurovascular fascia separated from the urethra. This fascial layer, which is adherent to prostatic substance, may be preserved or sacrificed in accordance with the extent of disease.*

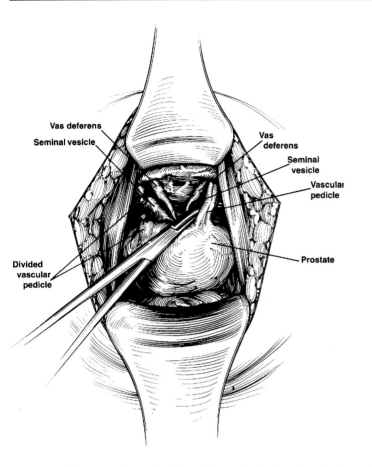

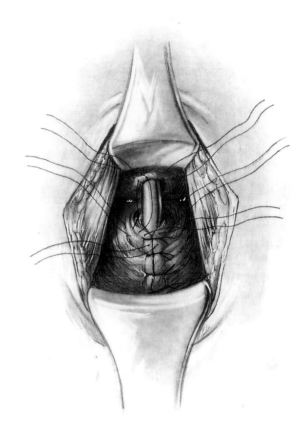

Figure 7. *The seminal vesicles bilaterally are the landmarks which the surgeon uses to identify the plane for control of the vascular pedicles of the prostate. A right-angled clamp may be passed lateral to the seminal vesicles and medial to the vascular pedicle. This tissue is divided sharply and vascular control established either mechanically or with electrocautery.*

Figure 8. *The anastomosis between the urethra and bladder neck, closed previously from 6–12 o'clock with interrupted 0 absorbable suture, is accomplished by 4–quadrant sutures of 00 absorbable sutures. The direct anastomosis is supported by Dees' modification of the Vest sutures in which 0 absorbable sutures, at each quadrant neck closure, are brought through the perineal body and secured anterior to anterior, posterior to posterior.*

(All figures published with permission from: Paulson DF. Controversies surrounding the management of radical perineal prostatectomy. In: *Principles and Practices in Genitourinary Oncology*, Raghavan, Scher, Liebel, Lange (Eds), Philadelphia: JB Lippincott, 1995)

External Genitalia

V

Feminization in Female Pseudohermaphroditism

J.E. Altwein
Department of Urology,
Hospital Barmherzigen Brüder,
München, Germany

Comment

This concrete contribution describes clearly the therapeutic strategy in female pseudohermaphroditism. In particular it calls attention to the necessity for a precise diagnosis in patients with palpable gonadal tissue in a hernia. The anatomy can be determined by the described radiologic, sonographic and endoscopic diagnostic tools.

Clitoris reduction plasty is the preferred technique in female pseudohermaphroditism. This procedure saves sexual stimulability and leads to excellent cosmetic results. It protects from painful erections, which are a major cause of morbidity in these patients if erectile tissue is not resected but placed with numerous stitches under the symphysis to protect against irritation of the ventral skin. In contrast, clitoris reduction plasty allows both preservation of the dorsal neurovascular bundle and adequate removal of the erectile tissue. The author stresses that the outer margins of the glans should be modelled to achieve an optimal cosmetic result.

The described vaginoplasty procedures correspond to the present gold standard and, in the hands of an experienced surgeon, give excellent functional and cosmetic results. Vaginoplasty should be performed shortly before puberty to reduce to a minimum the potential danger of stenosis.

David T. Mininberg, New York

Feminization in female pseudohermaphroditism

Introduction

Overvirilization of a female individual leads to female pseudohermaphroditism. This intersex state can be classified into the different forms of adrenal hyperplasia (adrenogenital syndrome, AGS) and various nonadrenal forms (simple hypertrophy of the clitoris with or without persistent cloaca, with or without bone malformation). Congenital adrenal hyperplasia (CAH) is found in 1 5000 to 15 000 births. Males and females are equally affected, but males rarely present with genital anomalies. CAH is caused by the autosomic recessive transmission of an enzyme defect: lack of 21-hydroxylase produces deficient catabolism of progesterone and 17α-hydroxyprogesterone to 11-deoxycorticosterone. Deficient synthesis of hydrocortisone then results in excessive formation of ACTH; this causes an increased synthesis of pregnenolone and finally a high level of adrenal androgens. In females, this produces AGS. This hormonal constellation disturbs the differentiation of female external genitalia between weeks 9 and 17 of pregnancy leading to fusion of the urogenital sinus and hypertrophy of the clitoris. Prader identified five different grades of masculinization of female genitalia (Figure 1). This classification determines the operative technique and suggests the probability of a salt loss.

The defect of 11β-hydroxylase is comparatively rare; in our own series of 53 patients, treated between 1979 and 1989, we found only one 11β-hydroxylase defect. Female adrenal pseudohermaphroditism was also observed in only one case.

It is important to pay attention to the hereditary pathway in children with a 21-hydroxylase defect because of the chance of prenatal diagnosis by detecting an increase of 17α-hydroxyprogesterone and 4-androstenedione in the amniotic fluid. If a child is affected there is a 25% possibility of transmission of CAH. CAH can be suppressed by prenatal dexamethasone therapy.

Preoperative evaluation

The cause of female pseudohermaphroditism must usually be determined before planning feminization. Where these are palpable scrotal or inguinal gonads the diagnosis must be verified. For determination of the grade of disease (Prader classification), ultrasonography, intraoperative endoscopy and most important, preoperative genitography are necessary. In our institution we observed 64% Prader grade IV and 24%

Prader grade III. Vesicoureteral reflux is often found incidentally in the course of genitography.

Operative indications and preparation

There is no need for operative correction in Prader I AGS without marked fusion of the perineum. Feminization is also contraindicated if AGS-female individuals have been educated as males and the diagnosis has been established only in adolescence. Of 11 apparent male hermaphrodites who underwent masculinization, we observed three AGS-individuals, aged 17, 24 and 25 years, for whom feminization was not possible for psychiatric reasons. The ideal age of surgery is between 6 and 18 months; feminization after 30 months is not possible because it causes psychological problems.

On anesthesia induction, a bolus injection of hydrocortisone (35 mg/m^2) will be given followed by 15 mg/m^2 hourly until the end of the procedure. In the first 12 hours after operation, 36 mg/m^2 i.v. are given at 2-hour intervals, then the same dose 4 times at 3 hour intervals. In an uncomplicated postoperative course 35 mg/m^2 hydrocortisone i.v. is given every 4 hours on days 1 and 2. On day 3, hydrocortisone (35 mg/m^2) can be given per os. Between days 4 and 7, hydrocortisone is given in maintenance doses (20 mg/m^2 per day).

Operative technique step by step

The aim of the operation is the cosmetic reconstruction of the vulva and the functional preservation of the clitoris. Somatosensitive evoked potentials measure the functional sensitivity of the clitoris.

We present the nerve-sparing shaft-recizing feminization procedure that we applied in 29 of 53 patients with AGS; this operation represents the best compromise between the Kumar[5] and the Praetorius[13] techniques.

- The skin of the clitoris shaft is split just in front of the ventral commissure of the labia majora; lateral glans segments are included within the incision line. It is useful to mark the incision line before cutting, and to fix a sagittal glans stay suture. There is no need for subcutaneous injection of hemostyptic solution; even the use of tourniquets for clitoral ischemia is usually not necessary. Magnifying glasses (with 5.5 × magnification, for example) are required. The prepared skin segments are stabilized by a Scott ring retractor

- Preparation of the clitoris shaft with protection of the neurovascular bundle between the fascias of Colles and Buck. The prepared glans cheeks will be inverted together, and accessory foreskin segments used to cover the vestibule of the vagina later. The suspensory ligament of the clitoris inserts near the point of division of the corpora cavernosa. Excision and preparation of a trapezoid perineal wide pedunculated flap on the velar side. Release the dorsal neurovascular bundle after incision of Buck's fascia carefully form tunica albuginea. Isolating of the corpora cavernosa on the velar side from the front wall of the urogenital sinus. The glans is thus isolated from the neurovascular bundle dorsally and from the urogenital sinus in front. Both corpora cavernosa are removed by a piercing-suture ligature with 3/0 Vicryl (Ethicon, Edinburgh, UK). The corpora cavernosa are dissected leaving a small tunica albuginea edge near the glans. Normally bleeding is minimal. The glans itself is pedunculated twice and therefore well vascularized

- After preparation of the trapezoid perineal flap of the vaginal back wall, the vestibule can be demonstrable even in Prader VU AGS. Sometimes a 6 Fr catheter in the urethral is helpful. The vaginal back wall is split with scissors at 6 o'clock (the 'cut back' principle) until the vestibule of the vagina has a breadth of nearly 7 mm. For fast hemostasis, the trapezoid perineal flap is sutured with single 6/0 polydioxanone sutures in the V-shaped incision of the vaginal back wall. The glans clitoris should be well vascularized and of appropriate size

- The neurovascular bundle is pushed, folded, under the anterior labial commissure, and the glans is fixed near the infrapubic arch with subcutaneous sutures. (The top of the glans should be recognizable.) This raises the mons pubis (mons plastic). Then removed skin areas are united with single sutures. Glans segments are sutured in the angle between the trapezoid perineal flap and the velar glans pedicle; they enlarge the vestibule and should prevent its shrinkage due to elasticity. A 6 Fr catheter and vaginal tamponade are left until the compression bandage is removed

Postoperative complications

If this procedure is performed carefully it is well tolerated in children aged 6–12 months. Reintervention was necessary because of postoperative hemorrhage in one of 29 children operated on using this technique. Wound dehiscence in the vestibular area was seen in two other children, who were treated without secondary suture. There was no glans necrosis. In one child who had been operated on before, a rectal lesion was made accidentally during preparation and dorsal expansion of the stenotic vagina; after bilaminar suture and careful preparation of the vaginal back wall there were no postoperative problems.

If, in cases with a large phallus, clitoris shaft skin is used to form the lateral aspect of the vestibule of the vagina, it may produce an unsightly skin tongue near the newly created labia minora, However, after postoperative edema is eased, the symmetric skin fold is not a problem. The folds disappear, as the child grows, with good hormonal therapy.

Prader V AGS

Nerve-sparing clitoris reduction plasty is adequate for the lower Prader grades. Vaginal reconstruction is the main problem. This operation is usually postponed until after puberty. A perineal pull-through vaginoplasty has been used in the past in children under 1 month of age, but its cosmetic and functional results have been criticized. One of the reasons is that the newly formed vestibule lies in the perineum and is visible as an isolated hole in the perineum distant to the urethal meatus. Stenosis requiring bougienage usually follows. Bolkenius and Daum[2] report a negative impact on the psychological development of the girl.

On the basis of Monfort's experience,[8] Passerini-Glazel[11] developed a new one-stage procedure maintaining the opening of the urogenital sinus and dividing the vagina near the confluence using a transvesical approach. The vagina is finally unified using reversed penis shaft skin, tubularized by using the distal urethral plate behind the bladder. The cosmetic and functional results of this procedure, used by Passerini-Glazel in four cases, are unclear. The main apprehension is that the reversed skin tube will retract even if augmented with urethral mucosa. In one of the four reported cases a nearly untreatable vaginourethral fistula appeared. Further experience with long-term follow-up is needed to evaluate this procedure definitively.

Our experience is based on two of 29 children with Prader V AGS with opening of the meatus at the top of the glans. Velar opening of the urethra and resection of the corpora cavernosa precede stabilization of the vestibule by a trapezoidal flap. This avoids the occurrence of hydrocolpocele or hemocolpocele. After puberty, relocalization of the growing vagina is planned.

Bibliography

1. Altwein JE, Walz PH. Urologische Behandlung der Intersexualität. In: Hohenfellner R, Zingg EJ (eds) *Urologie in Klinik und Praxis*, Vol. 2. Stuttgart: Thieme (1983) 1114–34.
2. Bolkenius M, Daum R. Verbesserte Methode zur operativplastischen Korrektur der Klitoris bei Pseudohermaphroditismus femininus. *Z Kinderchir* 20 (1977) 71–6.

3. Fortunoff S, Lattimer JL, Edson M. Vaginoplasty technique for female pseudohermaphrodites. *Surg Gynecol Obstet* **118** (1964) 545–8.

4. Hendren WH, Crawford JD. Adrenogenital syndrome: the anatomy of the anomaly and its repair. Some new concepts. *J Pediatr Surg* **4** (1969) 49–59.

5. Kumar H, Kiefer JH, Rosenthal IE, Clark SS. Clitoroplasty: experience during a 19-year period. *J Urol* **111** (1974) 81–4.

6. Master WH, Johnson V. *Human Sexual Response.* Boston: Little, Brown (1966).

7. Money J, Hampson JG, Hampon JL. Hermaphroditism: recommendations concerning assignment of sex, change of sex and psychologic management. *Bull Johns Hopkins Hosp* **97** (1955) 284–300.

8. Monfort G. Transvesical approach to utricular cysts. *J Pediatr Surg* **17** (1982) 406–9.

9. Nihoul-Fékété CL. Traitement chirurgical des anomalies de différentation de la vulve et du sinus urogénital chez l'enfant. 1. Europäisches Symposium für Kinder- und Jugendgynäkologie, 19–21 March 1981. Wissenschaftliche Information Milupa, Friedrichsdorf *1* (1982) 219–35.

10. Opsomer RJ, Guerit JM, Wese FX, von Cangh PJ. Pudendal cortical somato-sensory evoked potentials. *J Urol* **135** (1986) 1216–18.

11. Passerini-Glazel G. A new 1-stage procedure for clitorovaginoplasty in severely masculinized female pseudohermaphrodites. *J Urol* **142** (1989) 565–8.

12. Prader A. Der Genitalbefund beim Pseudohermaphroditismus femininus des kongenitalen Syndroms. *Helv Pediatr Acta* **9** (1954) 231–48.

13. Praetorius M. Zur Korrektur des AGS-Genitales bei stärkeren Virilisierungsformen (Prader III–V). *Z Kinderchir* **33** (1981) 343–9.

14. Schwab KO, Kruse K, Dörr HG, Horwitz E, Spingler H. Effekt einer mütterlichen Dexamethasonbehandlung nach der 12. Schwangerschaftswoche auf die fetale Genitalentwicklung bei Adreno-Genitalem Syndrom. *Monatsschr Kinderheilkd* **137** (1989) 253–306.

15. Shapiro E. Santiago JV, Crane JP. Prenatal fetal adrenal suppression following *in utero* diagnosis of congenital adrenal hyperplasia. *J Urol* **142** (1989) 663–6.

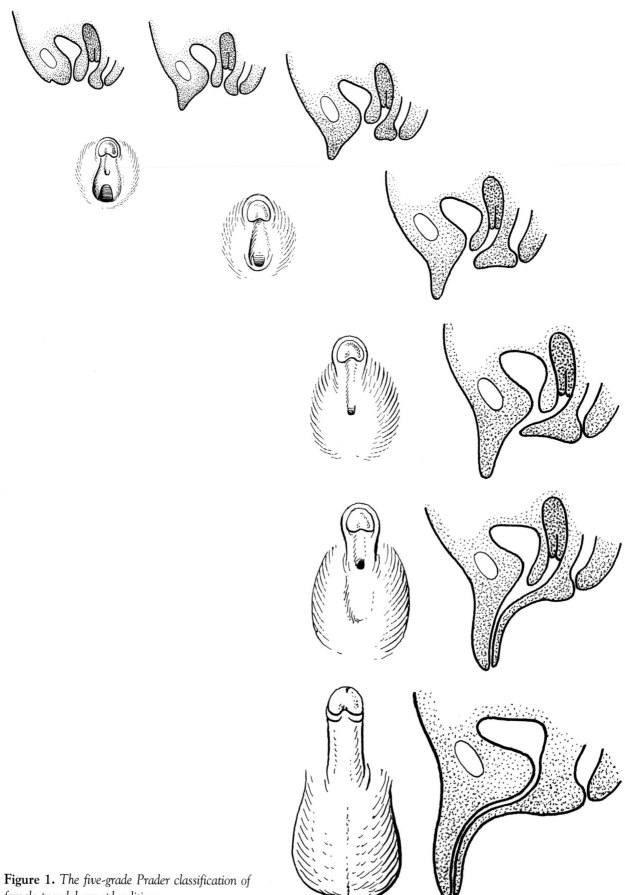

Figure 1. *The five-grade Prader classification of female pseudohermaphroditism.*

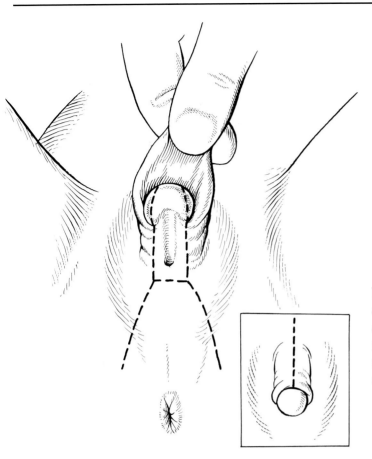

Figure 2. *Prader IV AGS. The incision line is marked. The clitoris shaft skin is then incised dorsal to the ventral labial commissure, with extension of the incision on the lateral segment of the glans. Further incision on the velar segment of the shaft parallel to the urethral line. The velar flap (Young flap) preserves the blood supply of the glans.*

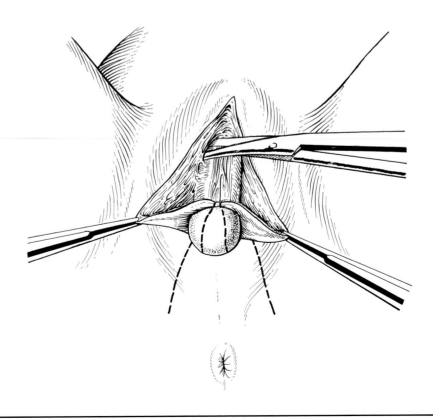

Figure 3. *Preparation of the clitoris shaft skin in the plane between the subcutaneous tissue and Colles fascia to avoid damaging the dorsal neurovascular bundle. On the dorsal side of the glans the incision line bifurcates on the coronary groove. After mobilization of the Young flap, occasional bleeding from the lateral part of the glans is easy to control.*

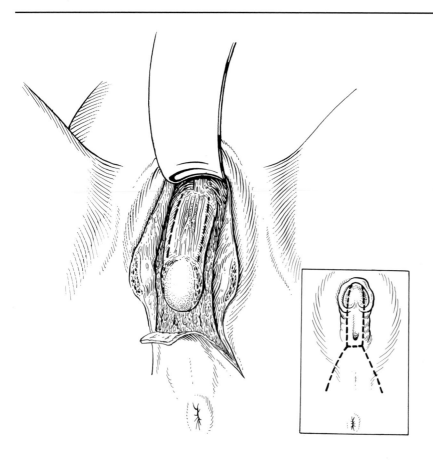

Figure 4. *Incision and insertion of the Young flap between Buck's fascia and the tunica albuginea. Separation of the lateral parts of the glans, which remain as a triangle on top of the mobilized shaft skin. Incision of Buck's fascia. Under 5.5 × magnifying glasses, separation of Buck's fascia and the neurovascular bundle from the tunica albuginea. This simple step is also used on the intercavernosal septum.*

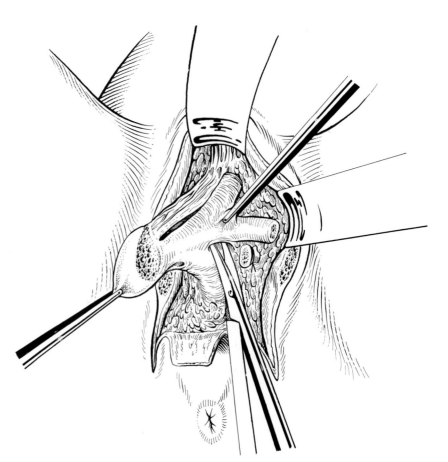

Figure 5. *The bifurcating crura of the corpora cavernosa are ligated by a piercing stitch on the ascending segment of the pubis. This is followed by preparation of the surrounding tissue from its tunica and separation of the crura from the glans on the coronary groove.*

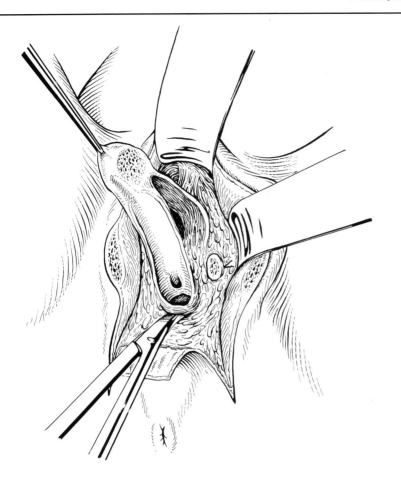

Figure 6. *Dorsal colpotomy after preparation of the perineal flap is difficult in higher Prader grades. Marking using ureteral catheter renders this step easier. Dorsal colpotomy is performed until the vestibule of the vagina is accessible to at least 7 mm. The perineal island flap is sutured by single stitches to the dorsal vaginal edge (similar to the Bengt-Johannson technique).*

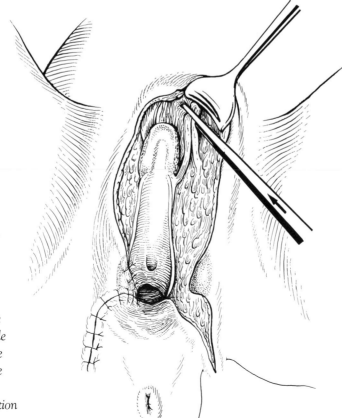

Figure 7. *Internalization of the lateral glans segments with single stitches in the angle between the perineal flap and the base of the Young flap. Folding of the neurovascular bundle and insertion below the mons pubis.*

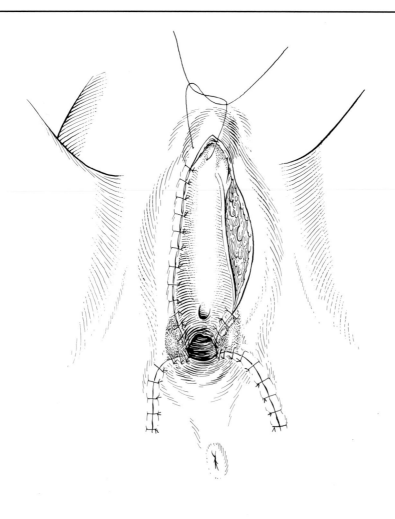

Figure 8. *Folded suturing of the clitoris under the newly formed anterior labial commissure to emphasize the mons.*

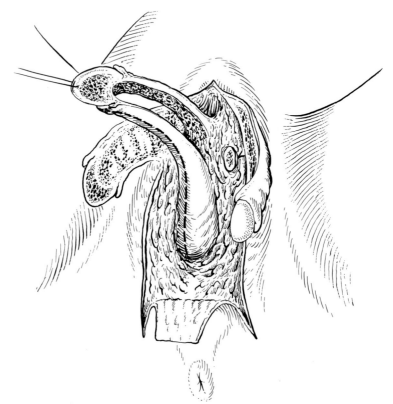

Figure 9. *Prader V AGS after phallus amputation and glans reduction. The glans is pedunculated dorsally by the neurovascular bundle and anteriorly by the still closed urethra. Suturing of the lateral glans segments is as shown in Figure 7.*

Single-Step Operation for Severe Hypospadias

S. Perović
Department of Urology,
University of Belgrade,
Belgrade, Serbia

Comment

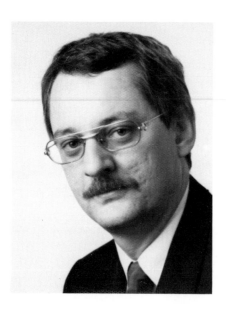

Treatment of simple distal hypospadias (glanular, coronal and subcoronal) without accompanying penile deviation, by Magpi's procedure, Mathieu's technique or other surgical options, achieves excellent functional and cosmetic results with low complication rates. However, severe hypospadias with penile deviation represents a challenge because after chordectomy and erection of the penis a long segment of the urethra must be replaced. In these cases there is no available gold standard technique and the operative strategy needs to be individualized; this is reflected in the countless reported techniques of hypospadias correction.

In primary hypospadias with abundant dorsal preputial skin an island flap technique, such as the Asopa–Duckett technique, in experienced hands offers excellent cosmetic and functional results. (High complication rates characterize the outcome in patients operated on by inexperienced surgeons.)

In cases with missing prepuce and unbalanced skin distribution on the ventral penis shaft, long urethral defects can be replaced by free transplants of bladder or buccal mucosa. However, these procedures are characterized by 30–50% of minor complications.

Perović presents a modification of the Hodgson and Devine technique, forming the new urethra using a well-vascularized pedunculated island flap from the dorsal penis shaft skin. This attractive and interesting technique represents an alternative treatment for severe hypospadias and hypospadia cripple. Exact isolation and preservation of the dorsal penis skin vessels is mandatory: the island flap has to be adapted to the course of these vessels. Reconstruction of the urethra has to be performed using an optimal vascularized island flap; the residual vascularization of the covering skin of the penis shaft is of minor importance. The buttonhole maneuver certainly minimizes the risk of twisting of the penis (which is a problem in the Asopa-Duckett technique), but I doubt whether it can also reduce the danger of recurrent chordee.

The main disadvantage of the technique presented here is limitation of the length of the new urethra, even if a spiral-shaped skin flap is prepared. A different operative procedure has to be considered if the meatus, after chordectomy, lies proximal to the penoscrotal angle. However, this technique shows satisfying results in selected patients: Perović reports an 85–90% functional and cosmetic success rate in a large series of patients.

Our own experience is that local application of dihydro-testosterone ointment, especially in the hypoplastic and often previously surgically treated penis, stimulates skin growth and improves the local skin distribution and vascularization. If 6/0, 7/0 or 8/0 sutures are used there is no need for an operative microscope: magnifying glasses are sufficient. There is controversy as to whether splinting of the reconstructed urethra is necessary. We splint the reconstructed urethral segment to the proximal edge of the anastomosis of the original urethra with a perforated urethral splint for 6–8 days. This guarantees optimal drainage of urethral secretions. Urinary drainage by subrapubic catheter is continued for 8–10 days. We leave the circular elastic compression bandage at the penis shaft for only 5–6 days. To avoid postoperative edema, we use antiphlogistics.

The timing of the operation depends on the length of penis and the local skin proportion; in some cases it is possible to operate in the first year of life. In our experience there is no need for early operative correction.

Efforts to develop a one-stage operation should not allow the operation in two steps, with its low complication rate and good results (especially in complicated cases and hypospadias cripples), fall into oblivion.

H. Riedmiller, Marburg, Germany

Single-step operation for severe hypospadias

Introduction

High-grade hypospadias with serious penile deviation represents a surgical challenge. The main problem is reconstruction of a new urethra. Satisfactory results can be achieved only by experienced surgeons and success is based on the possibility of continuous training on a large number of patients.

Indications

- High-grade hypospadias with absent or severely injured foreskin
- Congenital short urethra
- Hypospadias with penoscrotal transposition
- Hypospadias cripple
- High-grade hypospadias with intact foreskin

Age at operation

Improved microsurgical techniques enable the experienced surgeon to operate on patients in their first year of life if the penis is of adequate length.

Preoperative work-up

- Grading of the hypospadias and of the penis deviation
- Verification of the vascularization of the skin of the penis and scrotum
- Exclusion of intersex status in high-grade hypospadias and of cryptorchism
- Testosterone ointments to stimulate the growth of the penis and improve the vascularization of the skin
- Removal of adhesions of the foreskin at least 2 months before the operation and treatment with local antiseptic ointments

Instruments

- Microsurgical instruments and magnifying glasses (4 × mag-

nification) to enable the surgeon to examine small vessels; operating microscope if necessary (its use will prolong the operation)

- Absorbable synthetic suture: 6/0 for the new urethra and penile skin, 7/0 or 8/0 for the glans
- Bipolar diathermy forceps
- Tourniquet for the glans-groove technique
- Suprapubic cystostomy tube (14 Fr in adults, 10 Fr in infants)
- Self-adhesive pressure bandage

Operative technique step by step (Figures 1–16)

There is no universal operative strategy to treat different kinds of hypospadias. The grade of the hypospadias and penis deviation are critical factors in the individualization of the operative procedure.

The new urethra and the skin of the shaft are formed by well-vascularized dorsal penis skin:

- The skin of the penis is mobilized and divided into three flaps
- The new urethra is then modeled with the best-vascularized island flap (distribution and prominence of the vessels of the penis skin determine the position and form of the skin flap necessary to shape the new urethra)
- The island flap is displaced ventrally in place of the missing urethra, using the buttonhole transposition technique, and sutured to form a tube and anastomosed proximally to the hypospadiac urethra

Two methods are available to adapt the urethra at the top of the glans, depending on the configuration of the glans: the glans-channel technique and the glans-groove technique. Rotation of the remaining two skin flaps permits the reconstruction of the shaft skin. It is possible to utilize the inner layer of the foreskin to construct the subglandular part of the shaft skin.

A successful hypospadias correction must be individualized by additional procedures:

- Correction of penile deviation by chordectomy and, if necessary, corporoplasty using the Schroeder and Essett or the Nesbit procedure
- Maximal mobilization of the hypospadiac urethra
- In bipartite scrotum or penoscrotal transposition, scroto-

plasty with mobilization of the testis and contralateral fixation (interorchiopexy)

- In a cripple excision of the subcutaneous fibrous tissue to improve the elasticity of the skin

Advantages and disadvantages

- In contrast to techniques that use vacularized island flaps (transverse preputial island flap, double-faced preputial island flap, onlay island flap), there is no need for an intact foreskin. The dorsal shaft skin is used, even if damaged, to construct the new urethra

- To optimize blood flow, the position and form of the island flap are adapted to the longitudinal vessels in the penis skin

- The shaft skin is reconstructed with two vascularized skin flaps

- Ventral displacement of the new urethra is easy using the buttonhole transposition

- Dorsal traction of the island flap reduces the risk of recurrent penis deviation in patients with congenital short urethra and hypospadias with penoscrotal transposition

- The new urethra is completely surrounded by vascularized subcutaneous tissue

- Symmetric division of the flap base reduces the propensity of the penis to rotate

- A substantial disadvantage is the limited length of the new urethra. For larger defects, free skin and bladder mucosa transplants can be used (with their known advantages and disadvantages)

Technical tricks

- Preoperative irrigation of the hypospadiac urethra with mucosal disinfectant

- Stay sutures to help atraumatic preparation with micro-surgical instruments

- Closure of the urethra over a well-fitting catheter, which is changed to a smaller one after the operation to protect the suture and make urinary drainage possible

Postoperative care

- For the first 12–14 days urinary drainage has to be by suprapubic cystostomy; micturition is then possible through the new urethra

- A self-adhesive pressure bandage surrounds the penis shaft for 5 weeks (to prevent urethral kinking and diverticula). The pressure bandage has to be changed only for hygienic and physiotherapeutic reasons

- If necessary the new urethra, especially the glanular segment, can be bougied (even minimal obstructions can cause diverticula)

- Scars are prevented by application of antiscarring ointment and physical therapy of the scar

Complications

- Skin flap necrosis (very rare)

- Fistula (mostly spontaneous occlusion)

- Strictures in the meatal and anastomosis regions

- Urethral diverticulae

- Persisting penis deviation (mostly ventral)

- Chronic lymphedema of the subcutaneous tissue with secondary fibrosis

- Wound infection (especially in adolescents and adults, rarely in childhood)

The complication rate is below 15%.

Results

Satisfying anatomic and functional results are obtained in 85–90% of patients. The success rate is similar whether patients are being treated for the first time or have undergone operation before, and is independent of grade of hypospadias.

Bibliography

1. Asopa R, Asopa HS. One-stage repair of hypospadias using island preputial skin tube. *Indian J Urol* **1** (1984) 41–3.
2. Duckett JW. Hypospadias. In: Gillenwater, Grayback, Howards, Duckett (eds) *Adult and Pediatric Urology*, Vol. 2. Chicago: Year Book Medical (1987) 1880–1910.
3. De Sy W, Oosterlinck A. One-stage hypospadias repair by free full-thickness skin graft and island flap techniques. *Urol Clin North Am* **8** (1981) 491–502.
4. Firlit FC. The mucosal collar in hypospadias surgery. *J Urol* **137** (1987) 80–2.
5. Hendren WH, Crooks KK. Tubed free skin graft for construction of male urethra. *J Urol* **123** (1980) 858–62.

6. Hodgson NB. A one-stage hypospadias repair. *J Urol* **104** (1970) 281–4.

7. Juskiewenski S, Vaysse P, Moscovici J. A study of the arterial blood supply to the penis. *Anat Clin* **4** (1982) 101–7.

8. Perović S. Schwere Hypospadieformen – Einzeitiges Korrekturverfahren. *Akt Urol* **14** (1983) 310–15.

9. Perović S, Talic B, Sremcevic D, Scepanovic D, Harn-röhrenplastik nach Perović-Technik und Ergebnisse. *Verh Dtsch Ges Urol* **40** (1988) 94–7.

10. Perović S, Scepanovic D, Sremcevic D, Krstic Z. Einzeitige Korrektur von penoskrotaler Transposition mit Hypospadie. *Akt Urol* **21** (1990) 94–6.

11. Reda EF, Hendren WH. Tubed bladder mucosa graft for construction of the male urethra. *J Pediatr Surg* **21** (1986) 189–92.

12. Standoli L. One-stage repair of hypospadias: Preputial island flap technique. *Ann Plast Surg* **9** (1982) 81–8.

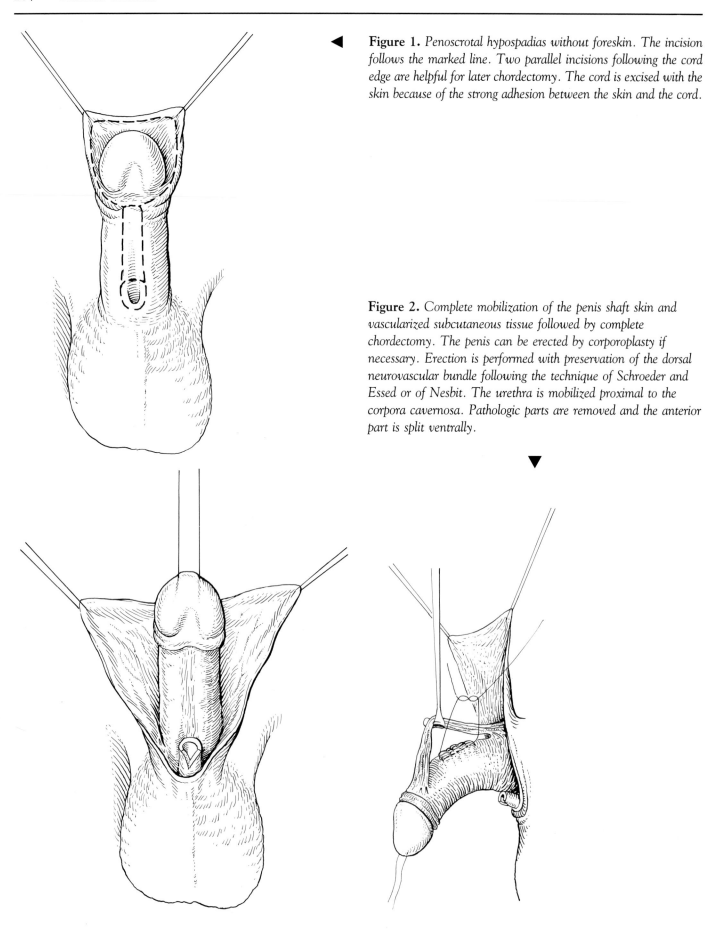

◀ **Figure 1.** *Penoscrotal hypospadias without foreskin. The incision follows the marked line. Two parallel incisions following the cord edge are helpful for later chordectomy. The cord is excised with the skin because of the strong adhesion between the skin and the cord.*

Figure 2. *Complete mobilization of the penis shaft skin and vascularized subcutaneous tissue followed by complete chordectomy. The penis can be erected by corporoplasty if necessary. Erection is performed with preservation of the dorsal neurovascular bundle following the technique of Schroeder and Essed or of Nesbit. The urethra is mobilized proximal to the corpora cavernosa. Pathologic parts are removed and the anterior part is split ventrally.*

▼

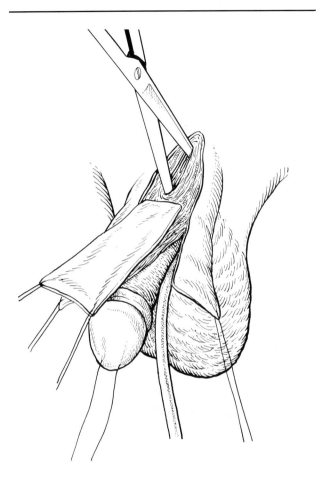

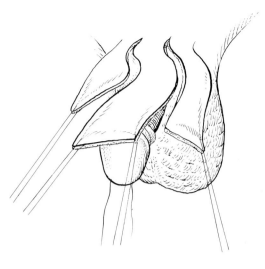

Figure 3. *The dorsal penis shaft skin is stretched by stay sutures and an asymmetric oblique skin flap is prepared for the new urethra. By mobilization of the superficial fascia of the lateral penis shaft skin good vascularization is ensured. Then the island flap is split in the medial line. If a very long new urethra is necessary, the island flap is prepared in spiral manner.*

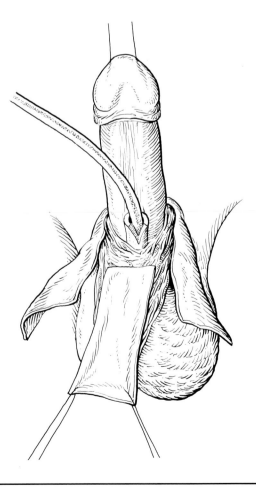

Figure 4. *The penis is moved dorsal by incision of the skin flap. Now the skin flap is on the ventral side of the penis.*

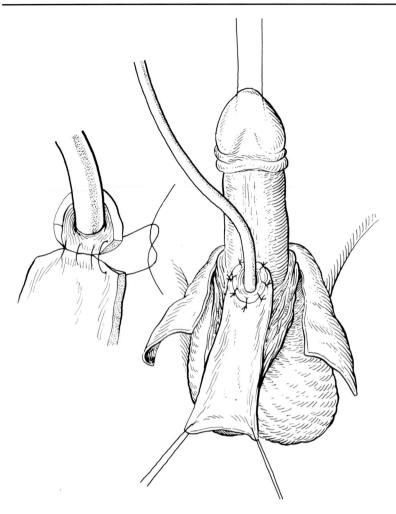

Figure 5. *Anastomosis of the urethra to the new urethra is started at the base of the urethral stump and is completed with single sutures on both sides. After positioning of the catheter, the anastomosis is on the dorsal side. In this way a good conversion between the urethra and the new urethra is obtained.*

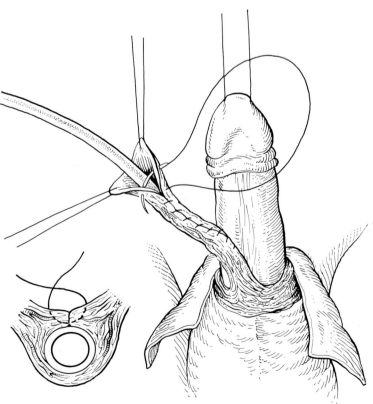

Figure 6. *The island flap is fashioned into a tube and closed by continuing the dorsal suture. The anastomosis of the urethra is covered by subcutaneous tissue. Subepidermal sutures border on the corpora cavernosa.*

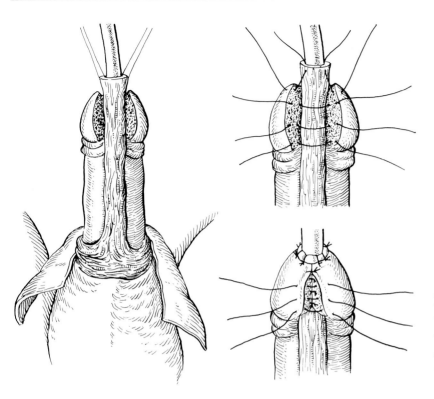

Figure 7. *Anastomosis between the new meatus and the glans top in a glans-groove technique. To prevent urethral stenosis the two parts of the glans are carefully mobilized. Closure of the glans is done in two layers without tension.*

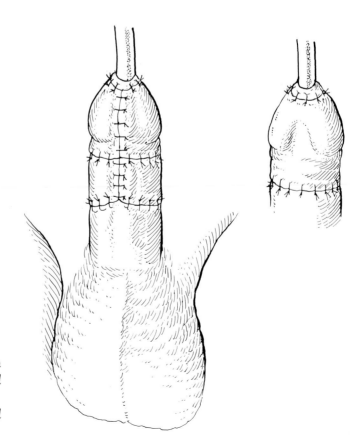

Figure 8. *Reconstruction of the penis shaft skin with the rotation flaps. The new urethra should be covered by vital skin. It can be adapted to the glans top depending on the shape of the glans in a glans-channel technique.*

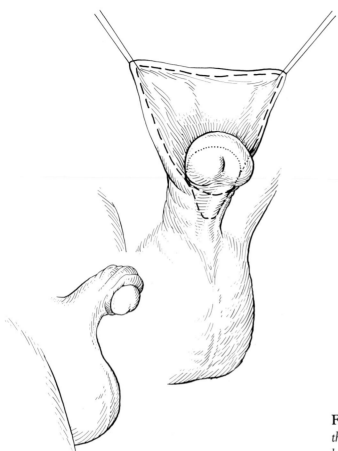

Figure 9. *Congenital short urethra. A ventral incision is started in the middle of the penis. The distal anastomosis is covered by skin between the new urethra and the urethral stump to prevent fistulas.*

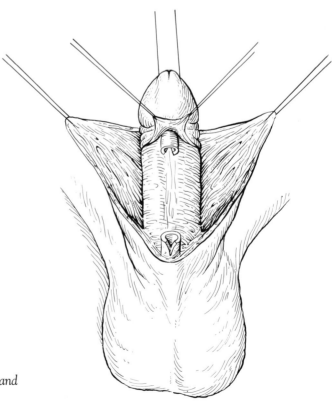

Figure 10. *Complete mobilization of the penis shaft skin and dissection of the urethra. The penis is erect.*

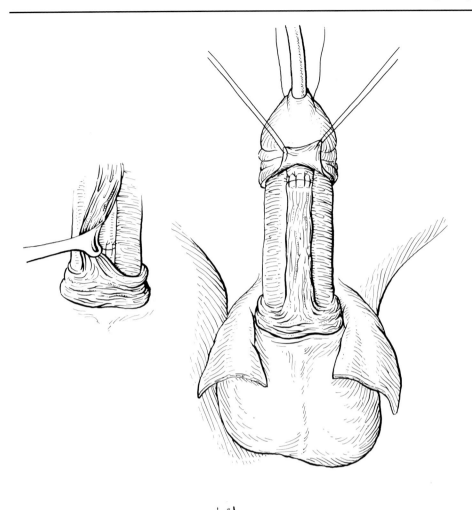

Figure 11. *The new urethra is created from a vascularized island flap and anastomosed to the original urethra on both sides. The proximal connection is covered by subcutaneous tissue and the distal by vital skin.*

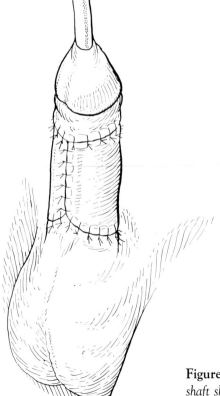

Figure 12. *Inner foreskin is used for the subglanular segment of penis shaft skin (mucosal-collar technique). Both lateral island flaps build the proximal penis shaft.*

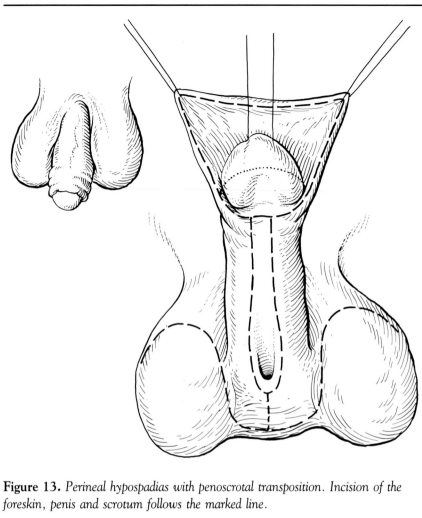

Figure 13. *Perineal hypospadias with penoscrotal transposition. Incision of the foreskin, penis and scrotum follows the marked line.*

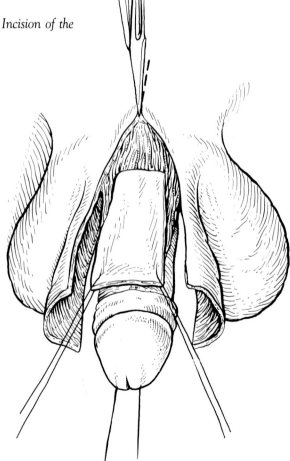

Figure 14. *After complete mobilization of the penis shaft and scrotal skin, including chordectomy, an island flap is constructed of dorsal penis shaft skin to form the new urethra. Preparation of two lateral island flaps to cover the penis shaft. Cranial transposition of the penis is done by incision in the direction of the symphysis.*

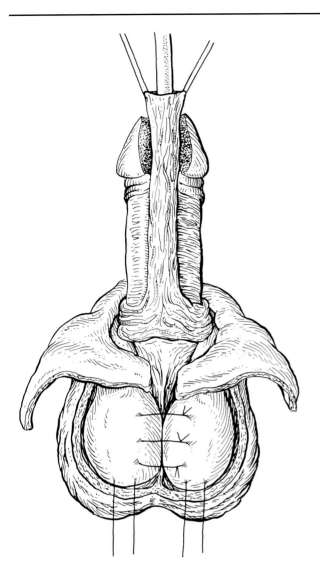

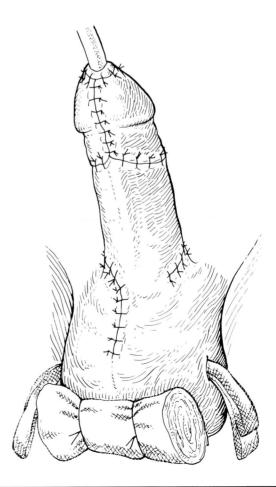

Figure 15. *Ventral transposition of the island flap by a buttonhole technique and anastomosis of the new urethra to the original urethra. Adaptation of the new urethra to the glans top in a glans-groove technique. Enhancement of cranial transposition of the penis by complete mobilization of the scrotum and fixation in the median line (interorchiopexy).*

Figure 16. *The subglanular segment of the penis shaft is reconstructed of inner foreskin using the mucosal-collar technique. The proximal penis shaft skin is built of both lateral island flaps, and the scrotum reconstructed in a Z-flap technique. Positioning of a scrotal drainage tube.*

Orchiopexy and Hydrocelectomy

M. Hohenfellner, A. Lampel, J.W. Thüroff
*Department of Urology,
Barmen Clinic,
Wuppertal-Barmen, Germany*

Comment

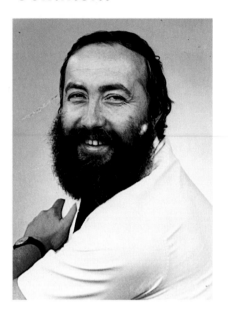

This chapter presents the undescended testis as essentially an endocrine problem in spite of the presence of a congenital malformation. Biopsies in young patients substantiate this view. Analysis of the primordial germ cells during the first 180 days after birth in patients with unilateral or bilateral undescended testis showed the marked influence of low testosterone levels influenced by hypogonadotropism. For this reason, treatment with gonadotropin releasing hormones and intramuscular human chorionic gonadotropin (HCG) is advised.

When this therapy proves ineffective, testicular biopsy is recommended. Intraperitoneal testes often show epididymal malformations and are associated with high rates of sterility. This group is very challenging to urologists.

F. Hadziselimovic, Basel

Orchiopexy and hydrocelectomy

Introduction

The testes at the second month of fetal life are located at the level of the kidneys. They then start a caudal progression, at the sixth month reaching the internal inguinal ring, at the seventh month occupying a position in the inguinal canal and finally at the eighth month reaching the scrotum. We define as testis *dystopia* postnatal localization of the testis outside the scrotum. When the testes are placed somewhere on their normal developmental route we call it testis *retention* (cryptorchism), and when outside its physiological route testis *ectopia*.

The pendular testis is generally palpable at the superficial inguinal ring and can be brought manually to the scrotum although it returns spontaneously and immediately to its former position due to its short funiculus. The retractile testis has a normal funiculus but a noticeably hyperreflexive cremaster muscle, which explains its dystopia.

Testis dystopia has a six times higher incidence in preterm infants than in those born at term. After 1 year of life about 1.8% of these children have testis dystopia, and unilateral dystopia carries the risk of exocrine dysfunction of both testes, torsion and development of neoplasia. Surgery is carried out in the second year of life to avoid compromise of reproductive function. If the condition is diagnosed after puberty, the dystopic testis should be removed.

Diagnosis

- The dystopic testis is palpable in 90% of cases

- When the testis is not palpable, sonography, computed tomography and magnetic resonance imaging are indicated in this order

- Laparoscopy is the most effective method of diagnosis of abdominal testis, but is invasive and should be used only when other methods prove inconclusive

- Conservative treatment with β-hCG (< 5 years 2500 IU; >5 years 5000 IU) for 1 or 2 months can be tried before surgery is indicated

Operative technique step by step

- Inguinal incision (Figure 1) about 1 cm parallel and cranial to the inguinal line in the distal two-thirds between the pubic tubercle and the anterior superior iliac spine. Careful sharp dissection of the subcutaneous tissue, looking for the testis

- Identification of the external inguinal ring and the external oblique muscle. In most cases the testis is found close to the superficial inguinal ring. If not, the roof of the inguinal canal (external oblique) must be opened to search for the testis cranially

- Blunt dissection and section of the adjacent fat surrounding the testis until a hemostat can be placed on the gubernaculum for traction and the cord can be looped (Figure 2)

- The tunica vaginalis is opened and the testis and epididymis are inspected, looking for testicular appendices that may be coagulated avoiding posterior torsion. Also the presence of an inguinal hernia may be excluded. If there is a hydrocele, the excess of tunica vaginalis is resected and inverted. The tunica is closed with a running 4/0 polyglycolic acid suture (Figure 3)

- Using fine scissors, the posterior wall of the peritoneum is mobilized from the cord structures inferiorly. The hernia sac is ligated cranially after excluding the presence of a bowel loop. A fixation suture may be inserted in the proximal stump below the internal oblique according to Bastianelli in older boys (Figure 4).[1] The distal stump should not be ligated to avoid the formation of cord cysts

- Sharp and blunt dissection is used to skeletonize the spermatic vessels and the vas, which may be looped. The fibrous attachments and the cremasteric fibers are loosened and vessels and vas can be then entirely mobilized. The cord should be long enough to bring the testis to the scrotum without tension. Fixation can be accomplished with a single suture on its lower pole (Figure 5) or according to the Shoemaker technique[2]

- In the Shoemaker technique (Figures 6–10) the index finger of the surgeon is inserted through the inguinal incision to the level of the scrotum and a small incision is made through the epidermis and dermis. A darts pouch is then created and the testis is brought to it without the necessity of fixation

- The wound is closed in layers

Special situations

- The testicular vessels (commonly) and the vas (rarely) may limit the mobilization of the testis. In these cases the incision may be extended cranially. Section of the transversalis fascia and epigastric vessels (Prentiss technique) allows better medial mobilization of the cord (Figure 11)

- When the vessels are very short they can be divided according to the Fowler–Stephen technique; the testis will be adequately supplied through collaterals. This procedure does not always allow enough mobilization of the testis

References

1. Bastianelli. Chirurgie der Brüche des Erwachsenen. In: Baumgarth F, Kremer K, Schreiber HW eds *Spezielle Chirurgie für die Praxis*, Vol 2, Part 3. Stuttgart: Thieme (1972) S. 6.
2. Shoemaker J. Über Kryptorchismus und seine Behandlung. *Chirurgie* **4** (1932) 1–3.

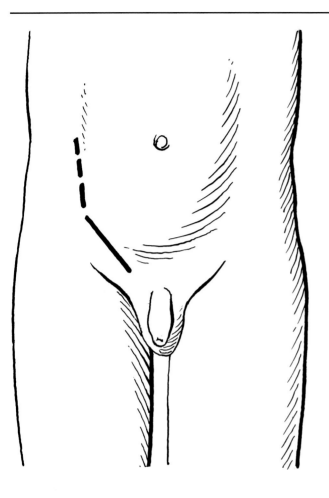

Figure 1. *The retroperitoneum can be exposed by a cranial prolongation of the inguinal incision into a pararectal incision.*

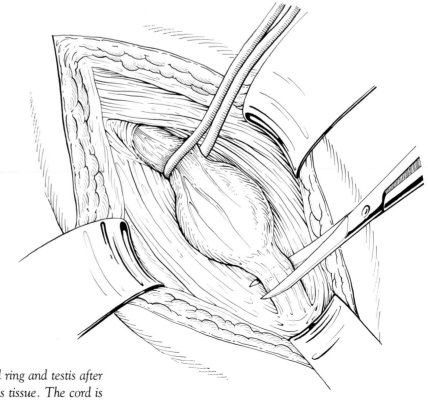

Figure 2. *Exposure of the superficial inguinal ring and testis after sharp and blunt dissection of the subcutaneous tissue. The cord is looped and the gubernaculum sectioned.*

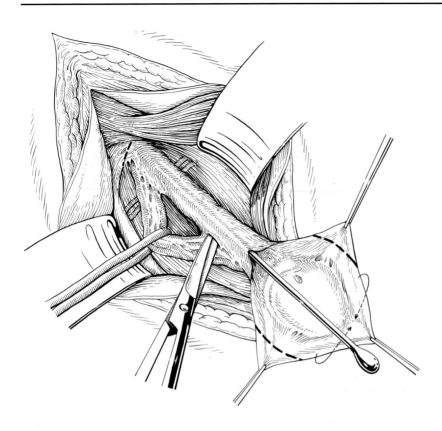

Figure 3. *The anterior wall of the inguinal canal (external oblique) is opened as well as the tunica vaginalis. The testicular vessels and the vas are isolated, and hydroceles are treated by resection of the excess of tunica vaginalis and its inversion.*

Figure 4. *Complete resection of the internal and external spermatic fascia and cremaster muscle. The testicular vessels and the vas are then skeletonized. Inset: Bastianelli suture of the proximal stump below the internal oblique.*

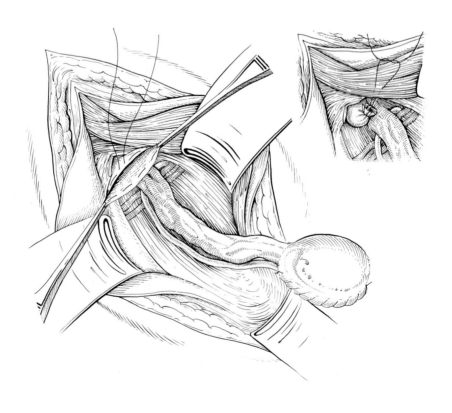

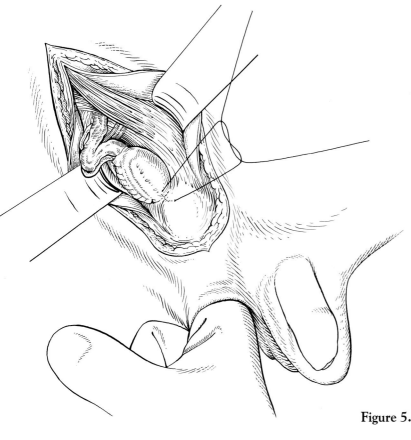

Figure 5. *Fixation of the testis in the scrotum with a single suture.*

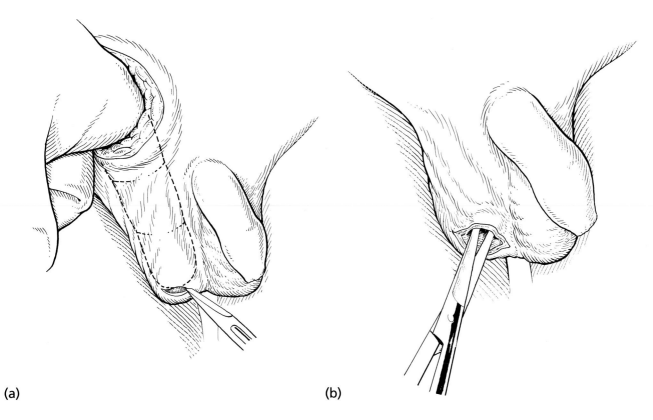

(a)   (b)

Figure 6. *Shoemaker technique. (a) Skin incision sparing the dartos fascia. (b) Creation of a dartos pouch between the skin and the dartos fascia.*

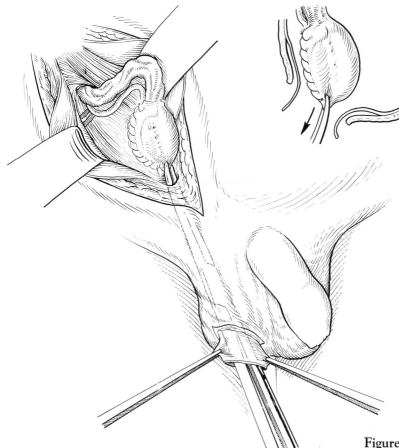

Figure 7. *The dartos fascia is incised and the testis is brought to the pouch with a fine instrument.*

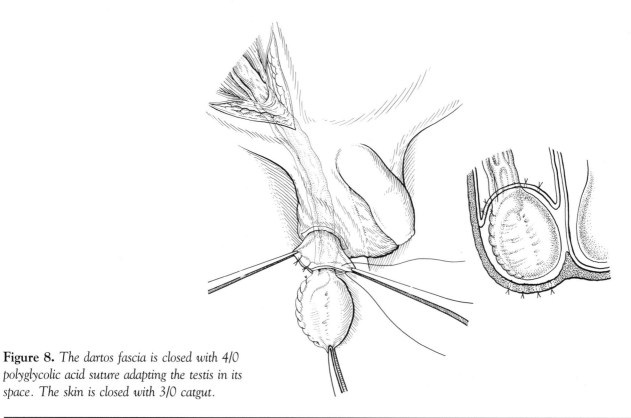

Figure 8. *The dartos fascia is closed with 4/0 polyglycolic acid suture adapting the testis in its space. The skin is closed with 3/0 catgut.*

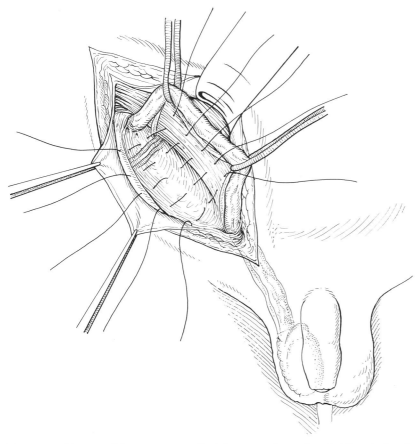

Figure 9. *Closure of the posterior wall of the inguinal canal with 2/0 polyglycolic acid sutures, involving cranially the transversalis fascia, the transversus abdominis muscle fascia and the internal oblique muscle and caudally the inguinal ligament.*

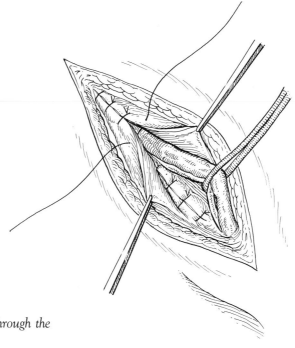

Figure 10. *The anterior wall is closed by a suture through the external oblique muscle fascia.*

Prentiss technique

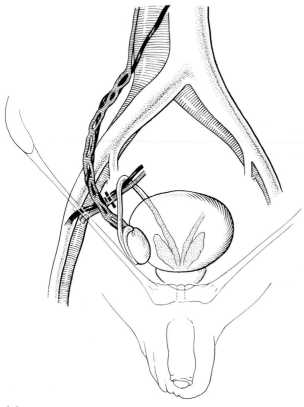

(a)

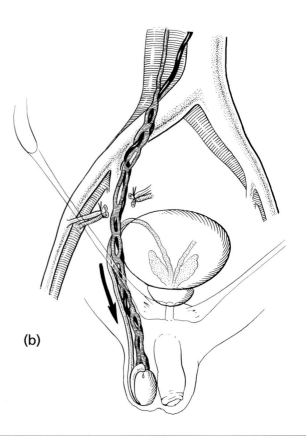

(b)

Figure 11. *(a) Division of the epigastric vessels. (b) Mobilization of the testicular vessels medially.*

Combined Retropubic and Perineal Urethrectomy

C.B. Brendler
Department of Urology,
Johns Hopkins University School of Medicine,
Baltimore, Maryland, USA

Comment

Urethrectomy is an important procedure and, when performed prophylactically, prevents many unnecessary deaths.

The technique described by Brendler (Chapter 5.4) is very similar to my own. I have never used the prepubic approach (Chapter 5.5), nor does it appeal much to me because it would not be possible to ligate the arteries to the bulb. However, whereas most urologists would consider these significant vessels, most orthopedic surgeons, I suspect, would divide them without a second thought and, like these authors, would merely apply a pressure dressing.

Both articles advocated removal of the whole urethral mucosa, including that within the meatus. I agree that, just as the intramural part of the ureter should be removed for tumors of the upper urinary tract, so the fossa navicularis should be removed for tumors of the lower tract; ten cases of meatal recurrence have been described when it was left behind.[1,2]

By far the most important feature of these two presentations is the demonstration by Brendler that potency can be preserved if urethrectomy is performed in the manner he describes. This is a great advance and removes one of the last arguments against prophylactic urethrectomy.

There are three observations I wish to make:

- Any patient may develop urethral recurrence after cystectomy for tumor

- If urethral recurrence develops, the chances of the patient surviving are slim

- Some patients have unsuspected tumors or carcinoma *in situ* in the urethra at the time of cystectomy

Although urethral recurrence is more common in patients with multiple tumors, tumors around the bladder neck or diffuse carcinoma *in situ*, it may occur in patients with solitary tumors nowhere near the bladder neck – three of my eight patients with urethral recurrence after cystectomy fell into this category.[3]

Although such recurrence may be diagnosed during follow-up by urethroscopy or cytological methods, by the time it is discovered it is almost always too late. As with transitional tumors invading the prostate, the majority of these patients will be dead within 2 years in spite of excision. These are totally unnecessary deaths – prophylactic urethrectomy would have prevented them.

If the urethra is removed prophylactically some patients will be found to have totally unsuspected tumors or carcinomas *in situ* within the urethra, which has not been discovered even on repeated urethroscopy. Once again, the prognosis for these patients is extremely poor.

Few urologists would remove the bladder for tumor in a woman and leave the urethra behind. Why should it be any different for men? With modern methods of preserving continence after cystectomy, and now Brendler's excellent method of preserving potency after urethrectomy, the only argument for keeping the urethra is to use it to connect a pouch, so that a man may still have the pleasure of passing urine through his urethra.

A patient's chief desire after cystectomy for invasive tumor is to survive. To be continent and to be potent are both added bonuses and neither carries any special risk. To pass urine through the urethra is a luxury and, like smoking, carries a definite risk.

References

1. Schellhammer PF, Whitmore WF. Urethral meatal carcinoma following cystourethrectomy for bladder carcinoma. *J Urol* **115** (1976) 61–4.
2. Zabbo A, Montie JE. Management of the urethra in men undergoing radical cystectomy for bladder cancer. *J Urol* **131** (1984) 267–8.
3. Clark PB. Urethral carcinoma after cystectomy: the case for routine urethrectomy. *J Urol (Paris)* **90** (1984) 73–9.

Philip Clark, Leeds, UK

Combined retropubic and perineal urethrectomy

Introduction

Recent studies have shown that extension of tumor to the prostatic urethra is the main risk factor for urethral recurrence, especially when the tumor has infiltrated the prostatic stroma. In 124 patients (median follow-up 67 months) secondary urethrectomy had to be performed in none with a single tumor in the bladder neck, in 1.5% of those with multifocal tumor, in 4.5% of those with diffuse extensive carcinoma *in situ*, and in 17% of those with a tumor limited to the prostate.[1] Tumor infiltration in the prostatic urethra is therefore the most convincing indication for simultaneous urethrectomy. Orthotopic bladder reconstruction with connection to the urethra is possible in patients with multifocal tumors or carcinoma *in situ* if they have careful follow-up with urethral irrigation cytology.[2]

Indications

- Multifocal bladder tumor
- Tumor in the bladder neck
- Diffuse carcinoma *in situ*
- Infiltration of the prostatic urethra

Anatomy

Lepor *et al.*[3] and Schlegel and Walsh[4] described in detail the topographic relationship between the cavernous nerves, prostate and bladder. New anatomic studies of the prostate membranous urethra have shown that nerves leading to the corpora cavernosa during passage through the urogenital diaphragm follow the membranous urethra posterolaterally. These nerve branches diverge distal to the membranous urethra into the crura of the penis and are then difficult to separate from the surrounding muscle tissue. Intraoperative mobilization of the membranous urethra causes nerve lesions leading to impotence. The retropubic technique allows careful dissection of the membranous urethra from the urogenital diaphragm with maintenance of the nerves and potency.[5]

Operative technique step by step (Figures 1–9)

- The patient is placed in the Trendelenburg position with the legs horizontal and the operating table extended at the level of the umbilicus for radical cystoprostatectomy with preservation of the cavernous nerves according to the technique of Schlegel and Walsh

- Ligation and dissection of the dorsal vein of the penis

- Ligation of the urethra with a silk suture (1/0) to avoid urine flow alongside the catheter

- Careful cranial retraction of the urethra with a rubber rein and preparation of the urethra from the urogenital diaphragm with a cotton swab

- Resection of the mucosa and smooth urethral muscle; striated muscle of the urogenital diaphragm is left

- The neurovascular bundle, which is located immediately posterolateral to the membranous urethra, is pushed carefully aside with a cotton swab

- Dissection is continued until the membranous urethra is completely free from the urogenital diaphragm

- Dissection and cranial displacement of the urethra and catheter

- Dissection of the remaining connective tissue bridges and withdrawal of the cystoprostatectomy preparation

If urethrectomy is planned and tissue from the urethral edges is free from tumor on immediate microscopic examination, we delay urethrectomy for 2 weeks. Destructive perineal and pelvic mobilization of the cavernous nerves is thus avoided. One-stage urethrectomy is performed if immediate microscopic examination shows that the tissue is positive for tumor:

- Lithotomy position with flexion of the legs at the hip joint (legs at 60°) and complete flexion of the legs at the knee joints

- The perineal operation field is painted with iodine and a curved 24 Fr metal bougie inserted in the urethra to the level of urogenital diaphragm

- Vertical or U-shaped incision. Alternatively we use a Y-incision, which gives excellent exposure of the bulbar urethra

- Dissection of subcutaneous tissue and insertion of a perineal Turner-Warwick retractor

- Exposure of the bulbar urethra by a medial incision in the bulbocavernosus muscle

- The bulbar urethra is dissected from the connecting tissue. This is assisted by palpating the metal bougie in the urethra

- The metal bougie is exchanged for a 20 Fr indwelling catheter. This is fixed on the glans penis with suture until complete dissection of the penile urethra

- Incision of Buck's fascia on both sides and preparation of the penile urethra from the corpora cavernosa. Accidental damage to the corpora cavernosa can lead to severe bleeding and is therefore to be avoided

- Inversion of the penis renders dissection of the urethra to the top of the glans problem-free. Preparation is arrested at this point and the penis is repositioned in its normal anatomical place

- To further isolate the intraglanular urethra, sharp dissection of the external meatus and a ventral T-shaped incision to the coronary groove are needed. Bleeding can be controlled by positioning a tourniquet at the base of the penis

- After complete isolation of the urethra the whole penile urethra is brought out from the perineal incision; a drain is placed in the urethral bed

- The glans penis is finally reconstructed with 4/0 absorbable suture and the tourniquet is removed

For dissection of the bulbar part of the urethra, sharp excision of the avascular tissue between the urethra itself and the symphysis is done first. This mobilization allows optimal exposure of the arteries that enter the bulb of the penis posterolaterally which reduces the danger of accidental damage to these vessels. Electrocautery of these arteries is often followed by injury to the internal pudendal artery and should therefore be avoided. Otherwise, the result is insufficient arterial supply to the corpora cavernosa. We prefer ligation of the bulbar arteries with mechanical hemoclips. Because of the primarily cranial dissection of the membranous urethra, the perineal preparation can be completed without problems. In any case, accurate dissection of the proximal urethra is of most importance; residuals of bulbomembranous urethra represent a high risk for recurrence.

If urethrectomy is carried out in combination with cystectomy or 2 weeks after this procedure, removal of the bulbomembranous urethra presents no difficulties. A transurethral catheter can be placed in the pelvic cavity only up to 2 weeks after cystectomy; an interval of several weeks between the two procedures is therefore to be avoided. Exposure of the tip of the catheter during secondary urethrectomy is sufficient to render complete removal of the urethral stump possible. After a 2-week period, transurethral positioning of a catheter in the pelvic cavity is extremely difficult; the membranous urethra is by this time fixed to the surrounding tissue, so that traction could rupture the stump with consequent incomplete removal of the specimen. In delayed urethrectomy a careful and slow preparation is therefore mandatory.

Postoperative bleeding is minimal if the bulbar urethral arteries are adequately ligated. Smaller veins should be intraoperatively cogulated or ligated. A Jackson–Pratt drain is placed in the proximal urethral bed and bulbocavernosus muscle is adapted in the midline by a continuous absorbable suture (3/0) with superficial perineal fascia. The skin is sutured with absorbable continuing stitches (4/0). We use a spraying surgical dressing or, in severe postoperative bleeding, a T-shaped dressing. To avoid ischemia the penis is bandaged completely with gauze, leaving the glans visible to control blood flow.

Postoperative care

The penile and perineal drain is removed 24–48 hour after the operation. Antibiotic therapy is needed only if an abdominal procedure is performed at the same time. After urethrectomy alone, the patient can eat and drink from day 1. Mobilization occurs at day 1 or 2, and the patient is discharged on day 5. Bathing should be avoided for 1 week after the operation.

References

1. Levinson AK, Johnson DE, Wishnow KI. Indications for urethrectomy in an era of continent urinary diversion. *J Urol* **144** (1990) 73–5.
2. Hickey DP, Soloway MS, Murphy WM. Selective urethrectomy following cystoprostatectomy for bladder cancer. *J Urol* **136** (1986) 828–30.
3. Lepor H, Gregerman M, Crosby R *et al.* Precise localization of the autonomic nerves from the pelvic plexus to the corpora cavernosa: a detailed anatomic study of the adult male pelvis. *J Urol* **133** (1985) 207–12.
4. Schlegel PN, Walsh PC. Neuroanatomical approach to radical cystoprostatectomy with preservation of sexual function. *J Urol* **138** (1987) 1402–6.
5. Brendler CB, Schlegel PN, Walsh PC. Urethrectomy with preservation of potency. *J Urol* **144** (1990) 270–3.

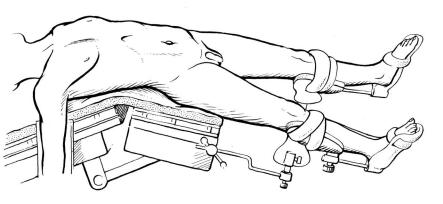

Figure 1. *(a) Patient in the Trendelenburg position with legs horizontal and the operating table extended at the level of the umbilicus.*

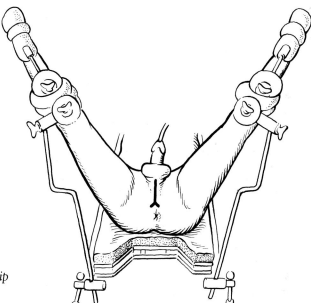

Figure 1. *(b) Lithotomy position with flexion of the legs at the hip joint (legs at 60°) and complete flexion of the legs at the knee joints.*

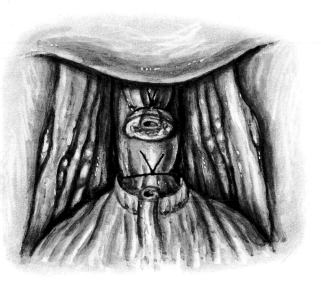

Figure 2. *(a) Ligating the urethra silk suture (1/0) avoids urine flow alongside the catheter.*

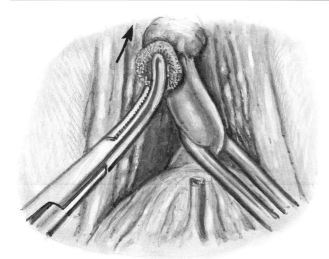

(b)

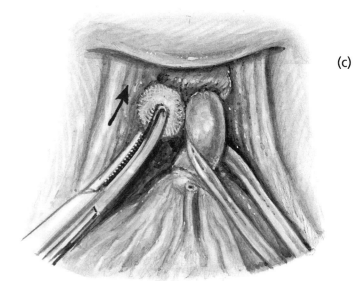

(c)

Figure 2(*b*) *and* (*c*). *Careful cranial retraction of the urethra with a rubber rein and preparation of the urethra from the urogenital diaphragm with a cotton swab.*

(d)

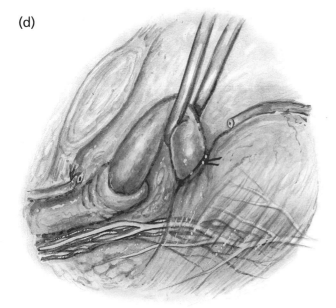

Figure 2. (*d*) *Lateral view of the completely mobilized membranous urethra with its posterolateral neurovascular bundle.*

(e)

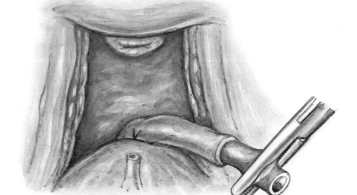

Figure 2. (*e*) *Dissection of the urethra and catheter with preservation of the neurovascular bundle, and cranial displacement.*

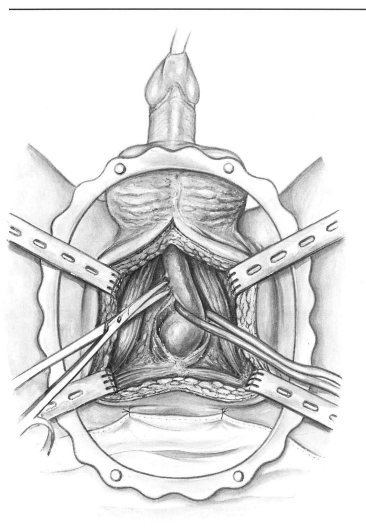

Figure 3. *Insertion of a perineal Turner-Warwick retractor and exposure of the bulbar urethra by a medial incision in the bulbocavernosus muscle.*

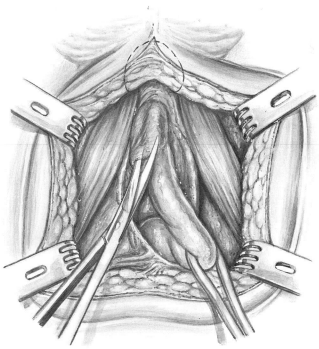

Figure 4. *Incision of Buck's fascia on both sides and preparation of the penile urethra from the corpora cavernosa.*

(a)

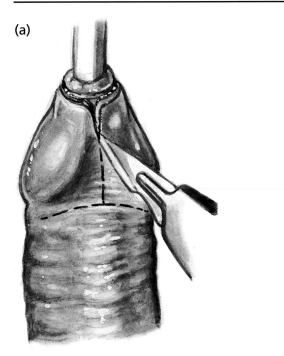

(b)

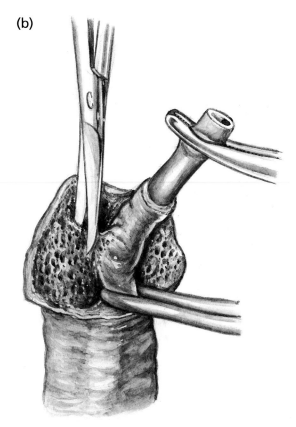

Figure 5(a) and (b). *Sharp dissection of the external meatus and a ventral T-shaped incision to the coronary groove to further isolate the intraglanular urethra.*

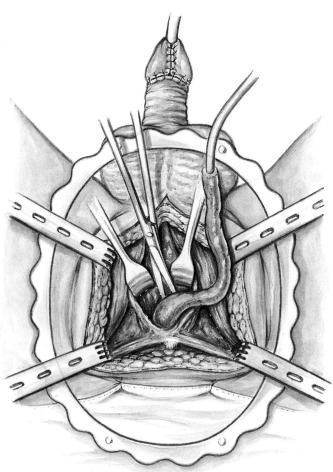

Figure 6. *Sharp dissection of connective tissue ventral to the bulbar urethra facilitates exposure and control of the posterolateral urethral bulbar arteries.*

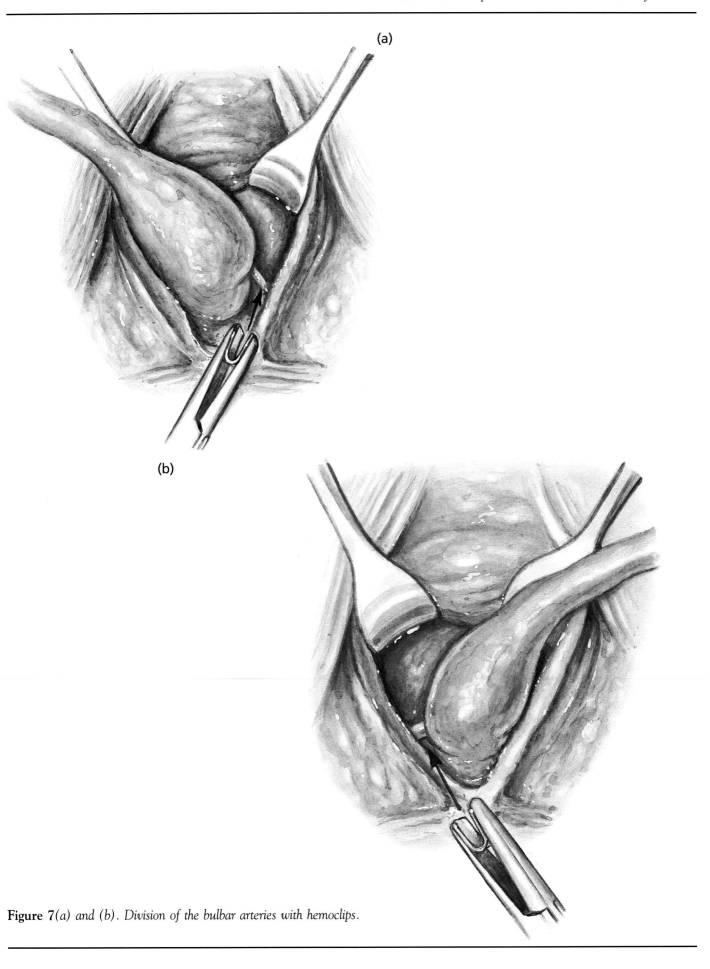

Figure 7(a) and (b). Division of the bulbar arteries with hemoclips.

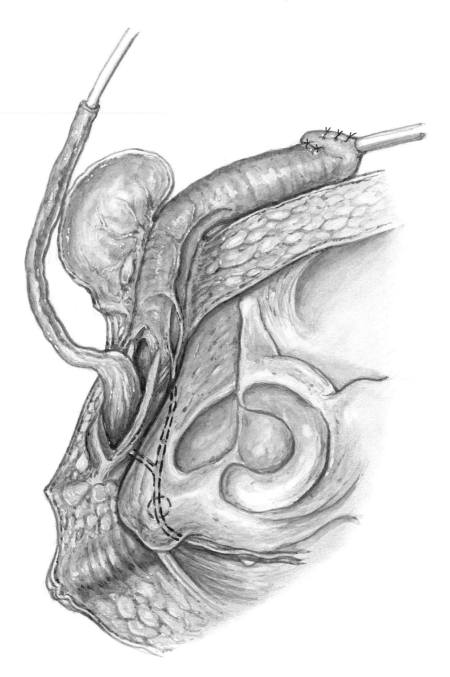

Figure 7. (c) Anatomical relationships of the internal pudendal artery, bulbar arteries and inferior branch of the pubic bone. Coagulation of bulbar arteries should be avoided to prevent the risk of injury to the internal pudendal artery.

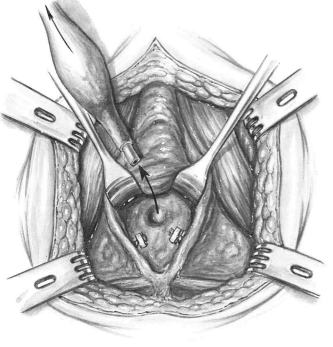

Figure 8. *Primary cranial mobilization of the membranous urethra facilitates complete dissection of the bulbar urethra.*

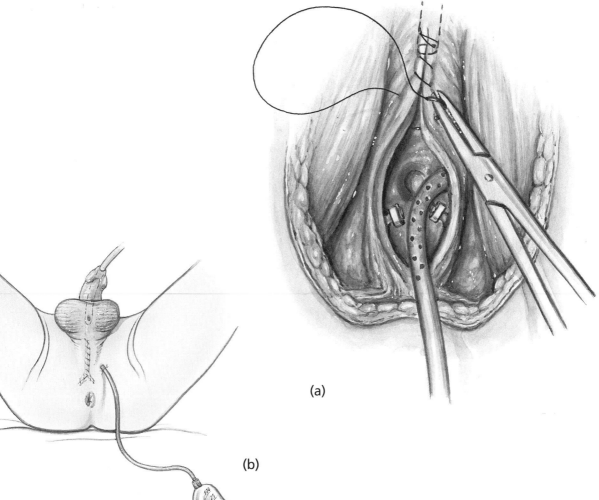

(a)

(b)

Figure 9(a) **and** (b). *Positioning of a Jackson–Pratt drain and closure of the perineal incision.*

Prepubic Urethrectomy

H. Van Poppel, L. Baert
Department of Urology,
Catholic University of Leuven,
Leuven, Belgium

Introduction

The risk of urethral recurrence in patients undergoing cystectomy for transition cell carcinoma without simultaneous urethrectomy is estimated[1] at 4–18%. The risk factors for urethral recurrence are carcinoma *in situ*, multifocal disease and tumors at the bladder neck or extending into the prostatic urethra.

In recent years, much progress has been made in the development of bladder substitution techniques; these can be proposed only when the urethra is not at risk for urethral recurrence. Therefore, cytology of the first voided urine and urethroscopy are applied to detect urethral recurrence in these patients. When there is no bladder substitution and the urethra is left in place, regular barbotage cytology is recommended.[2] When, however, there is transition cell carcinoma in the prostatic urethra invading the prostatic stroma, the risk of subsequent urethral recurrence is too high.[3] These patients should not undergo bladder substitution and should have the urethra removed at the time of the cystoprostatectomy.

Simultaneous perineal urethrectomy is common, but is time consuming for the surgeon and uncomfortable for the patient because of perineal pain, which hinders postoperative mobilization. A urethrectomy performed through the same abdominal incision in the prepubic area has therefore been developed.[4]

Indications

Because every remnant of urethra after cystoprostatectomy for bladder cancer carries a risk – however small – for urethral recurrence, a simultaneous urethrectomy can be advocated in all patients who are not suitable for bladder substitution. The simultaneous urethrectomy is imperative in patients with involvement of the prostatic urethra by carcinoma *in situ* or transition cell carcinoma invading the prostatic stroma.

Special instruments

- Small diver retractors or deep Langenbeck retractors for exposure of the prepubic urethra

Operative technique step by step (Figures 1–10)

- The patient is in the supine position; the incision is prolonged caudally to the penile base
- The membranous urethra is dissected bluntly through the pelvic floor musculature, reaching the bulbous urethra in the prepubic area

- Traction on the cystoprostatectomy specimen should be applied cautiously to avoid avulsion of the unsupported membranous urethra
- Through the caudally prolonged incision the penile body is dissected free upon Buck's fascia and then encircled
- The penile skin is invaginated by traction on the penile body, which is brought into the hypogastric incision
- The corpus spongiosum is sharply dissected free of the corpora cavernosa after incision of Buck's fascia
- The urethra is dissected towards the glans penis, and inversion of the glans enables resection of the urethra up to the urethral meatus
- The dissection is then continued proximally towards the bulbous urethra both sharply and bluntly until the dissection plane is reached from above
- When possible, bleeding from the bulbar arteries is stopped by electrocautery or sutures
- The cystoprostatourethrectomy specimen is removed *en bloc*
- The dissection area is filled with gauze for hemostasis during the rest of the procedure
- The penis is everted and wrapped in a compressive bandage
- At the end of the operation a suction drain is placed in the prepubic area

Postoperative care

The suction drain can be removed after 48 hours. It is important to leave the compressive bandage in place for 48 hours as well. Hematoma formation will be avoided by these measures.

References

1. Stöckle M, Gökcebay E, Riedmiller H, Hohenfellner R. Urethral tumor recurrences after radical cystoprostatectomy: the case for primary cystoprostatourethrectomy? *J Urol* **143** (1990) 41–3.
2. Hickey DP, Soloway MS, Murphy WM. Selective urethrectomy following cystoprostatectomy for bladder cancer. *J Urol* **136** (1986) 828–30.
3. Hardeman SW, Soloway MS. Urethral recurrence following radical cystectomy. *J Urol* **144** (1990) 666–9.
4. Van Poppel H, Strobbe E, Baert L. Prepubic urethrectomy. *J Urol* **142** (1989) 1536–7.

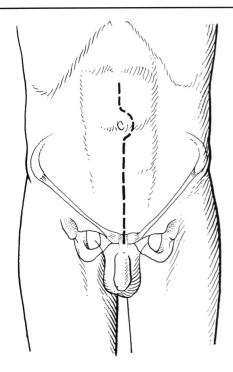

Figure 1. *The midline incision is prolonged towards the penile base.*

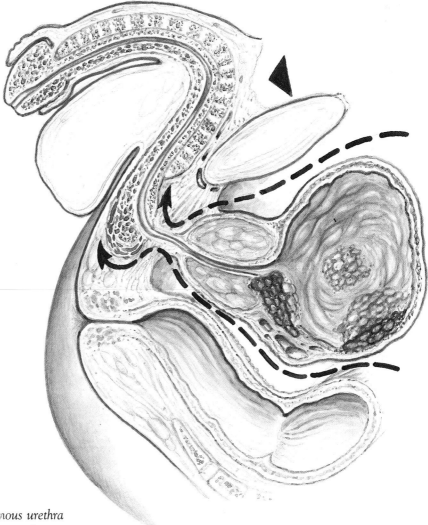

Figure 2. *Blunt dissection of the membranous urethra through the pelvic floor towards the bulbous urethra.*

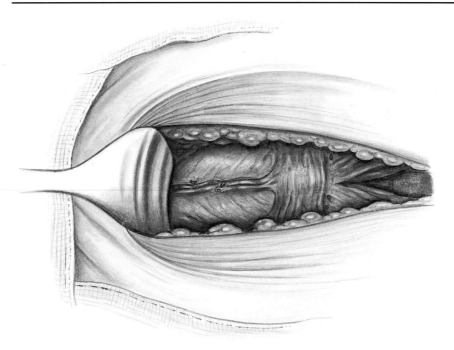

Figure 3. *Prepubic exposure of the penile body.*

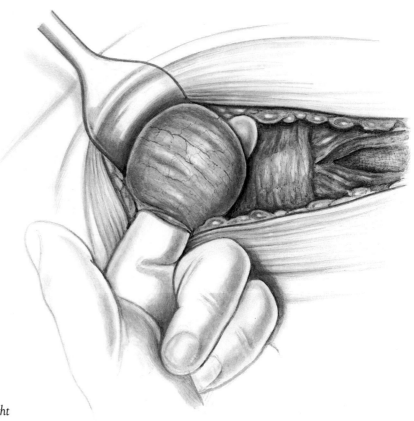

Figure 4. *The penile body is encircled and brought into the prolonged hypogastric incision.*

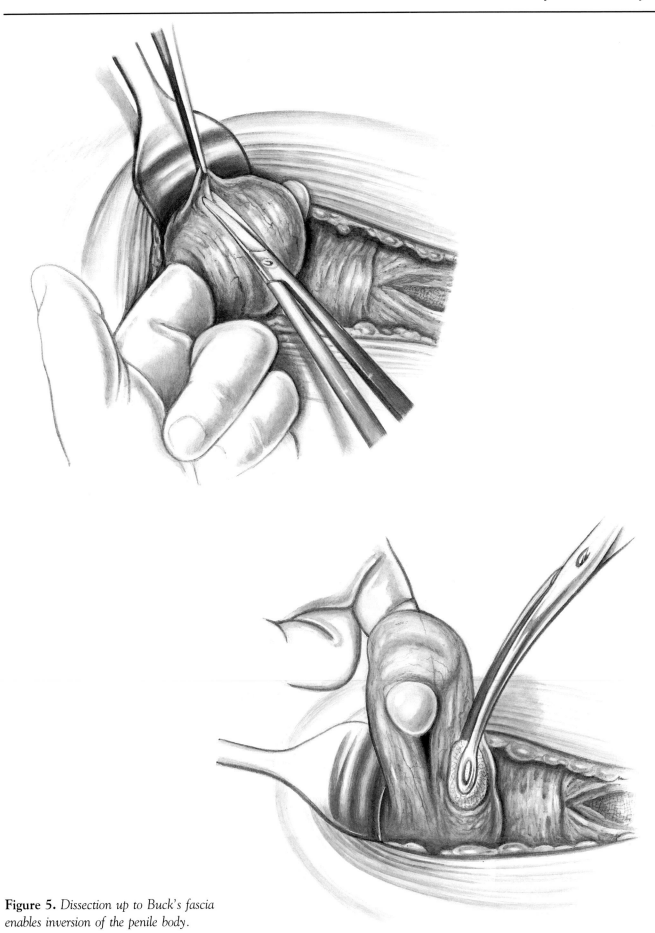

Figure 5. *Dissection up to Buck's fascia enables inversion of the penile body.*

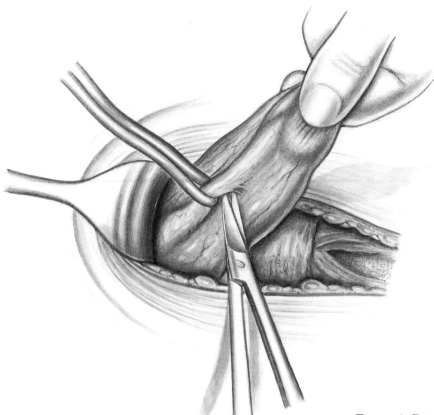

Figure 6. *Dissection between the corpus spongiosum and corpora cavernosa.*

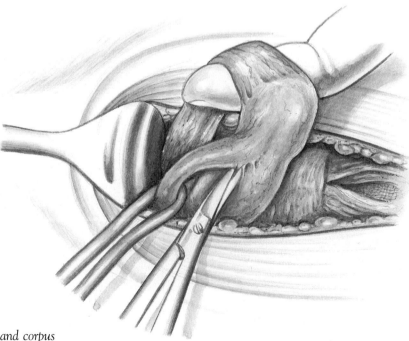

Figure 7. *Separation between urethra and corpus cavernosum towards the glans.*

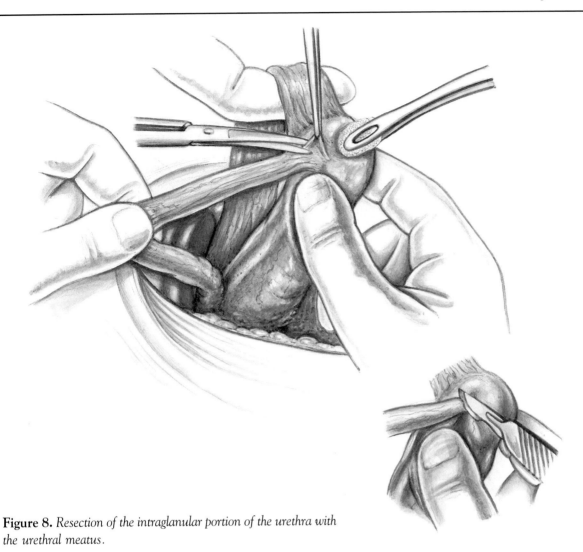

Figure 8. *Resection of the intraglanular portion of the urethra with the urethral meatus.*

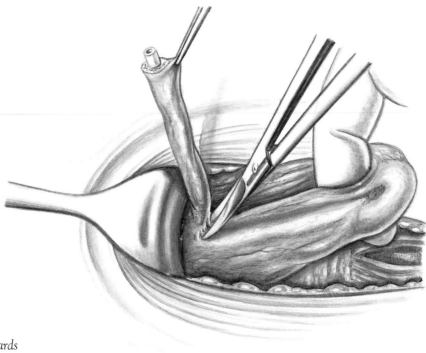

Figure 9. *Preparation of the urethra towards the bulbous urethra.*

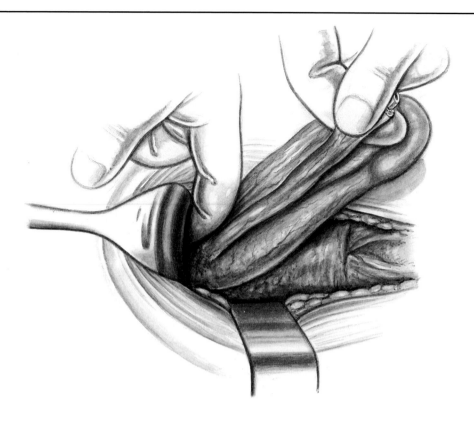

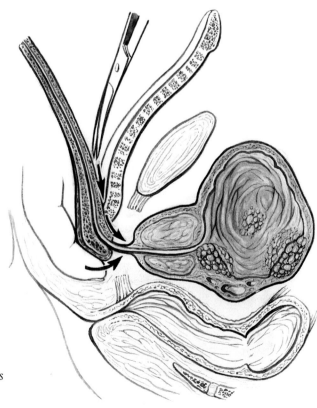

Figure 10. *Combined sharp and blunt dissection of the bulbous urethra reaching the dissection plane prepared from above.*

Surgery on the Female Urethra: Meatal Stenosis, Urethral Caruncle, Urethral Prolapse and Diverticulum

Th. Fritz, S.C. Müller, R. Hohenfellner
Department of Urology,
University of Mainz School of Medicine,
Mainz, Germany

Comment

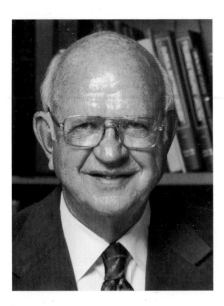

It is a privilege to comment on the modern approach to operations on the female urethra so well described and illustrated here. I find nothing of significance with which to differ.

Because they are not life-threatening the conditions addressed here are often overlooked, but they cause chronic symptoms of a most annoying nature in females of all ages. Furthermore, when they are detected in a quiescent state, it is difficult to determine whether operative treatment is or is not indicated.

Meatal stenosis

Recurrent urinary tract infections, in the past attributed to such fanciful concepts as 'bladder neck organic obstruction', 'mid-urethral ring', etc., may find their answer in simple meatal stenosis. (In the young, vesical outlet dysfunction of a behavioural pattern should be kept in mind.) In *true* meatal stenosis the operative procedure shown well in Figures 1 and 2 is appropriate. Use of an electrosurgical needle for the incision may obviate the need for sutures.

Caruncle

This benign, reddish, polypoid vascular mass of varying size at the lower lip of the meatus is found in adult women as their years advance. It is often completely asymptomatic (when it is best left alone). If troublesome irritative symptoms or postcoital or spontaneous 'spotting' of blood become worri-

some, shrinkage of the lesion by the application of a silver nitrate stick may be tried for a time. Most often, however, the operation depicted in Figure 4–6 is required. Certainly the admonition that the excised tissue be examined histologically must be heeded; clinical observation alone cannot exclude a malignancy of the urethra, which can masquerade as a caruncle but demands more radical treatment.

Prolapse of the urethra

Before embarking on operative correction it is essential, particularly in infants and young girls, to make sure that the presenting lesion is not a prolapsed ureterocele emerging from the meatus. This may require both cystourethroscopy and urography.

Fortunately the messy procedure of the past wherein a necrosing ligature proximal to the mass was tied around an indwelling catheter and followed by a wait of several days for sloughing to occur, has been supplanted by the clean surgical technique well illustrated in Figures 7–9.

The author emphasizes the necessity for measures to prevent retraction of the healthy mucosa as the prolapsed portion is excised. To this end I have found it helpful to begin the circumferential incision at 6 o'clock with the diathermy needle electrode and proceed upward by steps approximating normal urethral mucosa to adjacent vaginal lining by fine interrupted sutures. This affords hemostatic visualization of an anatomic closure requiring only brief catheter drainage.

Diverticulum of the female urethra

I am grateful for the author's accurate description of the technique proposed by J. Duckett and myself over 20 years ago. I can add nothing to his account. Our contribution, looked on askance at the time, has held up well over the years.

Of course, complete extirpation of the intact sac with severence and accurate closure of its opening into the urethra constitutes the desideratum, but more often than not this cannot be achieved and the frustrated surgeon becomes lost in a morass of blood, pus and shredded tissue with absence of all landmarks.

In 1970 I found myself in such a situation when attempting conventional removal of a multilocular pus-filled sac ramifying about the bladder neck and base in an elderly diabetic. To at least ensure drainage, I simply unroofed all pockets and slit the floor of the urethra from the meatus to the mouth of the diverticulum, which lay distressingly close to the vesical neck (through which a catheter was inserted). To my surprise, convalescence was smooth and, despite my fears, continence was complete after removal of the catheter at 5 days.

In this case and in the many patients both in our own and other centers where the saucerization principle has been employed, relief of symptoms and absence of complications has been the rule.

Postoperative voiding cystourethrograms have uniformly shown a strong trajectory of the stream, no vaginal puddling and, most noteworthy, a substantial length of proximal urethra still present even though preoperative endoscopy had revealed the orifice of the diverticulum to have been disturbingly close to the bladder neck. Furthermore, the *few* instances of stress leakage were all attributable to factors unrelated to the Spence procedure.

I have made a few other observations over the years:

- Dyspareunia should arouse suspicion of a diverticulum, as should exquisite tenderness on palpation with or without the appearance of a drop of pus at the meatus

- Voiding cystourethrography may be relied on almost exclusively to show the presence, as well as the size and extent, of diverticula

- Small crypts on the floor of the urethra, when they retain purulent material, may be managed successfully by transurethral incision with the knife blade of the resectoscope

Harry M. Spence, Dallas, USA

Meatal stenosis

Congenital meatal stenosis is rare. The increased incidence after the menopause indicates a hormonal influence. Loss of elasticity and formation of a fibrotic ring lead to higher micturition pressures and turbulences in the proximal segment of the urethra, with following dilatation of the paraurethral excretory ducts. Ascending bacterial invasion and multiplication lead to urethral syndrome and dysuria.

Urethral calibration

In childhood, the diameter of the urethra should be the age (in years) plus 10 Fr; in adults it should be at least 26–28 Fr.

Therapeutic options

Therapeutic options include urethral bougie, and internal or external meatotomy. High recurrence rates characterize urethral bougie. Bleeding requiring operative revision is common after internal meatotomy. External meatotomy has fewer complications and lower recurrence rates.[1]

Special instruments

- Bougie á boule set
- Diathermy needle
- Catgut 4/0

Operative technique (Figures 1–3)

- The patient is placed in the lithotomy position
- The labia minora are fixed with stay sutures on the thigh
- Bougies of increasing size are inserted into the meatus until one withdraws a white annular scar
- Meatal incision at 6 o'clock on the convexity of the scar
- Hemostasis by positioning of two to four single sutures (catgut 4/0) along the margins
- Positioning of a 24 Fr indwelling catheter, to be left for 1–2 days

Urethral caruncle

Older women are mostly affected by urethral caruncles. They originate from the dorsal circumference of the distal urethra and spread in the vestibule of the vagina. Histologically, the broad-based excrescence of the urethral mucosa shows hypervascularization and leukocytic infiltration. Recurrent bleeding and inflammation are caused by mechanical irritation. Inspection of the vulva and sounding of the urethra are the only diagnostic tools needed.

Special instruments

- Small bougie
- Wound hook
- Diathermy needle
- Catgut 4/0

Operative technique (Figures 4–6)

- Inspection of the external urethral meatus with the aid of a small bougie to localize the caruncle and to exclude the presence of a meatal stenosis
- Spreading of the meatus with a wound hook for better visualization of the operative field
- Grasping of the caruncle with forceps and excision at its base with a diathermy needle
- Closure of the mucosal defect with single sutures (catgut 4/0)
- Larger defects may be closed with an anterior vaginal wall pedunculated flap
- To exclude malignancy, histological examination of the specimen must follow

Urethral prolapse

Congenital weakness of the submucosal connective tissue of the urethra and sudden increases of intra-abdominal pressure (e.g. in coughing) are responsible for the development of a urethral prolapse.[2] Its incidence is highest in coloured girls (< 6 years) followed by postmenopausal women. The presenting symptom is urethral bleeding; voiding difficulties are relatively rare.

Inspection reveals an inflamed, sometimes gangrenous, circular mucosal bulge with the external urethral meatus at its centre.

Conservative measures such as repositioning and insertion of an indwelling catheter seldom show long-term success.

Various operative techniques have been developed, ranging from simple ligation of the mucosal protrusion on a catheter to fixation of the bladder and urethra to the symphysis and to the rectus abdominis muscle. Circular excision of the prolapsed urethral mucosa is a simple surgical procedure and necessitates short-term hospitalization. Complications (recurrence, meatal stenosis and stress incontinence) are extremely rare.[3,4]

Special instruments

- Diathermy needle
- Catgut 4/0

Operative technique (Figures 7–9)

- To avoid internal slipping of the mucosa, a piercing ligature (catgut 4/0) is inserted through the prolapsed urethra proximal to the resection line
- Circular excision of the prolapsed urethral mucosa with the diathermy needle
- Pulling out a loop from the centre of the piercing stitch and cutting it at this site
- Adaptation of the resection margins by knotting of the two resulting sutures and placement of additional hemostatic stitches

Urethral diverticulum

The main location of isolated or multiple female urethral diverticula is between the urethra and the anterior vaginal wall. Etiologically we can divide congenital diverticula from those originating from infection and secondary dilatation of the paraurethral ducts. Presenting symptoms are dysuria, recurrent urethrocystitis, purulent urethral discharge and dyspareunia. Postvoid dripping of urine is characteristic.

Preoperative evaluation

History and inspection of the outer genitalia with a speculum are most important. In case of larger diverticles a reponable mass on the anterior vaginal wall can be detected.

Diagnosis will be made by voiding cystourethrography (the positioning of one finger at the meatus to increase resistance is helpful), retrograde urethrography using a double-balloon catheter or urethroscopy. Concretions and malignancies can sometimes be found in the diverticulum. The only indication for operative correction is a symptomatic infected diverticulum.[5,6]

Special instruments

- Urethrocystoscope
- Catgut 4/0

Operative techniques (Figures 10–17)

Surgical procedures including complete transvaginal diverticulectomy and reconstruction of the anterior urethral and vaginal walls are mostly used.[7,8] Although rarely used, they are characterized by a high rate of postoperative complications (urethrovaginal fistula, incomplete resection of the diverticulum, stress incontinence and meatal stenosis).[1,2,6] Diverticula located in the middle and distal third of the urethra are best treated by the technically simple procedure first introduced by Spence and Duckett in 1970.[10] The patient must be informed that she will void through the vagina as a consequence of the artificial hypospadic urethra. This procedure is contraindicated for proximal diverticula to avoid the high risk of postoperative stress incontinence.[2]

- Urethroscopical localization of the diverticulum outlet.
- Transection of the distal urethra from the external urethral meatus to the diverticulum neck
- Sounding of the diverticulum and prolongation of the incision to the base of the diverticulum
- In larger diverticula, additional incision to provide abundant mucosal margins
- Diverticulum and vaginal resection margins are sutured together by single stitches (catgut 4/0) as in marsupialization. A continent hypospadic urethra results
- In addition to an indwelling catheter a vaginal tamponade is placed during the night
- The marsupialized open diverticulum shrinks slowly postoperatively to a flat mould

References

1. Käser OF, Ikle A, Hirsch HA. Operationen an den Harnorganen. In: Käser OF, Ikle A, Hirsch HA (eds). *Atlas der gynäkologischen Operationen*, 19, 4th edn. Stuttgart: Georg Thieme (1985) S. 19. 1.
2. Lowe CF, Hill GS, Jeffs RD, Brendler CB. Urethral prolapse in children: insights into etiology and management. *J Urol* **135** (1986) 100–3.
3. Barros SD, Oscar De. Protrusion of the female urethra. *J Urol* **68** (1952) 617–19.

4. Devine PC, Kessel HC. Surgical correction of urethral prolapse. *J Urol* **123** (1980) 856–7.

5. Patanaphan V, Prempree T, Sewchand W, Hafiz MH, Jaiwatana J. Adenocarcinoma arising in female urethral diverticulum. *Urology* **22** (1983) 259–64.

6. Hanno PM, Wein AJ. Female urethral diverticula. In: Ball TB Jr (ed.) AUA Update Series, Vol. V (1986) Lesson 3.

7. Adolphs HD Weissbach L. Klinik des weiblichen Harnröhrendivertikels. *Akt Urol* **12** (1981) 107–10.

8. Davis B, Robinson DG. Diverticula of the female urethra: assay of 120 cases. *J Urol* **104** (1970) 850–3.

9. Davis HJ, Telinde RW. Urethral diverticula: an assay of 121 cases. *J Urol* **80** (1958) 34–9.

10. Spence HM, Duckett JW Jr. Diverticulum of the female urethra: clinical aspects and presentation of a simple operative technique for cure. *J Urol* **104** (1970) 432–7.

11. Abet L, Richter J, Kotolla H, Hegenscheid. Die Doppelballonurethrographie der Frau. *Z Urol Nephrol* **76** (1983) 19–28

12. Lyon RP, Smith DR. Distal urethral stenosis. *J Urol* **80** (1963) 414–21.

13. Miskowiak J, Lichtenberg MH. Transurethral incision of urethral diverticulum in the female. *Scand J Urol Nephrol* **23** (1989) 235–7.

14. Moore TD. Diverticulum of female urethra; an improved technique of surgical excision. *J Urol* **68** (1952) 611–16.

15. Owens SB, Morse WH. Prolapse of the female urethra in children. *J Urol* **100** (1968) 171–4.

16. Petri E, Marberger H. Erkrankung der weiblichen Harnröhre. In: Petri E (ed.) *Gynäkologische Urologie*, chapter 17, 1st edn. Stuttgart: Georg Thieme (1983) S. 161.

17. Wulff HD, Petri E. Gynäkologie für Urologen. In: Hohenfellner, Zingg (eds) *Urologie Klinik und Praxis*, 1st edn. Stuttgart: Georg Thieme (1983) S. 1181.

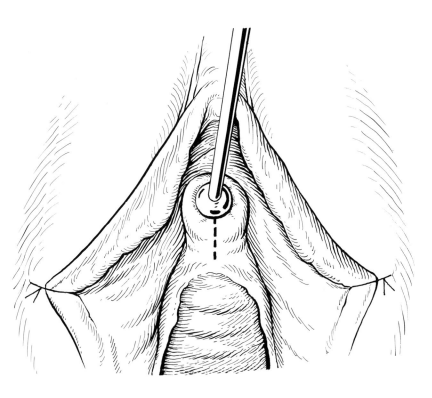

Figure 1. *Dilatation of the distal urethra with a bougie á boule and incision of the white inelastic annular scar at 6 o'clock.*

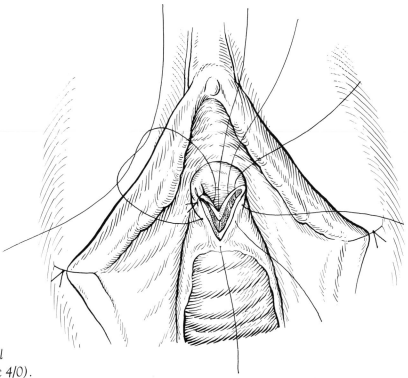

Figure 2. *Adaptation of urethral and vaginal mucosa with hemostatic single sutures (catgut 4/0).*

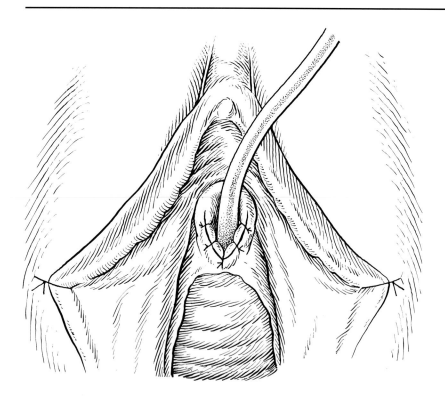

Figure 3. *Indwelling 24 Fr catheter for 1 or 2 days.*

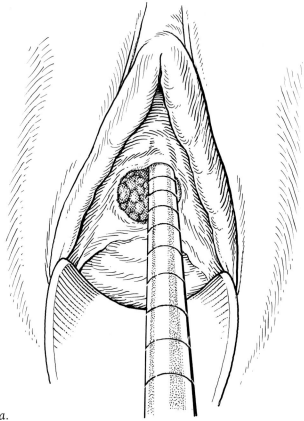

Figure 4. *Sounding of the urethra with a small bougie and localization of the caruncle on the dorsal wall of the distal urethra.*

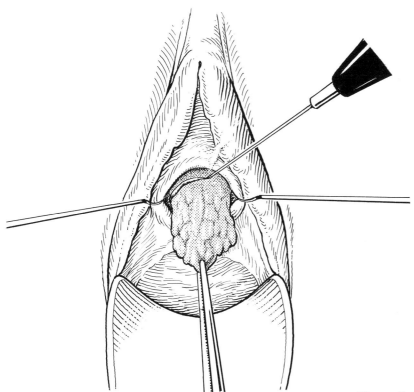

Figure 5. *Grasping of the caruncle with forceps and excision at its base with a diathermy needle.*

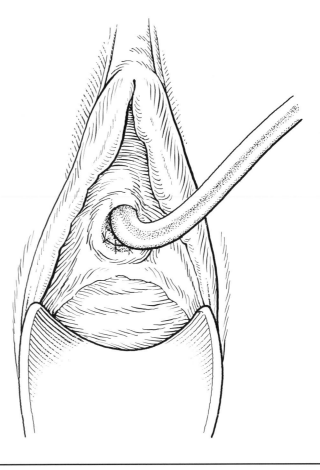

Figure 6. *Closure of the mucosal defect with single sutures (catgut 4/0).*

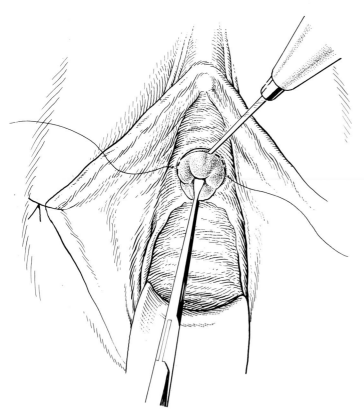

Figure 7. *Placing of a piercing ligature (catgut 4/0) through the prolapsed urethra proximal to the resection line. Circular excision of the prolapsed mucosa with a diathermy needle.*

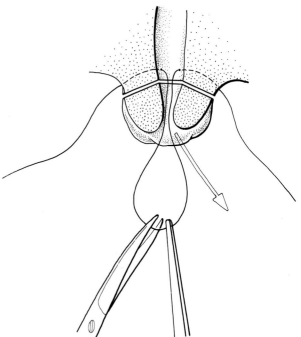

Figure 8. *Pulling out a loop from the centre of the piercing stitch and cutting it at this site. Adaptation of the resection margins by knotting the two resulting sutures.*

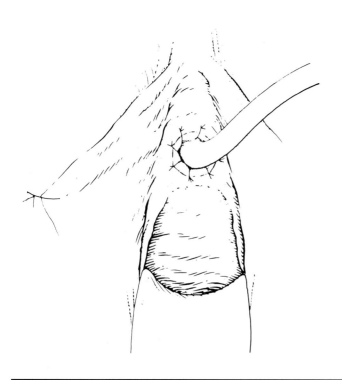

Figure 9. *Reconstruction of the meatus through an additional piercing stitch and positioning of a 24 Fr catheter.*

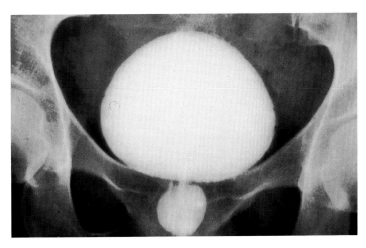

Figure 10. *Voiding cystourethrogram for detection of urethral diverticulum.*

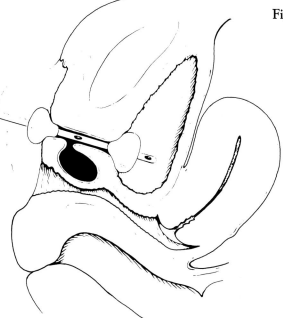

Figure 11. *Double-balloon catheter to visualize the urethral diverticulum.*

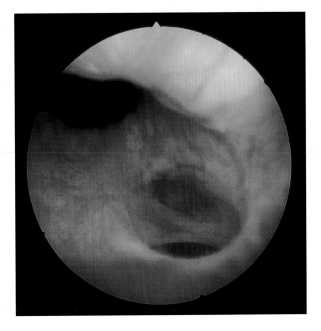

Figure 12. *Endoscopic image of the urethra. On the left is the bladder neck and on the right a septate diverticulum neck. The distance between the diverticulum entrance and the bladder neck appears endoscopically smaller than it is in fact.*

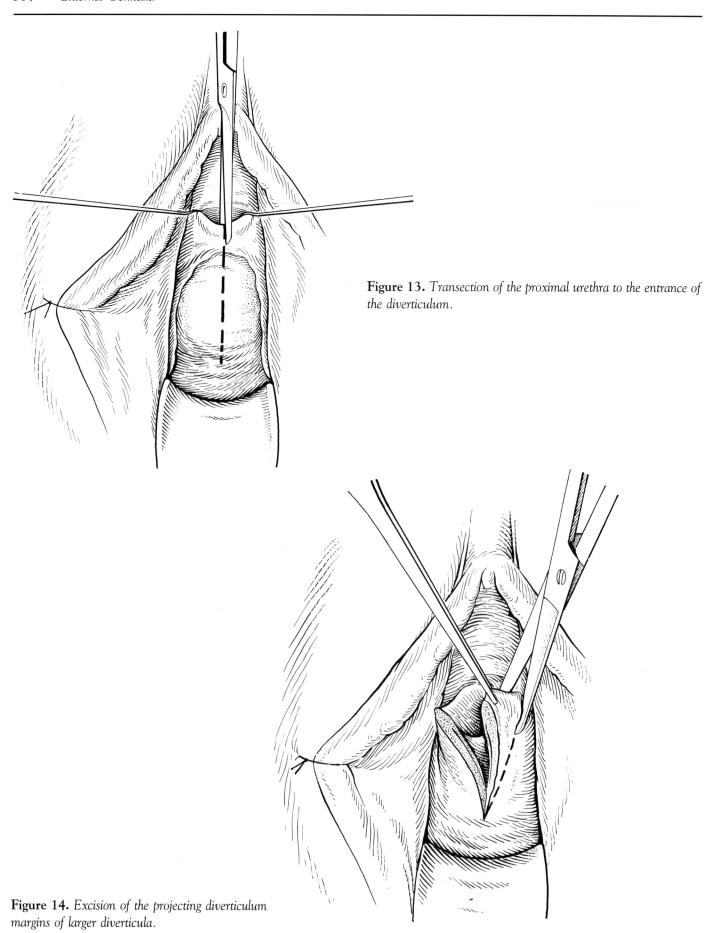

Figure 13. *Transection of the proximal urethra to the entrance of the diverticulum.*

Figure 14. *Excision of the projecting diverticulum margins of larger diverticula.*

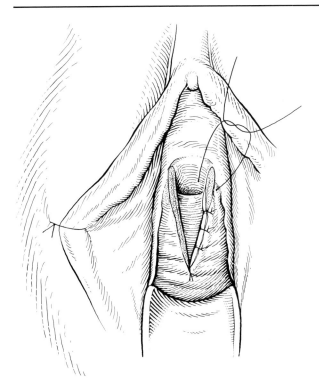

Figure 15. *Hemostatic single stitches (catgut 4/0) between the urethral and vaginal resection margins.*

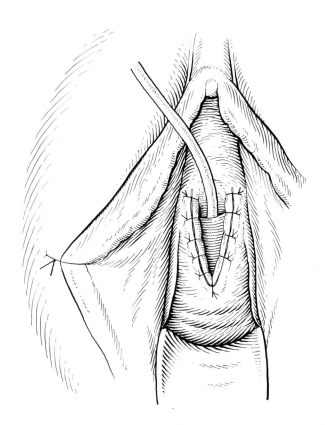

Figure 16. *A continent hypospadiac urethra and a marsupialized diverticulum.*

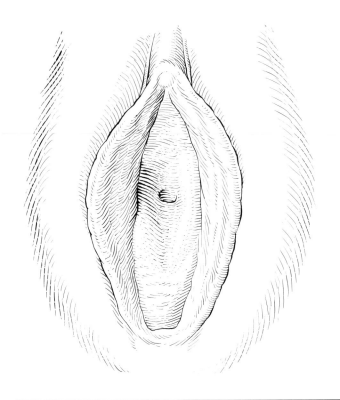

Figure 17. *Outcome of the Spence and Duckett operation some weeks after the operation.*

Surgery for Peyronie's Disease and Congenital Penile Deviation

V. Moll, E. Becht, M. Ziegler
Department of Urology,
University of Saarland,
Hamburg, Germany

Comment

I agree with the authors that the surgical treatment of penile deviation according to Nesbit is the treatment of choice and that the slight shortening of the penis due to the operation does not limit the usefulness of the method. Patients with Peyronie's disease already have a shortening of the penis at the site of the inflammatory fibrosis of the tunica albuginea, and correction of this deformity produces generally a very limited and well-accepted shortening of the penis.

Excision of the plaque and use of a homologous dermal patch allows better elasticity than the use of heterologous material. In large defects a functional cavernous insufficiency characterized by venous leakage could lead to impotence. For this reason we believe that surgery should be limited to patients who cannot have normal sexual intercourse because of the penile deviation.

Excision of the tunica albuginea is superior to the suture described by Essed and Schroeder. Also, the longitudinal incision of the penile skin described here is not as efficient as classic circumcision, especially because in the Buck's fascia there are neurovascular bundles that must be carefully dissected from the plaque. In dorsal deviation, the urethra is often completely mobilized from the tunica albuginea.

Radiotherapy does not have a positive effect in Peyronie's disease. In fact, it makes operation afterwards more difficult. Clinical results with potassium aminobenzoate are very similar with those obtained without any form of therapy. Surgery is the treatment of choice and the particular technique is chosen to suit the case: Nesbit's operation is preferred for congenital penis deviation, but there is still some controversy as to the best technique for Peyronie's disease.

F. Schreiter, Schwelm, Germany

Surgery for Peyronie's disease and congenital penile deviation

Introduction

Penile curvature can be congenital or acquired. Congenital curvature is generally associated with hypospadias but can also be present in isolation. The acquired form is Peyronie's disease.

The diagnosis is made from the history and confirmed by inspection of the erect penis or by a picture showing the deviation. Confirmation is essential before surgery. Other complaints, such as pain during sexual intercourse or incapacity of penetration, are also indications for the operation.

Surgical correction for Peyronie's disease should be done at a phase of stabilization of the disease to avoid postoperative progression of the disease.

Instruments

- Standard instruments for genital operations
- Suture material: polyglycolic acid 1/0 (children 2/0–3/0) and catgut 4/0 (children 5/0–6/0)

Operative technique step by step

- An artificial erection is produced by placing a tourniquet at the penis base and infusing a saline solution in the corpus cavernosus through a butterfly puncture. This procedure may be repeated as required during surgery

- The classic approach described by Nesbit (Figure 1)[1] involves circumcision and mobilization of the skin to the penis base. We use a simplified medial or paramedial approach (Figure 2) preserving the dorsal nerve bundles at the exact point of the compensating suture, but in complicated cases we still prefer the original approach

- In the original Nesbit technique (Figures 3 and 4), small windows of the tunica albuginea are removed from the convex site of the deviation. The site is closed using a nontraumatic needle and 1/0–3/0 polyglycolic acid suture. In dorsal deviation a ventral paraurethral suture is generally sufficient. Eventually, complete mobilization of the urethra from the corpora cavernosa is required

- In the modified technique, the suture is placed without removing the window (Figure 5). Before tying the knot, traction on the suture material allows control of the end result (Figure 6). A modification described by Essed and Schroeder is also based on this principle (Figure 7)[2]

Postoperative care

- A cystostomy tube should be placed and left for 1–2 weeks to reduce the number of erections

- The bandage should be left until day 4

- The patient should be sexually abstinent for 8 weeks

- The patients should be informed that there will be a slight shortening of the penis due to the operation

References

1. Nesbit RM. The surgical treatment of congenital chordee without hypospadias. *J Urol* **72** (1954) 1178–80.
2. Essed E, Schroeder FH. New surgical treatment for Peyronie disease. *Urology* **25** (1985) 582–7.

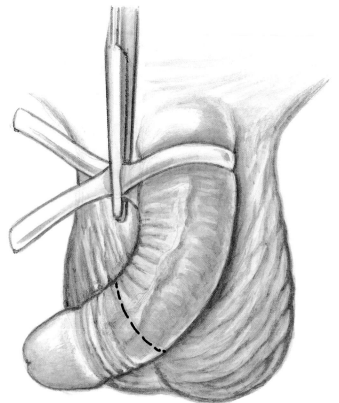

Figure 1. *Original approach described by Nesbit: circumcision and mobilization of the penile skin. A tourniquet is placed on the penis base to obtain an artificial erection.*

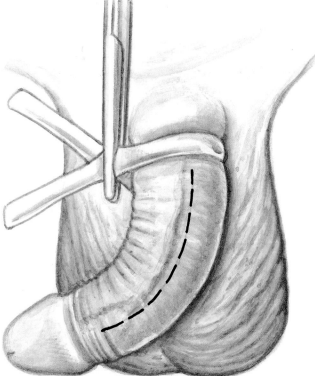

Figure 2. *Modified approach: longitudinal medial or paramedial dorsal incision.*

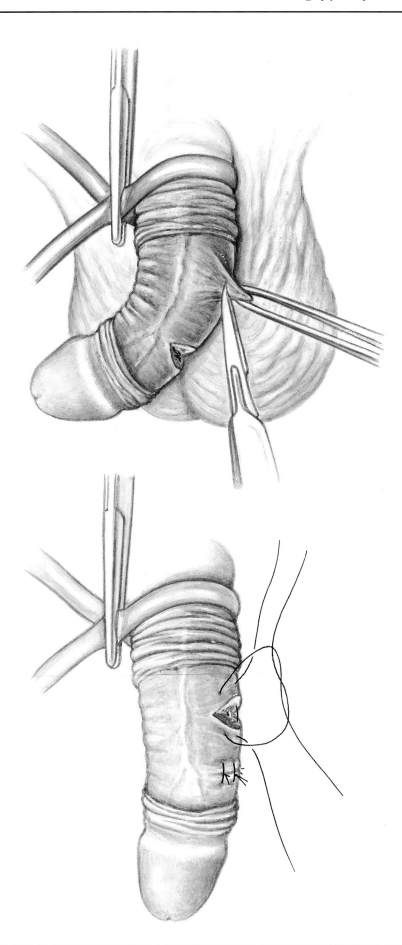

Figure 3. *Oval windows are removed from the tunica albuginea at the convex site of the deviation.*

Figure 4. *The wound is sutured.*

Modified Techniques

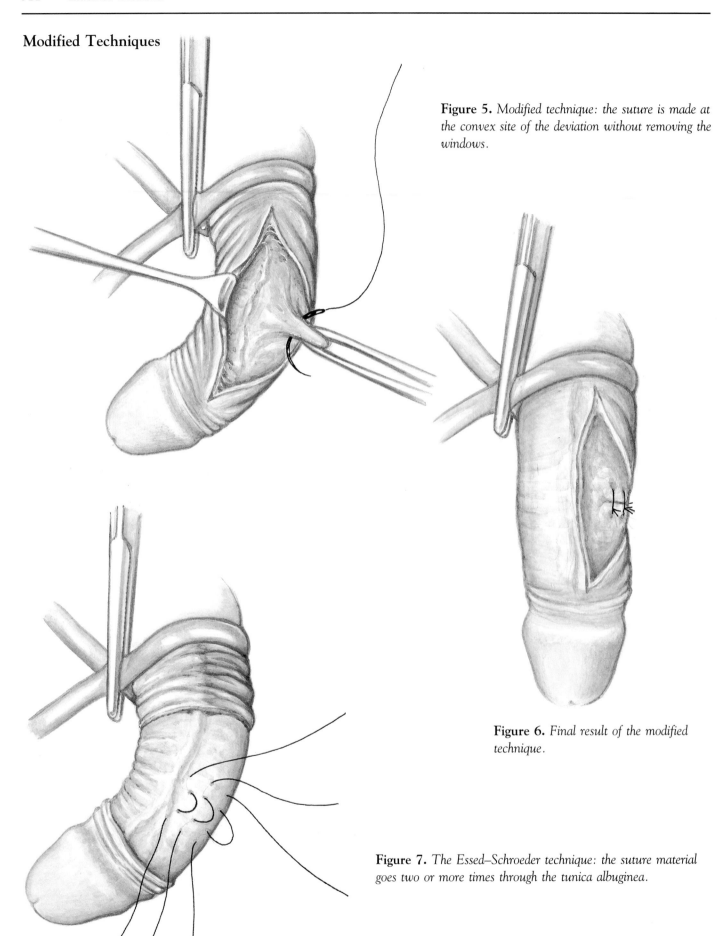

Figure 5. *Modified technique: the suture is made at the convex site of the deviation without removing the windows.*

Figure 6. *Final result of the modified technique.*

Figure 7. *The Essed–Schroeder technique: the suture material goes two or more times through the tunica albuginea.*

Carcinoma of the Penis

O. Seemann, J. Rassweiler, P. Alken[a]
Departments of Urology,
Stadtkrankenhaus Heilbronn,
Teaching Hospital of the University of Heidelberg,
Germany and
[a]Klinikum Mannheim,
Clinical Faculty of the University of Heidelberg,
Mannheim, Germany

Comment

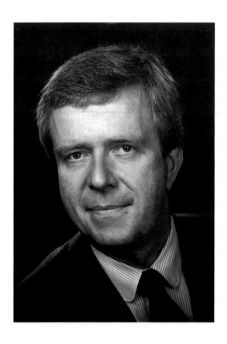

The principle of retaining function while operating as radically as necessary is particularly important in cancer of the penis. Surgery to preserve the organ can be justified, therefore, when carcinoma of the penis is diagnosed and treated early. The stage of the primary tumor and its degree of differentiation[1] are critical for the prognosis.

In superficial penis cancer of stage T1 and good differentiation (G1), inguinal lymph node metastases have not been observed, according to Pettaway et al.[2] In all higher stages and in undifferentiated penis carcinoma, the probability of lymph node metastases increases up to 94%. The findings from DNA flow cytometry proved to be significantly inferior prognostically because 37% of 38 patients with pN0 stage cancer and 31% of 13 patients with lymphogenetically metastasizing penis carcinoma were aneuploid.[2] Thus, ilioinguinal lymphadenectomy can be excluded only in stage T1G1. The value of lymphadenectomy, prognostically or therapeutically, could not be determined. Nevertheless, Johnson and Lo[3] found that early lymphadenectomy improved the 5-year survival rate by almost 50% in comparison with later lymphadenectomy. This has been confirmed by the study of Srinivas,[4] which showed that the survival rate was no different in patients with positive lymph nodes and those whose lymph nodes were free of metastases. Fossa et al.[5] came to the same conclusion. Thus, inguinal lymphadenectomy is justified in spite of complications. Here the Schildwächter lymph node is of only limited value in indicating the condition of the other inguinal lymph nodes.[7] In contrast, the 5-year survival rate[4] is only 12% in cases of bilateral positive inguinal lymph nodes so that in this unfavorable situation, without the assurance of therapeutic value at this stage, primary lymphadenectomy does not seem to help. It should be critically investigated whether in patients with stage pN2 cancer neoadjuvant chemotherapy with vincristine, bleomycin and methotrexate should be applied, as Pizzocaro suggests.[1] If the involved inguinal lymph node responded, specific removal of a lymph node would confirm the therapeutic result.

Organ-preserving methods of treatment such as biopsy, excision, laser ablation and circumcision are justified only when the indication is most critically determined. The tendency of penis carcinoma to metastasize early into the inguinal lymph nodes endangers the patient in the event of understaging or incomplete tumor removal. Baker's data,[6] therefore, do not indicate that a patient with new lymph node metastases because of a delayed lymph adenectomy would be worse off than a patient with primary tumor recurrence and secondary lymph node involvement. The recent opinion that lasers offer the optimal treatment for carcinoma of the penis surely cannot be endorsed.

References

1. Pizzocaro G, Piva L. Adjuvant home vincristine, bleomycin, methotrexate (VBM) in resected nodal metastases from squamous cell carcinoma of the penis. *J Urol* **145** (1991) 367A.
2. Pettaway CA, Stewart D, Vuitch F, Savino D, Ewalt D, McConnell JD. Penile squamous carcinoma: DNA flow cytometry versus histopathology for prognosis. *J Urol* **145** (1991) 367A.
3. Johnson D, Lo R. Management of regional lymph nodes in penile carcinoma: complications of groin dissections in penile cancer. *Urology* **24** (1984) 308–9.
4. Srinivas V. Morsel M, Herr H, Sogani P, Whitmore W. Penile cancer: relation of node extent of nodal metastasis to survival. *J Urol* **137** (1987) 880–2.
5. Fossa S, Hall K, Johannessen N, Urnes T, Kaalhus O. Cancer of the penis. *Eur Urol* **13** (1987) 372–7.
6. Baker BH, Spratt SS, Perez-Mesa C, Watson FR, Leduc RJ. Carcinoma of the penis. Analysis of therapy in 100 consecutive cases. *J Urol* **116** (1976) 458–61.
7. Perinetti E, Crane DB, Catalona WJ. Unreliability of sentinel node biopsy for staging penile carcinoma. *J Urol* **124** (1980) 134–50.

J.E. Altwein

Carcinoma of the penis

Introduction

Penile carcinoma in Europe and North America is an uncommon disease accounting for less than 1% of all malignancies in males, an incidence of 0.6–1.3 cases per 100 000 per year. It is most frequently located on the glans penis and the prepuce. Metastatic disease mainly affects the regional lymph nodes: lymphatic drainage of the penis proceeds from the superficial inguinal nodes to the deep inguinal nodes and from there to the pelvic nodes. Due to crossings of the lymph drainage, metastases may be found bilaterally in both inguinal areas.

Except in very small and distal lesions, the standard treatment is always partial or total penectomy. Treatment of regional lymph nodes is still a subject of controversy. In a large series, early lymphadenectomy shortly following treatment of the primary lesion significantly improved survival on comparison with cases where primary treatment without lymphadenectomy was performed.[1] On the other hand, morbidity after groin dissection is significant: major complications such as lymphedema, lymphocele, abscesses and wound breakdown are reported in up to 60% of cases. McDougal *et al.* found a 100% tumor-free survival rate in stage I patients after local excision without groin dissection and therefore suggested a wait-and-see strategy in these patients.[2] In addition, others stressed the significance of tumor grade and advocated early lymphadenectomy for moderately or poorly differentiated carcinoma regardless of tumor stage.[3,4]

Selective lymph node biopsy has been proposed by Cabanas, who found that a sentinel node adjacent to the superficial epigastric vein accurately predicts the presence of inguinal lymph node metastases.[5] Unfortunately, Perinetti *et al.* reported a patient who developed lymph node metastases within 6 months of negative bilateral sentinel lymph node biopsy – indicating the limitations of this approach.[6]

Indications

- Radical circumcision in small tumors which are confined to the prepuce

- Partial penectomy in distal tumors with residual penile length not less than 3 cm when divided with at least 2 cm of grossly tumor-free margin

- Total penectomy and perineal urostomy in larger and more proximal tumors

- Inguinal lymphadenectomy or selective sentinel lymph node biopsy in patients with tumor stage >pT1 and/or grade >G1

- Pelvic lymph node dissection when inguinal nodes are positive

Instruments

- Standard instruments
- Suture material: polyglycolic acid
- Clips

Exposure

- Single-incision approach for ipsilateral lymphadenectomy: an incision 1 cm below and parallel to the inguinal ligament allows access to the inguinal and pelvic lymph nodes

- Double-incision 'skin bridge' technique:[7] incision 3 cm below and parallel to the inguinal ligament for inguinal lymphadenectomy; a second incision above the inguinal ligament exposes the pelvic nodes for ipsilateral dissection

- Bilateral lymphadenectomy: inguinal exposure via an incision 3 cm below and parallel to the inguinal ligament; a lower midline incision for extraperitoneal pelvic lymph node dissection

Operative technique step by step

Partial penectomy (Figures 1–3)
- Exclusion of the tumor by a firmly affixed condom or glove; tourniquet; skin incision circumferentially 2 cm proximal to the gross tumor extent

- Division of the cavernous bodies; the urethra is divided and spatulated 1 cm distally but respecting the tumor margins

- Ligation of the dorsal vessels and closure of the cavernous bodies with interrupted sutures that include the septum (2/0 Dexon; Davis and Geck, Gosport, UK)

- Removal of the tourniquet and hemostasis if necessary; insertion of a Foley catheter

- Creation of a neomeatus by anastomosis of the spatulated urethra to the skin ventrally and approximation of the redundant skin to complete wound closure

Total penectomy (Figures 4–7)
- Isolation of the tumor with a condom

- Elliptic incision around the base of the penis, which is extended 2 cm dorsally in the midline and inferiorly along the scrotal raphe

- Ligation of the dorsal vessels and division of the suspensory ligament. Prepubic dissection including the fat and nodes in the specimen

- Incision of Buck's fascia ventrally and division of the urethra in the bulbar region

- Ligation of the deep arteries; clamping of both crurae of the cavernous bodies and division at the pubic rami. Closure of the crurae with mattress sutures (2/0 Dexon)

- For perineal urostomy a 2 cm elliptic skin incision is made at the perineum, and the urethral stump is pulled through a bluntly dissected tunnel

- The urethra is spatulated dorsally and anastomosed to the skin with interrupted 3/0 chromic catgut sutures

- Placing of two Penrose drains and transverse closure of the wound

Lymphadenectomy (Figures 8–15)

- The ipsilateral thigh is abducted and externally rotated; the scrotum is sutured to the opposite thigh. Prior to draping, the extent of the area to be dissected should be marked

Selective biopsy of the sentinel lymph node
- The fossa ovalis is exposed through an oblique 5 cm incision two fingerwidths lateral and caudal to the pubic tubercle

- The sentinel lymph node is found in the angle of the superficial epigastric vein and the external pudendal vein; all nodes in this area should be removed

- If frozen section examination is positive, the incision is extended laterally for inguinal and pelvic lymphadenectomy

Inguinal and pelvic lymphadenectomy: single-incision exposure
- Incision 1 cm below and parallel to the inguinal ligament from the anterior superior iliac spine to the pubic tubercle

- Skin flaps with only a few millimeters of subcutaneous tissues are sharply dissected within the marked area; the inguinal ligament is exposed cranially and the deep fascia of the thigh medially, laterally and caudally

- The dissection of the specimen starts laterally with incision of the deep fascia of the thigh over the sartorius muscle; small vessels and lymphatics are carefully ligated or clipped

- The deep fascia of the thigh with all overlying lymphatic and fatty tissue is now mobilized from the lateral to the medial side; the saphenous vein is reached inferomedially and should be preserved

- Mobilization of the fascia medially from the adductors toward the femoral sheath, leaving skeletonized femoral vessels and nerve in an empty fossa. The specimen is attached only at the femoral canal

- If pelvic lymphadenectomy is necessary, the external oblique fascia is incised 3 cm above the inguinal ligament and the iliac and obturator nodes are dissected and removed *en bloc* with the inguinal specimen. Alternatively, a laparoscopic pelvic lymphadenectomy can be performed

- Closure: the femoral nerve and vessels in the empty femoral trigone are covered by the sartorius muscle, which is divided at the anterior iliac spine. The muscle is placed over the nerve and vessels and sutured to the inguinal ligament with its cranial end. Laterally and medially it is tacked to the iliac muscle and the adductor muscle, respectively

- Two suction drains are inserted, ischemic skin margins excised and the wound closed without traction

Surgical tricks

- *Partial penectomy*: if sufficient penile skin is left after excision of a distal tumor, it can be folded to a neoprepuce, which covers the meatus, and a better cosmetic result is achieved. In this case, the neoprepruce is stabilized by subcutaneous plication sutures

- *Inguinal lymphadenectomy*: wound infection, slough or erosion of the femoral vessels may be prevented by gentle handling of the skin flaps. Unnecessary trauma must be avoided. The skin flaps should be kept covered with moistened sponges. Sharp skin hooks are preferable to Roux hooks for exposure. Devascularized skin must be excised; if tension-free closure is not possible, a split thickness graft should be applied. Careful ligation of lymphatics and preservation of the saphenous vein help to prevent lymphoceles and lymphedema

Postoperative care

- Prophylactic antibiotics

- Catheter removal 7 days after penectomy

- Elastic stockings and elevation of the leg are recommended after lymphadenectomy

References

1. Ornelias AA, Seixas ALC, Marota A, Wisnescky A, Campos F, de Moraes JR. Surgical treatment of invasive squamous cell carcinoma of the penis: retrospective analysis of 350 cases. *J Urol* **151** (1994) 1244–9.
2. McDougal WS, Kirchner FK Jr, Edwards RH, Killion LT. Treatment of carcinoma of the penis: the case for primary lymphadenectomy. *J Urol* **136** (1986) 38–41.
3. Horenblas S, van Tinteren H, Delemarre JF, Moonen LMF, Lustig V, van Waardenburg EW. Squamous cell carcinoma of the penis. III. Treatment of regional lymph nodes. *J Urol* **149** (1993) 492–7.
4. Fraley EE, Zhang G, Manivel C, Niehans G. The role of ilioinguinal lymphadenectomy and significance of historical differentiation in treatment of carcinoma of the penis. *J Urol* **142** (1989) 1478–82.
5. Cabanas MR. An approach for the treatment of penile carcinoma. *Cancer* **39** (1977) 456.
6. Perinetti E, Crane DB, Catalona WJ. Unreliability of sentinel node biopsy for staging penile carcinoma. *J Urol* **124** (1980) 734–5.
7. Fraley EE, Hutchens HC. Radical ilio-inguinal node dissection: the skin bridge technique. A new procedure. *J Urol* **108** (1972) 279–81.

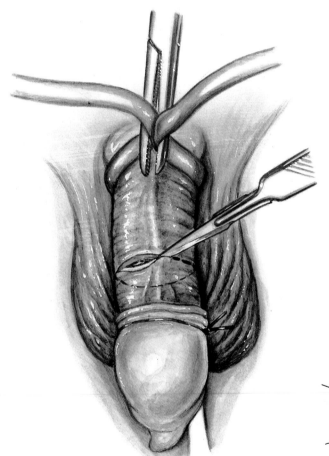

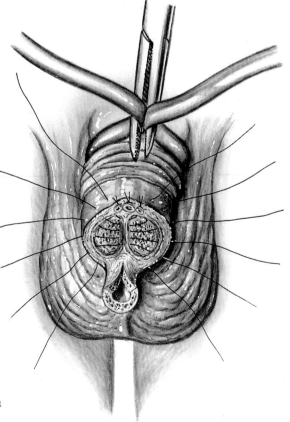

Figure 1. *Tumor margins are confirmed by biopsy specimen. Circumferential resection with a margin of 2 cm.*

Figure 2. *The cavernous bodies are divided. The urethra is transected with a 1 cm redundancy and dorsally spatulated. The dorsal vessels are ligated, and the cavernous bodies are closed with interrupted sutures that include the septum.*

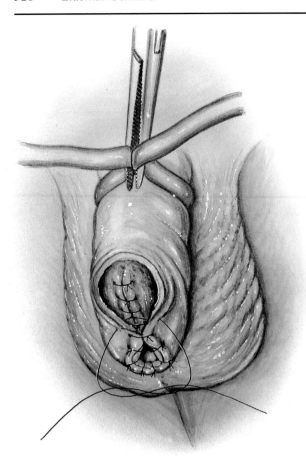

Figure 3. *Wound closure beginning ventrally. Skin-to-urethra anastomosis and adaptation of the redundant skin dorsally.*

Total penectomy

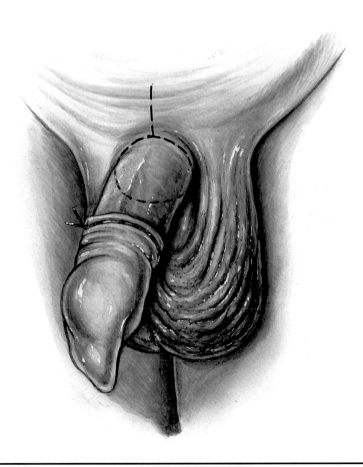

Figure 4. *Incision line for total penectomy.*

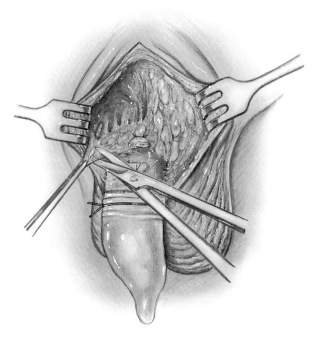

Figure 5. *Prepubic dissection of nodes and fatty tissue after division of the suspensory ligament. The dorsal vessels are ligated.*

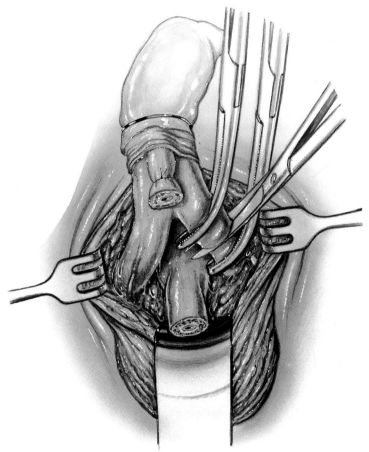

Figure 6. *The urethra is divided and the crura of the cavernous bodies are clamped and divided at the pubic rami. Closure of the crurae with mattress sutures.*

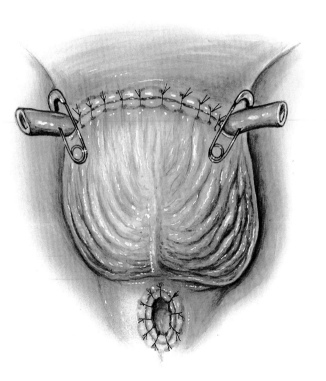

Figure 7. *Perineal urostomy and transverse wound closure.*

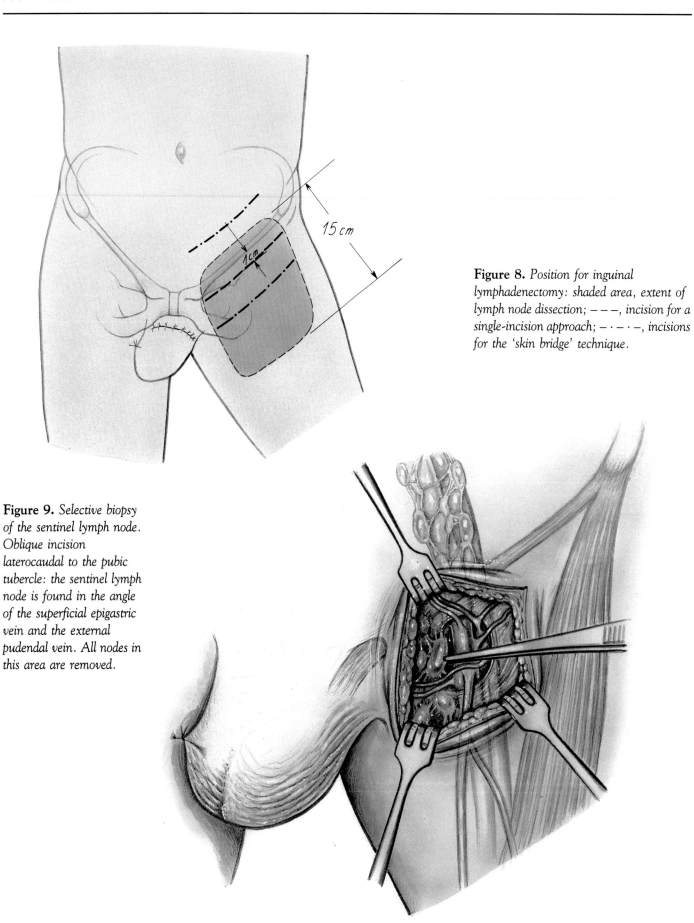

Figure 8. *Position for inguinal lymphadenectomy: shaded area, extent of lymph node dissection; – – –, incision for a single-incision approach; – · – · –, incisions for the 'skin bridge' technique.*

Figure 9. *Selective biopsy of the sentinel lymph node. Oblique incision laterocaudal to the pubic tubercle: the sentinel lymph node is found in the angle of the superficial epigastric vein and the external pudendal vein. All nodes in this area are removed.*

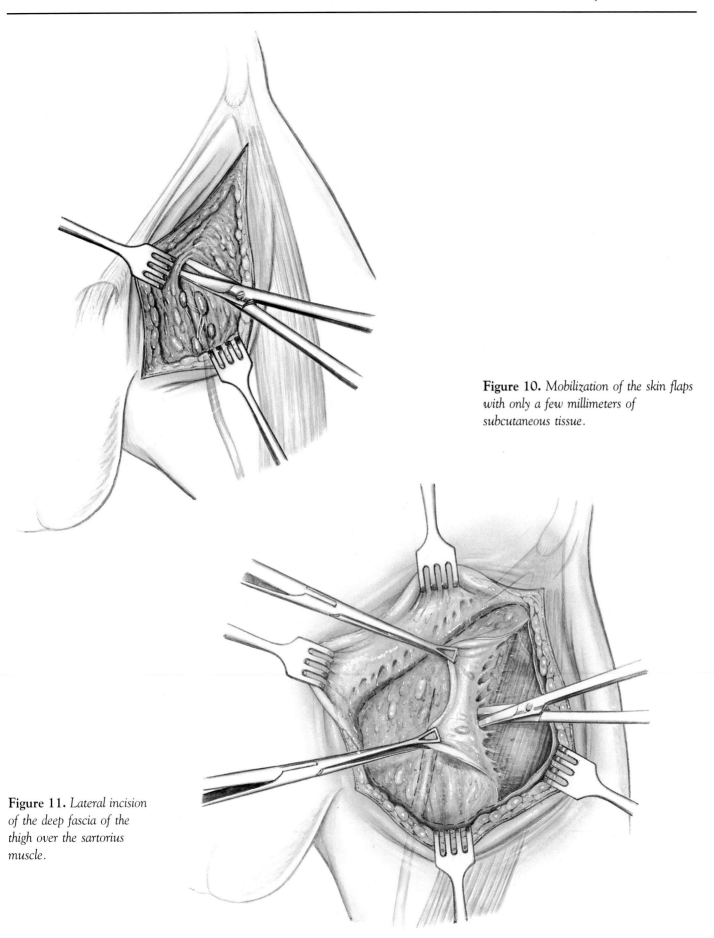

Figure 10. *Mobilization of the skin flaps with only a few millimeters of subcutaneous tissue.*

Figure 11. *Lateral incision of the deep fascia of the thigh over the sartorius muscle.*

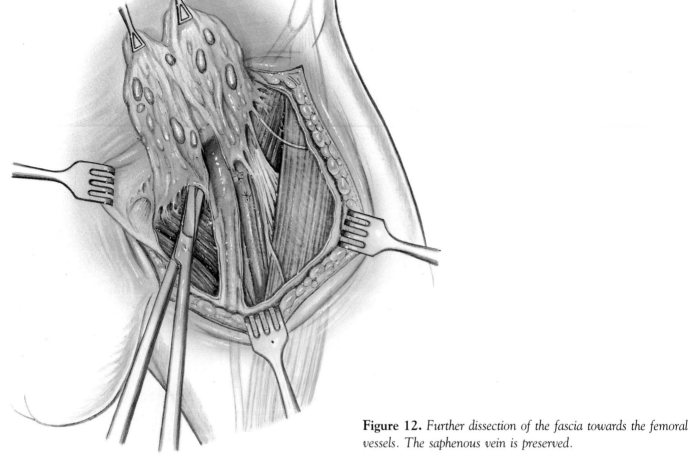

Figure 12. *Further dissection of the fascia towards the femoral vessels. The saphenous vein is preserved.*

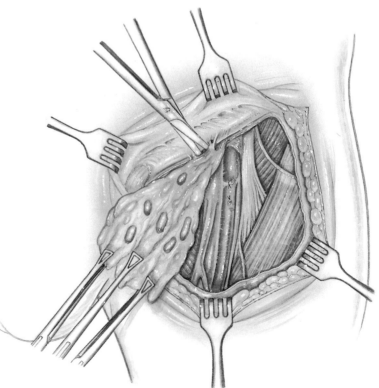

Figure 13. *The specimen completely dissected and only adherent at the femoral canal.*

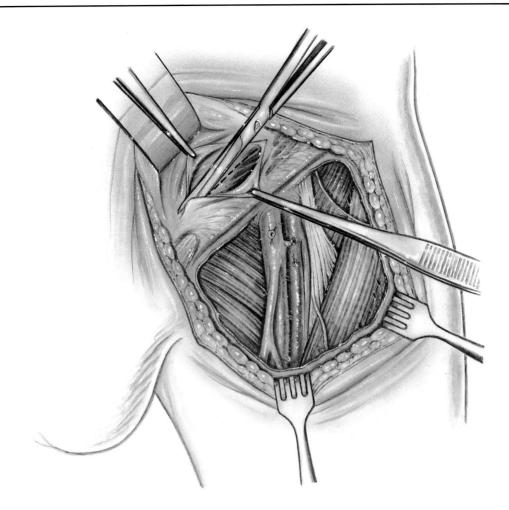

Figure 14. *Extraperitoneal access for pelvic lymphadenectomy through the same incision. The external oblique fascia is incised 3 cm above the inguinal ligament, and the iliac and obturator nodes can be dissected.*

(a)   (b)

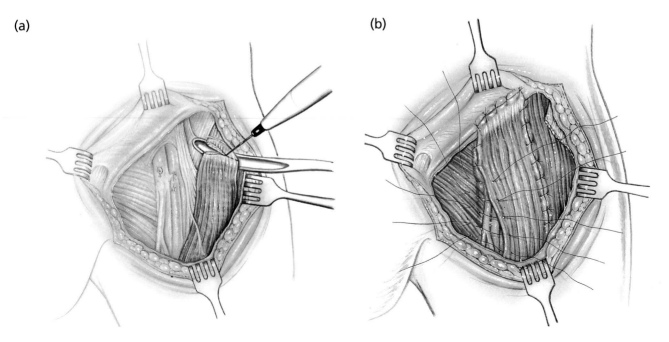

Figure 15. *The sartorius muscle is divided at the anterior iliac spine, placed over the femoral nerve and vessels, and sutured to the inguinal ligament with its cranial end. Laterally and medially it is tacked to the iliac muscle and the adductor muscle, respectively.*

Correction of Hypospadias: Denis Browne Technique

F. Ikoma, H. Shima
Department of Urology,
Hyogo College of Medicine,
Nishinomiya, Hyogo, Japan

Introduction

Hypospadias is seen at a frequency of about 1 in 300 male births, making it a major disorder among deformities of the external genitalia. One-stage repair is currently popular. However, complications such as fistula and stricture are relatively common in one-stage repair, especially in the correction of severe hypospadias because there is not enough dartos fascia across the entire penile ventral surface to be sutured for urethroplasty if chordectomy is complete. Two-stage repair is therefore still important, and offers reliable procedures for the correction of hypospadias. Simultaneous glanular urethroplasty at the time of chordectomy, and urethroplasty based on the technique of Denis Browne, are introduced here.[1-4]

Preoperative diagnostics

- Retrograde urethrocystography and micturating cystourethrography to find an enlarged prostatic utricle or male vagina, which are often associated with hypospadias[5]

- Chromosomal analysis to exclude intersex cases in a patient with severe hyospadias;[6] when intersex is suspected, endoscopic examination should be performed at the time of operation[7]

- Intravenous pyelography to find anomalies of the upper urinary tract, although their incidence is low[8]

Indications

- All forms of hypospadias with chordee

Special instruments

- Small optic scissors
- PDS sutures (5/0) (Ethicon, Edinburgh, UK)
- Bipolar fulguration for all procedures
- Prolene (Ethicon) or nylon sutures (5/0 or 6/0) for urethroplasty
- Diathermy to fulgurate the hair roots
- 10 ml saline for artificial erection

Chordectomy with reconstruction of the glanular urethra at 2–3 years

Operative techniques (two-stage procedures) step by step
Complete chordectomy is obligatory to make the penis straight after correction of hypospadias

- Placement of a stay suture (3/0 Prolene) in the glans penis (Figure 1a)

- The skin incision, in a U-shape, extending over the corone of the glans (Figure 1c)

- Bilateral ablation of the ventral skin (Figure 2); bleeding is controlled by bipolar fulguration

- Sharp dissection of the skin over the urethra (Figure 3)

- Longitudinal incision of the mucosal urethra until normal urethra in the corpus spongiosum appears (Figure 4a); the length of the ventral penis is measured (Figure 4b)

- The cord clamped with forceps at the glans corona (Figure 5)

- Sharp dissection of the cord with a knife (Figure 6a and b); after complete resection, the penis becomes straight, bends ventrally with ease, and measures the length of the ventral penis (Figure 6c)

- Confirmation of complete chordectomy by artificial erection with saline injected into the corpus cavernosum through the glans penis after tying the root of the penis with a Nélaton catheter

- A Nélaton catheter (10 Fr) is placed through the new meatus and fixed into the ventral skin with no. 3 silk (Figure 7). When an enlarged prostatic utricle or a male vagina is present, a sound must be used to assist insertion of the catheter into the bladder

- Circumcision is completed (Figure 8)

- A window is opened in the preputial skin (Figure 9a and b), and the preputial skin distal to this window moved to the ventral side of the penis by passing it through the glans (Figure 9c)

- The skin tube is formed with PDS (5/0) sutures, inverted, and turned upside down (Figures 10, 11 and 12)

- A ventral incision is made in the glans penis, and the neomeatus formed with 5/0 PDS sutures (Figure 13)

- A Penrose drain is placed in the ventral space, and a Nélaton catheter (8 Fr) in the glanular urethra, which is fixed on the glans with 3/0 Prolene (Figure 14)

- The wound is closed with 5/0 PDS sutures. A gauze pillow is placed behind the dorsal penis, the glans is pulled slightly cranially with a stay suture, and the stay suture is sewn to a small piece of gauze and taped to the lower abdomen

- If there is not enough dorsal skin to form the glanular urethra, orthodox skin suturing is applied[9]

Postoperative care
- Oral antibiotics are prescribed for 2 weeks

- Nebacetin powder (Yamanouchi Pharma, Heidelberg, Germany) is applied to the penile wound every day for 2 weeks to dry the wound

- The Nélaton catheter in the glanular urethra is removed after a few days

- The urethral catheter and stay suture on the glans penis are removed on day 7

- The patient is discharged on day 8

Urethroplasty (1 year after first-stage operation)

Operative technique step by step

- A stay suture is placed on the glans penis with 3/0 Prolene

- Hair roots of the ventral penis are fulgurated by diathermy

- An oval skin incision is made including the proximal meatus and the opening of the glanular urethra (Figure 15)

- The ventral skin of the penis is dissected between the dartos and Buck's fascias, using sharp and blunt dissection (Figure 16)

- The ventral skin around the proximal meatus and the opening of the glanular urethra is ablated (Figures 17 and 18)

- A Nélaton catheter (10 Fr) is placed through the glanular meatus into the bladder and the bilateral edge of the median skin belt is sutured over the Nélaton catheter with 5/0 PDS sutures (Figure 19). Complete tubularization is not necessary, if the skin is too tight. The suture knot is made on the inner side of the tube with continuous PDS sutures (5/0). Care should be taken not to suture the skin itself but to suture only subcutaneous tissue

- Bilateral skin flaps are adapted by water-tight continuous subcutaneous suturing of the dartos fascia with Prolene or nylon (5/0 or 6/0) in two layers (Figures 20 and 21)

- The third suture layer is skin adaptation using the same suturing technique (Figure 22a). The distal ends of the three Prolene sutures are brought out on the dorsal side of the glans, passed through a sponge fragment and fixed by a small lead fishing sinker. The proximal sutures are also passed through a piece of sponge and fixed by fishing sinker (Figure 22b). The two sponge fragments are used to prevent compression necrosis. The Prolene sutures on the side of the glans penis and the urethral catheter are fixed on the lower abdomen with bandage

Postoperative care

- Oral antibiotics are recommended for 2 weeks

- Nebacetin powder is applied to the penile wound every day for 2 weeks

- The urethral catheter is removed after filling the bladder with saline on day 5. A patient can void smoothly as soon as the urethral catheter is removed (Figure 23)

- The three Prolene sutures are cut between the fishing sinker and the sponge fragment on the glans side on day 10, and the sutures spontaneously fall off in a day

- The patient is discharged on day 11

Results

This technique was used on 420 patients with hypospadias between 1980 and 1990. Postoperative fistula formation was seen in only 18 (4.3%), stenosis in three (0.7%), and diverticulum in two (0.5%).

References

1. Crawford BS. The management of hypospadias. *Br J Clin Pract* 17 (1963) 273–80.
2. Ikoma F. Hypospadiekorrektur nach Denis Browne. In: Hohenfellner R (ed.) *Äusseres Genitale in Ausgewählte Urologische OP-Techniken. Einzeldarstellungen.* Stuttgart: Georg Thieme, pp. 4.77–4.90, 1994.
3. Hodgson NB. A one-stage hypospadias repair. *J Urol* 104 (1970) 281–3.
4. Mays HB. Hypospadias: a concept of treatment. *J Urol* 65 (1951) 279–87.
5. Ikoma F, Shima H, Yabumoto H. Classification of enlarged prostatic utricle in patients with hypospadias. *Br J Urol* 57 (1985) 334–7.
6. Yabumoto H, Fichtner J, Shima H, Ikoma F, Sakamoto H, Furuyama J. Chromosomen Störungen bei Hypospadien? Eine Analyse bei 131 Patienten. *Urologe A.* 31 (1992) 227–30.
7. Shima H, Okamoto E, Uematsu K, Ikoma F. True hermaphroditism: pre- and postoperative evaluation of gonadal function and the necessity of endoscopic examination for the search of cervix uteri at an early stage of diagnosis. *Int Urol Nephrol* 23 (1991) 495–502.
8. Shima H, Ikoma F, Terakawa T *et al.* Developmental anomalies with hypospadias. *J Urol* 122 (1979) 619–21.
9. Ikoma F, Shima H. Hypospadia Penis: Chirurgische Korrektur und Ergebnisse bei 272 Fällen. *Akt Urol* 9 (1978) 155–61.

First operation

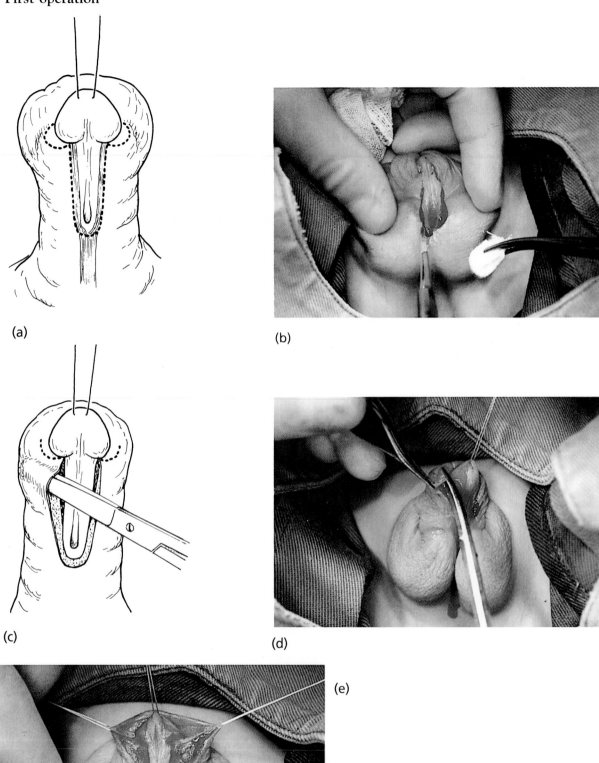

(a)

(b)

(c)

(d)

(e)

Figure 1. *A stay suture, U-shape skin incision and extension of the incision along the corona of the glans (dotted line).*

(a)

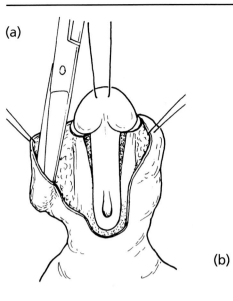

(b)

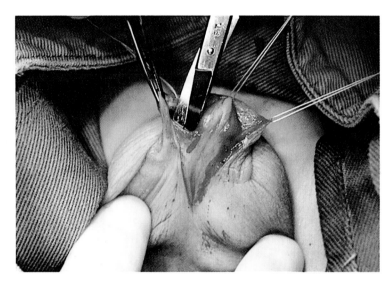

Figure 2. *Ablation of the ventral skin on both sides.*

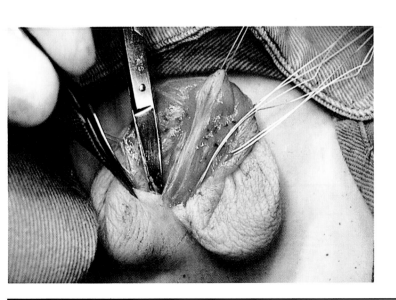

Figure 3. *Sharp dissection of the skin over the urethra.*

(a)

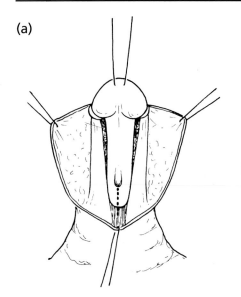

(b)

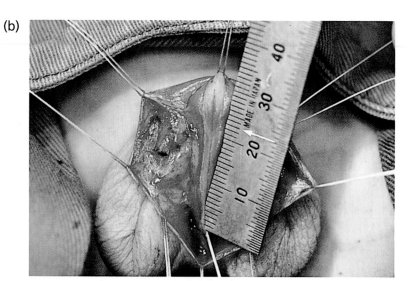

Figure 4. *Ablation of the skin around the meatus, and excision of the meatus back to normal corpus spongiosum tissue.*

(a)

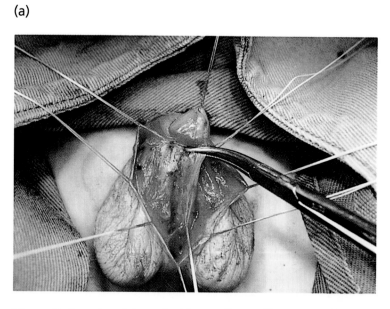

Figure 5. *Grasping of the cord with a small curved hemostat at the corona of the glans.*

(b)

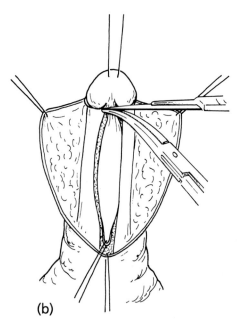

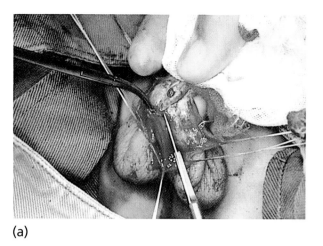

(a)

(c)

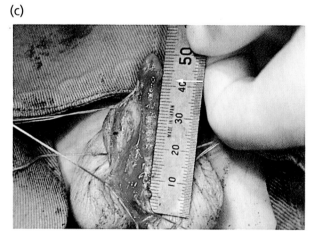

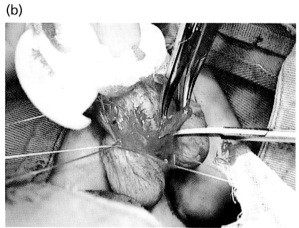

(b)

Figure 6. *Sharp dissection of the cord. An assistant pushes aside the dorsum of the penis.*

(a)

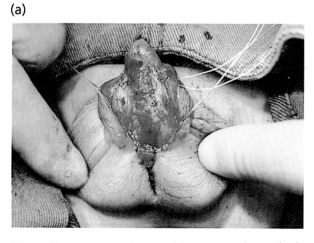

(b)

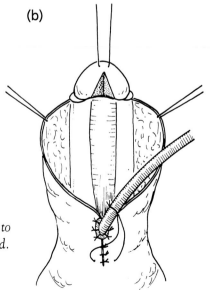

Figure 7. *The meatus is formed by suturing the urethral stump to penile skin with 5/0 PDS. A urethral catheter (10 Fr) is placed.*

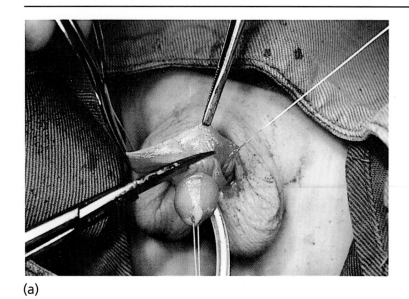

(a)

Figure 8. *Circumcision and stretching of the dorsal prepuce.*

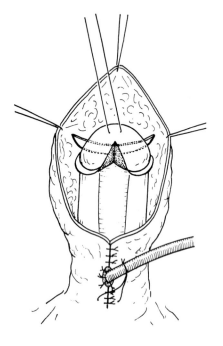

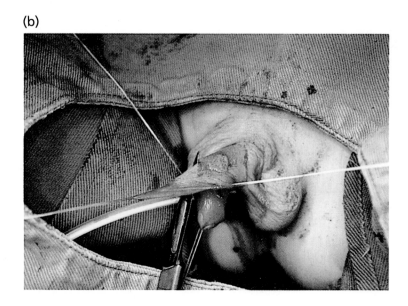

(b)

(c)

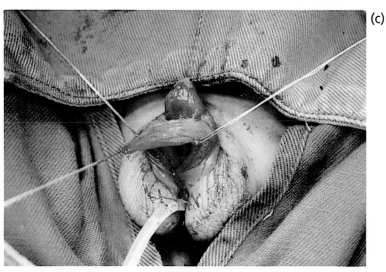

Figure 9. *An adequate window is made at the stretched prepuce. The glans penis is pulled through the window.*

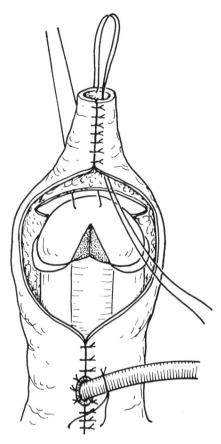

Figure 10. *Tubularization of the prepuce with a continuous 5/0 PDS suture.*

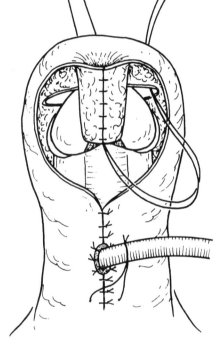

Figure 11. *The skin tube is turned inside-out by grasping the stay suture at the tube end.*

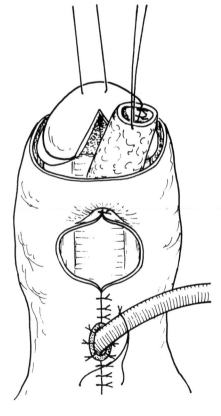

Figure 12. *The reversed skin tube is pulled out through the window.*

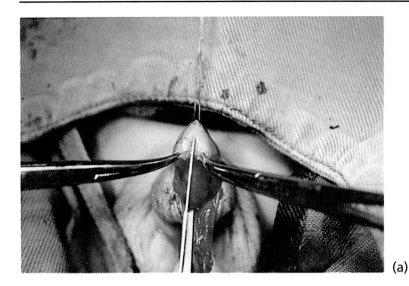

(a)

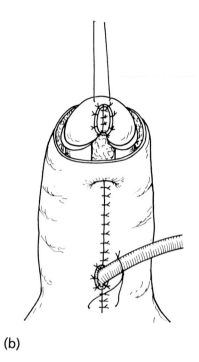

Figure 13. *An incision is made in the ventral side of the glans, and the skin tube is used to form the glanular urethra with 5/0 PDS suture.*

(b)

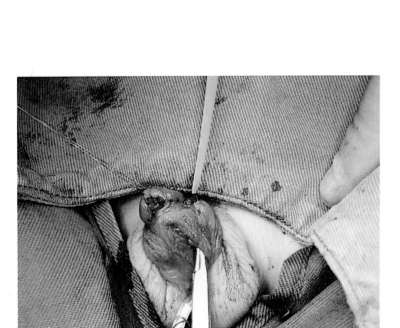

(a)

(b)

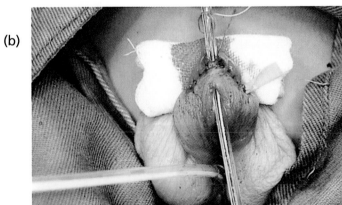

Figure 14. *Insertion of a Penrose drain in the wound, fixation of the glans penis to the lower abdomen, and insertion of a Nélaton catheter (8 Fr) in the glanular urethra.*

Second operation (after one year)

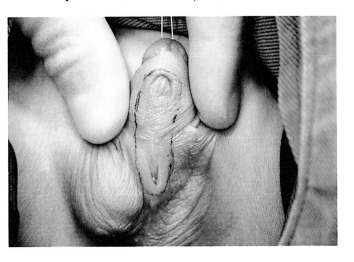

Figure 15. *Skin incision for urethroplasty (one year later). The median skin belt is about 10 mm in width. Electrofulguration of the hair roots around the urethral meatus is necessary. A deep skin incision, down to Buck's fascia, is important around the urethral meatus.*

(a)

(b)

(c)

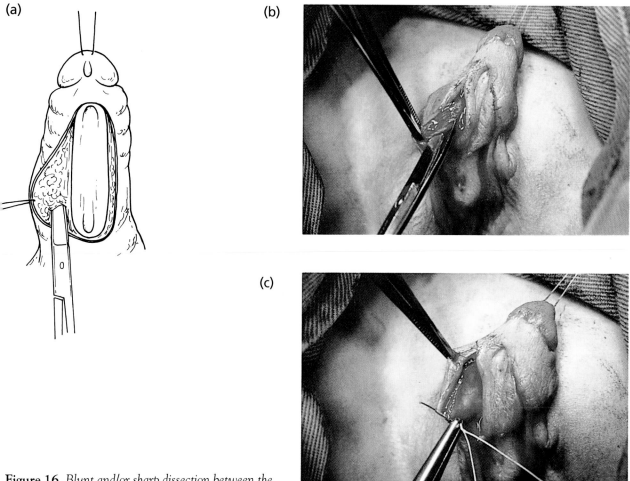

Figure 16. *Blunt and/or sharp dissection between the dartos fascia and Buck's fascia, and skin ablation.*

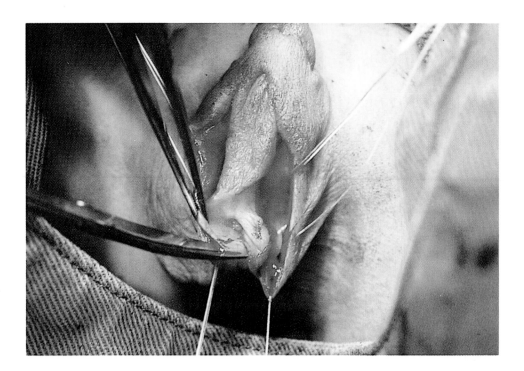

Figure 17. *Dissection between the dartos fascia and Buck's fascia around the urethral meatus.*

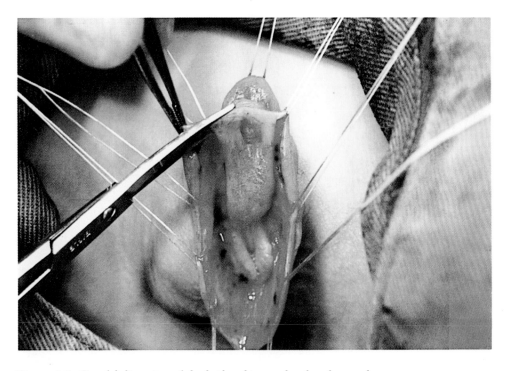

Figure 18. *Careful dissection of the bridge skin on the glanular urethra.*

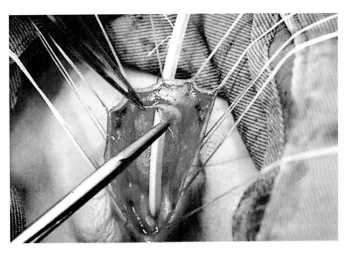

Figure 19. *Insertion of a urethral catheter (10 Fr) through the glanular urethra into the bladder, and tubularization of the buried median skin belt with 5/0 PDS suture. The suture knot is made on the inner side of the tubularized median skin belt. Care must be taken that tubularization over the catheter is not too tight.*

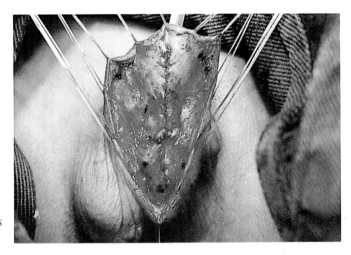

Figure 20. *The first layer of water-tight continuous subcutaneous suture with Prolene (5/0 or 6/0).*

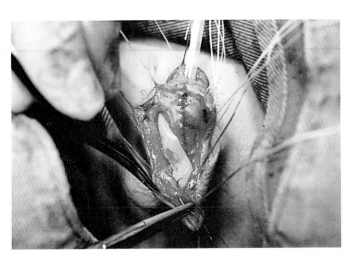

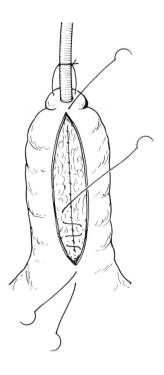

Figure 21. *The second layer of continuous subcutaneous suture with Prolene (5/0 or 6/0).*

(a)

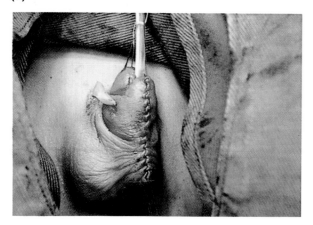

Figure 22. *The third layer is the suture of continuous adaptation of skin flaps. Three Prolene sutures are brought out on the dorsal side of the glans, passed through a sponge fragment, and fixed using a fishing sinker. The proximal part of fixed in the same way.*

(b)

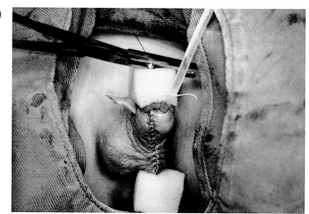

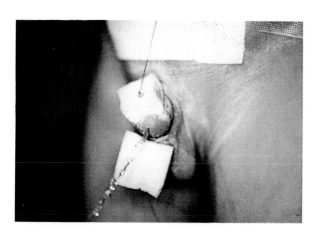

Figure 23. *Smooth voiding after removal of the urethral catheter on day 5.*

Microsurgical Vasovasostomy

R.A. Bürger, U. Witzsch, R. Stein,
L. Franzaring, U. Engelmann[a]
Department of Urology,
University of Mainz School of Medicine,
Mainz, Germany
[a]University of Cologne,
Cologne, Germany

Comment

All surgical progress is related to its results. Microsurgery not only opens up the surgical field but also shows astonishing success in terms of functional results. It is now possible to reattach phalanges and whole limbs, and to transplant nerves to treat unilateral paresis.

Microsurgical techniques are now standard in urology. Discussion on the means of and necessity for microscopic magnification were followed by experimentation. As always, when satisfying results are being achieved with existing knowledge and techniques, new techniques that are difficult to learn raise controversial discussion. They call for an individual interest in microsurgery, patience, a steady hand and an immense amount of practice. Progress means reaching even better than good results. However, microsurgery has opened up new dimensions for urogenital surgery. For example, it allows extracorporeal workbench surgery on the kidney, including vessel reconstruction techniques. Auto-transplantation of abdominal testicles is possible only with the use of an operating microscope. In plastic surgery of infants and in revascularization for erectile dysfunction, magnification guarantees an atraumatic preparation and exact adaptation. There is no question that vasovasostomy and epididymovasostomy performed in a microsurgical manner are the gold standard now. These frequent procedures, which have a dramatic influence on a patient's personal life and family planning, lead to a result-oriented optimization of operative techniques.

These authors show in a clear manner the microsurgical technique of vasovasostomy and epididymovasostomy. The procedure is easily followed step by step with the aid of excellent drawings. To learn and perform the new technique is basic for all modifications of handling and further developments.

An initial 9/0 all-layer stay suture at the 6 o'clock position for fixation of both vas deferens ends gives good visibility and exposure. From 6 to 12 o'clock adaptation of the mucosa with 10/0 single stitches under visual control and 9/0 single stitches in the muscular layer between the mucosal sutures complete the anastomosis. Instead of special vas approximators, Backhouse clamps can be used for approximation of both vasa deferentia ends via fixation at the connective tissue. Fixation of the vas deferens at the epdidymis is of major importance for adaptation of the mucosa in tubulovasostomies. The dissected vas deferens ends must be close to the prepared epididymal tubules for tension-free 11/0 single stitches. Good visibility of the vas and tubular mucosa must be guaranteed. Tying of the first suture opens the tubular lumen and aids positioning and tying of additional sutures. Experience generates confidence and leads to individual techniques being developed by each microsurgeon.

Microsurgical procedures on the human reproductive organ system are state of the art at a time when assisted reproductive techniques are developing and ICSI is giving new impulses to *in vitro* fertilization. Microsurgical operations aim for a natural adaptation of the germ cells, and microsurgical preparation and intervention techniques have an important role in specialized reproductive medicine.

Gunter Konrad, Mönchengladbach, Germany

Vasovasostomy: A Microsurgical Technique

Introduction

Most vasovasostomies are done after a previous vasectomy. Approximately 6% of vasectomized men desire reversal.[1] Other indications include localized congenital, inflammatory or traumatic occlusions of both ducts. Using microsurgical techniques a patency rate of nearly 70% is possible.[2,3] The use of an operating microscope guarantees atraumatic and vessel-sparing vas preparation. The two-layer technique[4] allows exact adaptation of lumina of different widths and a water-tight suture.

Preoperative diagnostics

- Semen analysis (azoospermia, pH >7)
- Ejaculate culture if more than 10 million white blood cells per ml (beware of secondary obstruction in ongoing infection)
- Hormone determination (follicle stimulating hormone and testosterone must be normal)

Counselling and consent

Patients should be informed of the following:

- There is a negative correlation between pregnancy rate and duration of occlusion
- Elevated sperm antibody titres are no contraindication
- There is a 4% incidence of postoperative secondary duct occlusion[5]

Anesthesia

- General anesthesia because of the operating time of 2–3 hours
- Regional anesthesia plus analgesia and sedation on cases where there is pulmonary or cardiac risk
- Before beginning anesthesia, a single shot of a second-generation cephalosporin should be given

Instruments and suture material

- Operating microscope, 200 mm lens 6–24 × magnification
- Standard microsurgical instruments
- Tendon forceps with guiding slot and special lancet (S & T Marketing, Neuhausen, Switzerland)
- Lacrimal probe (Aesculap, Tuttlingen, Germany)
- Teflon baby cannulas G26 (Critikon, Norderstedt, Germany)
- Microspike vas approximator (ASSI Corporation, Westbury, New York, USA)
- Mucosal suture: 10/0 nylon double-armed fishing-hook shaped (Sharpoint, Raguse, Ascheberg-Herbern, Germany)
- Musculature suture: 9/0 nylon tapered cut point

Operative technique step by step (Figure 1–8)

Macrosurgery
- 3 cm bilateral incision at the upper third of the scrotum
- If needed, inguinal elongation
- Alternative: infrapubic incision
- Exteriorization of the duct for a short defect
- Extrusion of the scrotal contents for a long defect or a vasectomy site close to the epididymis
- Preparation of the duct for 2 cm proximal and distal to the vasectomy site, taking care to preserve the vascular and nervous supply

Microsurgery
- Hold the vas with atraumatic tendon forceps
- Transection of the duct in a well-vascularized nonfibrotic area
- Microscopic examination of the harvested fluid
- If no fluid drips out spontaneously, massage of the epididymis or step-by-step transection up to the pars convoluta of the ductus deferens
- Vasovasostomy if sperm are evident
- Tubulovasostomy following epididymal exploration if sperm are not evident
- Vasovasostomy in azoospermia with clear liquid is possible (patency rate 60%, pregnancy rate 30%)[2]

- Proving the patency of the abdominal end with gentle injection of 5 ml normal saline

- If abdominal occlusion is suspected, vasography with low-viscosity contrast media

- Tension-free approximation of both ends of the duct with vasovasostomy clamps

- For long ductal defects, separation of the vas from the epididymis; in special cases, flipping the testis upside down with inguinal or pelvic mobilization of the ductus deferens

- Suture of the mucosal layer with 10/0 nylon for correction of the different luminal dilatations of the ends

- Exact suturing of the mucosa, stitching from the inside out using double-armed fishing-hook-shaped needles

- After tying the three or four anterior sutures flip the approximating clamps through 180°

- Exposure of the lumen by adjusting the angle of the approximating clamps

- Suture of the posterior wall

- Stabilization of the anastomosis with 10–12 9/0 nylon muscular sutures

- Insertion of an 8 Fr suction drain and closure of the wound layer by layer

Postoperative care

- Supportive underwear for 2 weeks

- No sexual intercourse or heavy work for 3 weeks

- Semen analysis at 6, 12, 24, 36 and 52 weeks

- If no sperm are seen after 6 months, occlusion of the anastomosis or epididymis must be suspected

- During the first postoperative year there is a continuing increase in sperm count

References

1. Engelmann U, Deindl F, Hertle L, Wilbert D, Senge T. Die Refertilisierungssituation in der Bundesrepublik Deutschland: Ergebnisse einer Umfrage. *Urologe B* **29** (1989) 29–33.
2. Belker AM, Thomas AJ Jr, Fuchs EF, Konnak JW, Sharlip ID. Results of 1469 microsurgical vasectomy reversals by the vasovasostomy study group. *J Urol* **145** (1991) 505–11.
3. Sharlip ID. What is the best pregnancy rate that may be expected from vasectomy reversal? *J Urol* **149** (1993) 1469–71.
4. Silber SJ. Perfect anatomical reconstruction of the vas deferens with a new microscopic surgical technique. *Fertil Steril* **28** (1977) 72–7.
5. Belker AM, Fuchs EF, Konnak JW, Sharlip ED, Thomas AJ Jr. Transient fertility after vasovasostomy in 892 patients. *J Urol* **134** (1985) 75–6.
6. Meinertz H, Linnet L, Fogh-Anderson P, Hjort T. Antisperm antibodies and fertility after vasovasostomy: a follow-up study of 216 men. *Fertil Steril* **54** (1990) 315–21.

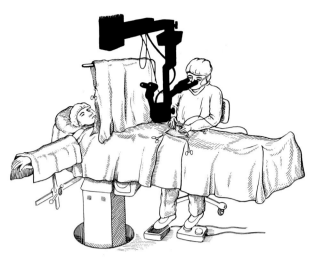

Figure 1. *Positioning the patient on a special operating table allows the surgeon and an assistant to sit comfortably with their knees under the table.*

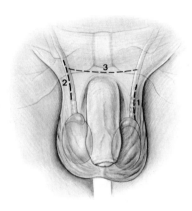

Figure 2. *The incision depends on the resection site (determined by palpation). Infrapubic incision after bilateral high resection.*

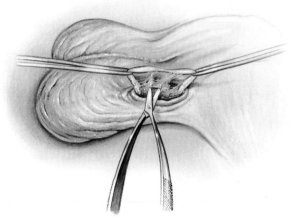

(a)

Figure 3. *(a) For short vasectomies with a mobile vas deferens, mobilization of the duct is sufficient. (b) Extrusion of the scrotal contents may be necessary in resections proximal to the epididymal opening of the tunica vaginalis.*

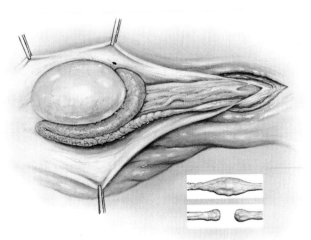

(b)

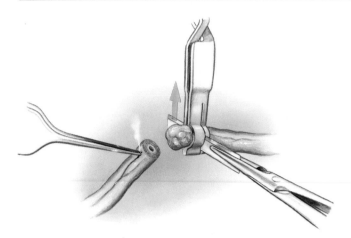

Figure 4. (a) Atraumatic fixation of the vas ends for well-vascularized areas with a smooth cross-section. Accurate coagulation with bipolar forceps.

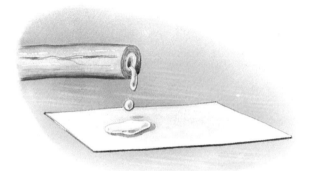

Figure 4. (b) Harvesting and immediate microscopic examination of the liquid dripping out of the distal stump.

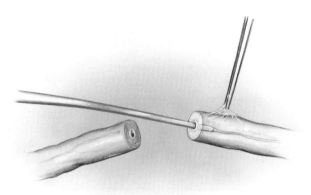

Figure 4. (c) Gentle dilatation of the proximal lumen with the lacrimal probe.

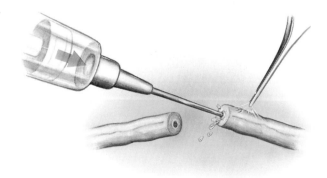

Figure 4. (d) Injection of 5 ml normal saline to test the patency of the cranial end.

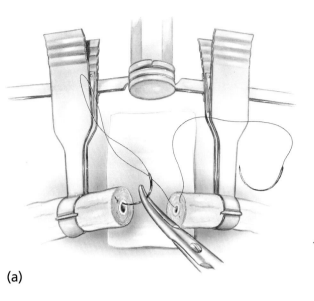

(a)

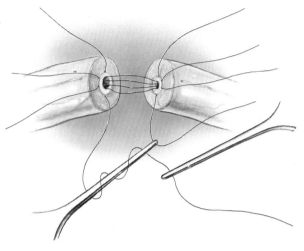

(b)

Figure 5. *Tension-free fixation of the vas ends. Anastomosis of the anterior wall with three or four mucosal sutures (nylon 10/0 double armed).*

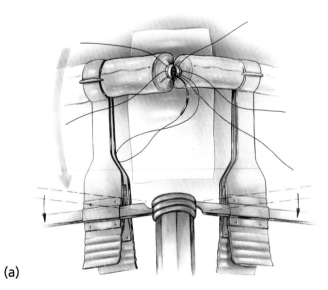

(a)

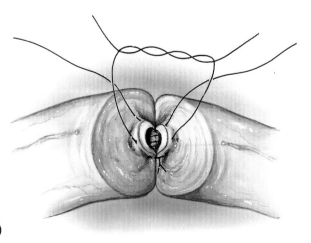

(b)

Figure 6. *Flipping of the approximating clamps and adjusting their angle for mucosal suturing of the posterior wall. Placing of all sutures, then tying.*

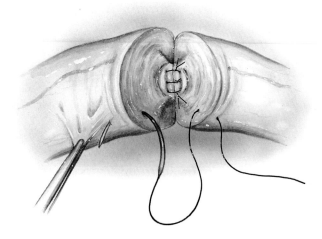

(a)

Figure 7. *Circular adaptation of the muscular layer of the vas deferens with 10–12 peripheral single stitches (nylon 9/0 taper needle).*

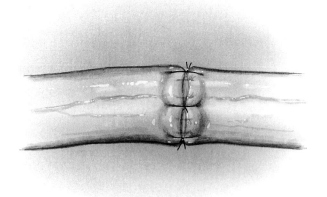

(b)

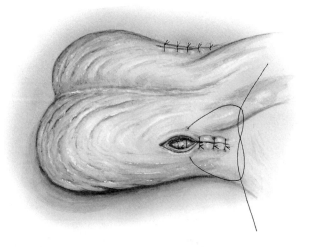

Figure 8. *Closure of the wound with single stitches (plain catgut 4/0).*

Microsurgical Vasoepididymostomy

R.A. Bürger, U. Witzsch, J. Leissner,
R. Stein, U. Engelmann[a]
Department of Urology,
University of Mainz School of Medicine,
Mainz, Germany
[a]University of Cologne,
Cologne, Germany

Introduction

Operating microscopes allow selective anastomosis between sperm-carrying epididymal tubules and the mucosa of the ductus deferens (vasotubulostomy). End-to-side and end-to-end techniques are possible and give patency rates of 70% and pregnancy rates of more than 40%. Results depend on the localization of the anastomosis: the outcome is best if the anastomosis is at the cauda epididymis.[1–3]

Preoperative diagnostics

- Palpation of ductus and epididymis (beware of aplasia)
- Semen analysis (azoospermia, pH >7, volume >1 ml)
- Ejaculation culture if more than 10 million white blood cells per ml are detected
- If the follicle stimulating hormone level is elevated more than three times, indicating irreversible damage of the testicular tubular tissue, no operation is indicated
- No preoperative vasography (secondary obstruction)
- Testicular biopsy if testicular size and follicle stimulating hormone levels are normal

Counselling and consent

Patients should be informed of:

- The incidence of secondary obstruction (13–40%)[1]
- The possibility of assisted reproduction techniques[4]

Anesthesia

- General anesthesia because of the operating time of 3–4 hours

Instruments and suture materials

- Operating microscope, 200 mm lens 6–24 × magnification
- Standard microsurgical instruments
- Tendon forceps with guiding slot and special lancet (S & T Marketing, Neuhausen, Switzerland)
- Lacrimal probe (Aesculap, Tuttlingen, Germany)
- Teflon baby cannulas G26 (Critikon, Norderstedt, Germany)
- Microspike vas approximator (ASSI Corporation, Westbury, New York, USA)
- Mucosal suture: 10/0 nylon double-armed fishing-hook-shaped (Sharpoint, Raguse, Ascheberg-Herbern, Germany)
- Musculature suture: 9/0 nylon tapered cut point
- 11/0 nylon suture for anastomosing the vas mucosa to the epididymal tubules

Operative technique step by step (Figures 1–10)

- Lateral scrotal vertical incision and extrusion of the scrotal contents
- Opening of the tunica vaginalis for inspection and gentle palpation of the ductus deferens and epididymis. In congenital disorders, anstomosis may not be possible
- In dilated epididymal tubules, section of the vas deferens at the beginning of the pars convoluta
- In normal epididymis, semicircular incision of the ductus close to the epididymis
- Aspiration of the liquid from the epididymal part and control of patency of the abdominal end (injection of 5 ml normal saline)
- If patency is proven at the abdominal end the problem should be in the epididymal part
- Total section of the vas deferens close to the epididymis

End-to-side anastomosis

If the dilated tubules are visualized, the covering tunica vaginalis is excised circularly (diameter approximately 5 mm). If no dilated tubules are microscopically detectable, the first tunica incision is located at the cauda epididymis. After preparation and longitudinal incision of a single tubular loop the extruding fluid is aspirated by a Teflon cannula and microscopically examined for complete spermatozoa. If no intact spermatozoa are seen, this procedure is repeated step-wise towards the caput epididymis until normal spermatozoa are found. Motility is not necessary. For a tension-free anastomosis, the ductal muscularis is fixated with two or three 9/0 nylon sutures at the lower margin of the tunica incision. Three to five 10/0 or 11/0 nylon sutures are used for the anastomosis between the tubule and the mucosa of the vas deferens. Then additional nylon 9/0 sutures complete the fixation of the muscularis to the epididymal tunica.

End-to-end anastomosis

After separation from the tunica vaginalis of the testis, the cauda epididymis is transected. The use of tendon forceps and a razor blade guarantees a smooth incision. After accurate bipolar coagulation, the transected epididymis is explored for secreting tubules. If no complete spermatozoa can be found, additional transections closer to the caput epididymis are necessary. A special approximator stabilizes the ductus and epididymal surface. The anastomosis is started with two posterior mucosa–tubule sutures (10/0 nylon double armed). Stitching from the inside out avoids accidental suture of the contralateral wall. Two or three additional anterior mucosal sutures are first positioned and then tied. Additional sutures (10/0 nylon with a taper-point needle) are placed between the muscular layer of the ductus and the epididymal tunica to stabilize the anastomosis.

Postoperative care

- Oral antibiotics for 5–7 days

- Supportive underwear for 3–4 weeks

- No sexual intercourse or physical work for 4 weeks

- Semen analyses after 6 and 12 weeks, then every 3 months until the first sperm are seen: there may be an interval of 9–18 months

- Increasing sperm counts are seen during the first 3 years

References

1. Kar JK, Phadke AM. Vaso-epididymal anastomosis. *Fertil Steril* **26** (1975) 743–56.
2. Lee HY. A 20-year experience with epididymovasostomy for pathologic epididymal obstruction. *Fertil Steril* **47** (1987) 487–91.
3. Palermo G, Joris H, Derde M-P, Camus M, Devroey P, van Steirteghem A. Sperm characteristics and outcome of human assisted fertilization by subzonal insemination and intracytoplasmic sperm injection. *Fertil Steril* **59** (1993) 826–35.
4. Bürger RA, Stein R, Witzsch U, Engelmann U. Vasovasostomie in mikrochirurgischer Technik. *Akt Urol* **25** (1994) Operative Techniken, chapter 5.11.
5. Schegel PN, Goldstein M. Microsurgical vasoepididymostomy: refinements and results. *J Urol* **150** (1993) 1165–8.

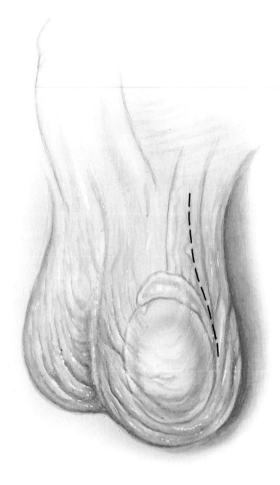

Figure 1. *Scrotal vertical incision for exploration of the ductus and epididymis.*

End-to-side anastomosis

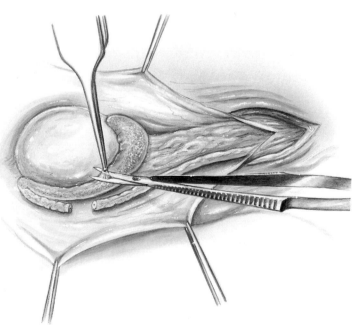

Figure 2. *Section of the vas deferens before the beginning of the pars convoluta and examination for patency in the proximal part. Circular fenestration of the tunica vaginalis in the area between the epididymal cauda and the corpus.*

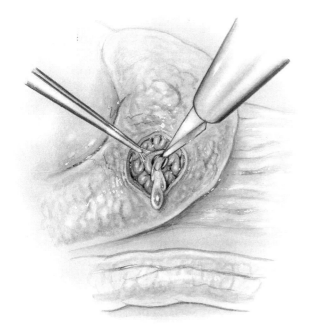

Figure 3. *Preparation and longitudinal incision of a single tubular loop.*

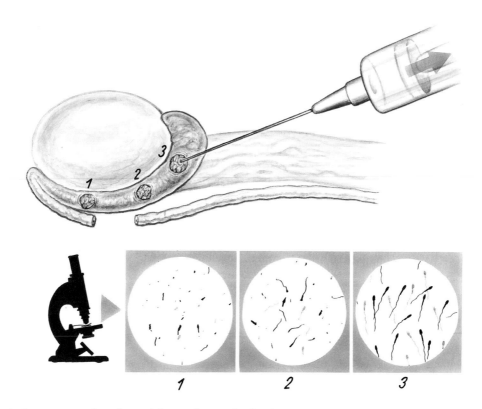

Figure 4. *Aspiration and analysis of the outflowing fluid. This step is repeated until complete sperms are detected.*

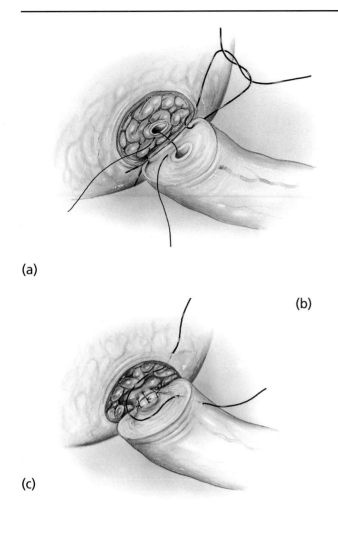

(a)

(b)

(c)

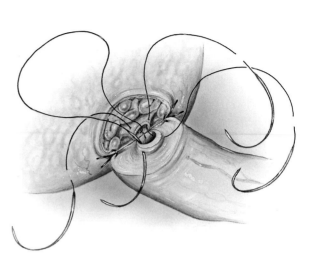

Figure 5. *(a,b) Adaptation of the muscular layer of the ductus deferens and tunica vaginalis of the epididymis with two or three single stitches (nylon 9/0). (c) Anastomosis between the tubular wall and the mucosa of the vas deferens (nylon 9/0).*

Figure 6. *Completion of the muscularis–tunica sutures (nylon 9/0).*

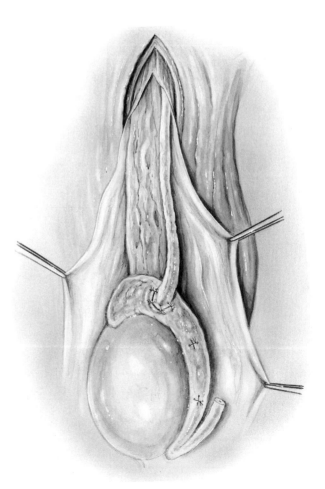

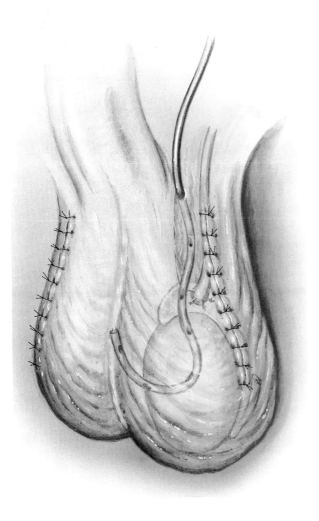

Figure 7. *Placing of an 8 Fr suction drain and closure of the wound layer-wise with plain catgut 4/0.*

End-to-end anastomosis

Figure 8. *Separation of the cauda epididymis. Horizontal incision for separation of the ductus from the epididymis.*

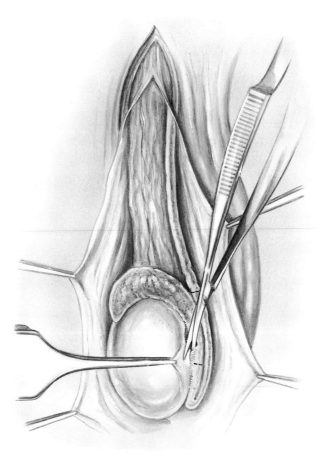

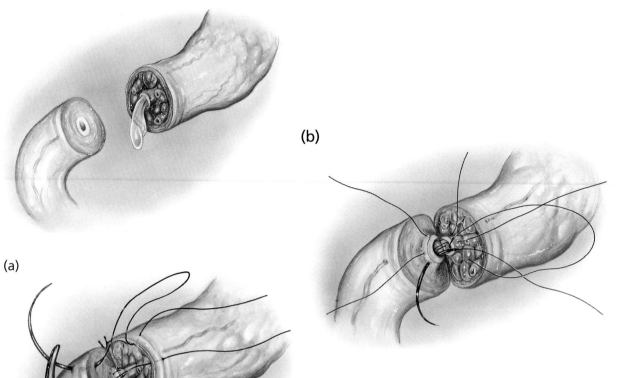

(a)

(b)

(c)

Figure 9. *(a) Identification of single tubules where fluid is dripping out. (b) Two-layer suture of the ductus and epididymis (four tubule–mucosa sutures (nylon 10/0) and (c) 12–16 tunica–muscularis sutures (nylon 9/0)).*

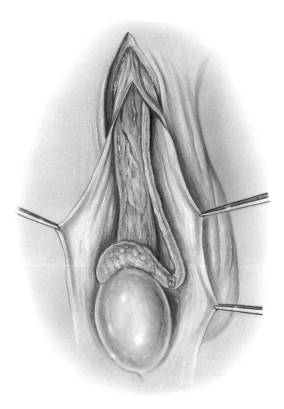

Figure 10. *After finishing the anastomosis, layered closure of the wound.*

Milling out of the Plaque and Modified Nesbit Procedure in Patients with Peyronie's Disease

R. Stein, S.C. Müller[a], R. Hohenfellner
Department of Urology,
University of Mainz School of Medicine,
Mainz, Germany
[a]University of Bonn,
Bonn, Germany

Introduction

Peyronie's disease[1] was first described in 1743. Spontaneous remission is possible, but conservative forms of treatment mostly fail.[2] Surgical intervention includes the Nesbit procedure at the contralateral site, excision of the plaque and filling with a dermal graft of lyophilized dura, tunica vaginalis, fascia temporalis, Dracon or GORE-TEX (W.L. Gore, Woking, UK).[2-6] After complete excision and filling of the defect there is a high risk of impotence, which can be corrected by penile prosthesis.[2,3]

Our technique consists of milling out the plaque without injury of the corpora cavernosa and, if necessary, with correction of the deviation by a modified Nesbit procedure.

Indications

- Failure of conservative treatment
- Inability to achieve intercourse
- Severe penile deviation associated with painful erection

Preoperative requirements

- Photographs of the erect penis in two planes are required
- The patient should be counselled that the procedure includes circumcision

Operative risks

- Impotence (prosthesis)
- Shortening of the penis
- Remaining or new deviation

Special instruments and materials

- Electric dental drill with face milling cutter (Storz)
- GORE-TEX suture CV-3
- Vessel loops
- Melolin nonadhesive dressing (Smith and Nephew, Hull, UK)

Anesthesia

- Insufflation anesthesia

Operative technique step by step (Figures 1–8)

- Supine position
- Placement of a stay suture at the glans
- Subcoronal (5 mm) circular incision of the inner layer of the prepuce (in circumcised men, along the old scar)
- Tourniquet at the penile basis (released every 20 minutes)
- Reflection of the skin to the base by blunt and sharp dissection between the layer of the dartos fascia (Scarpa's fascia) and the tunica albuginea of the corpora cavernosa (there is no bleeding in this space)
- Careful dissection of the dorsal arteries and nerves of the glans from the tunica albuginea 1–2 cm proximal and distal to the plaque (by slightly lifting with the vessel loops)
- Mobilization of the urethra (beware of injury followed by fistula or stricture)
- Marking of the plaque, and milling out of the hard plaque with the dental drill until the face milling cutter encounters elastic resistance at the bottom of the plaque (the fascia is thin, so beware of perforation of the corpora cavernosa); permanent cooling of the dental drill with 0.9% saline solution
- Artificial erection (0.9% saline); extension of the penis with the stay suture
- Lifting of the urethra (vessel loops) and gathering of the tunica albuginea with Allis clamps at the maximal part of the curvature and marking at both ends when the penis is straight
- Renewed artificial erection to demonstrate the extent of the penile deviation
- Oval excision of the tunica albuginea along the markings (over a length of 1 cm and 2–3 mm width)
- Placement of a double-armed GORE-TEX suture (CV-3) going from inside to outside; during tying (five knots), the knots should be made below
- Renewed artificial erection and if necessary renewed modified Nesbit procedure
- In patients with the plaque on the ventral side a mirror-image of this procedure is performed
- Final circumcision prevents edema and hematoma
- Adaptation of the skin with catgut 4/0
- Dexpanthenol and Melolin
- Nonadhesive wound dressing; the glans remains uncovered to maintain the circulation

Postoperative care

- Removal of the wound dressing 5 days after surgery

References

1. Peyronie F de la. Sur quelques obstacles qui s'opposent a l'elaculation naturelle de la semence. *Mem Acad R Chir* (1743) 425.
2. Benson GS. Peyronie's disease: editorial comment. *J Urol* **149** (1993) 1326.
3. Dalkin BL, Carter MF. Venogenic impotence following dermal graft repair for Peyronie's disease. *J Urol* **146** (1991) 849–51.
4. Devine CJ, Jordan GH, Schlossberg SM. Surgery of the penis and urethra. In: Walsh PC, Retik AB, Stamey TA, Vaughan ED (eds) *Campbell's Urology*, 6th edn. New York: W.B. Saunders (1992) 2957–3032.
5. Gelbard MK, Hayden B. Expanding contractures of the tunica albuginea due to Peyronie's disease with temporalis fascia free graft. *J Urol* **145** (1991) 772–6.
6. Nesbit RM. Congenital curvature of the phallus: report of three cases with description of corrective operation. *J Urol* 93 (1965) 230–2.
7. Kelâmi A. Autophotography in evaluation of functional penile disorders. *Urology* **21** (1983) 628–9.

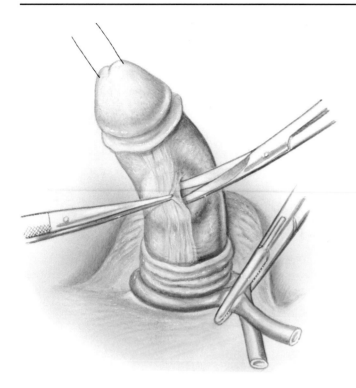

Figure 1. *Stay suture, circular incision, reflection of the skin including the dartos fascia (Scarpa's fascia) to the basis, and mobilization of the dorsal nerves and vessels.*

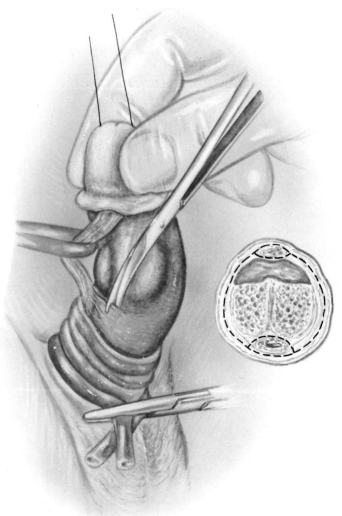

Figure 2. *Lifting of the dorsal vessels and nerves, and mobilization to the base and glans (1–2 cm away from the plaque).*

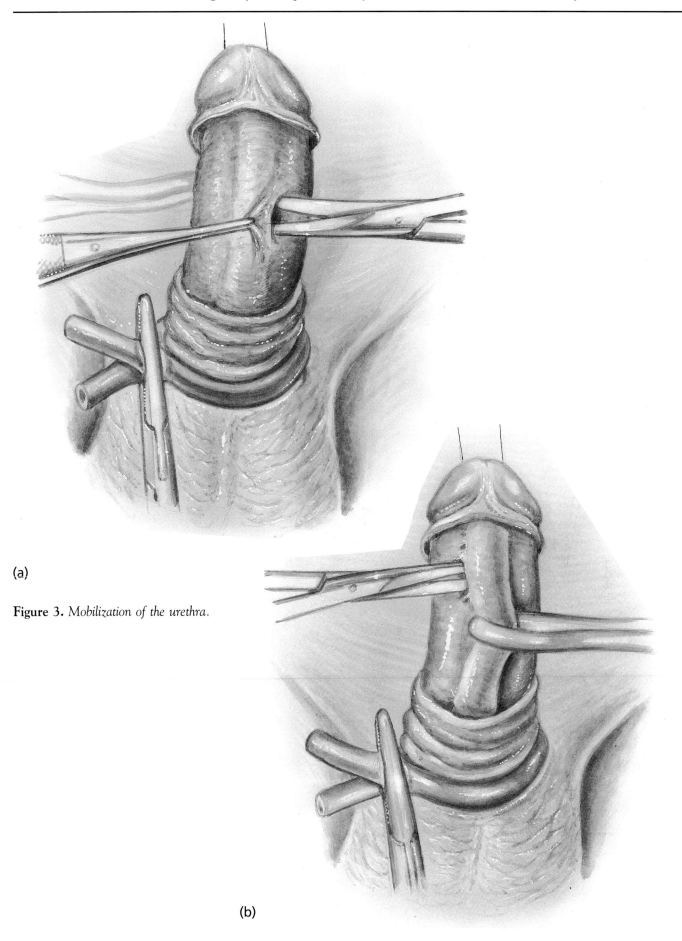

(a)

Figure 3. *Mobilization of the urethra.*

(b)

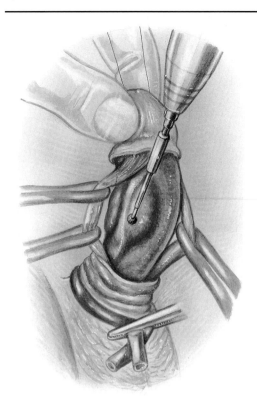

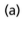

Figure 4. Milling out of the plaque (permanent cooling of the drill with 0.9% sodium chloride solution) until there is only a thin fascia over the corpora cavernosa.

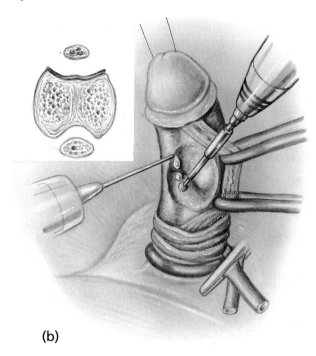

(b)

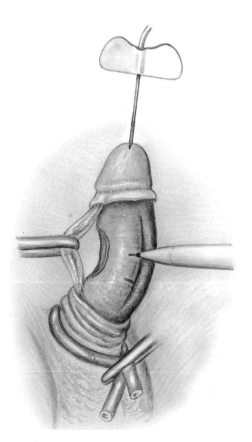

Figure 5. Artificial erection to demonstrate the remaining deviation, and marking of the Nesbit 'windows'.

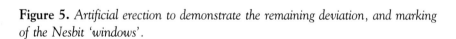

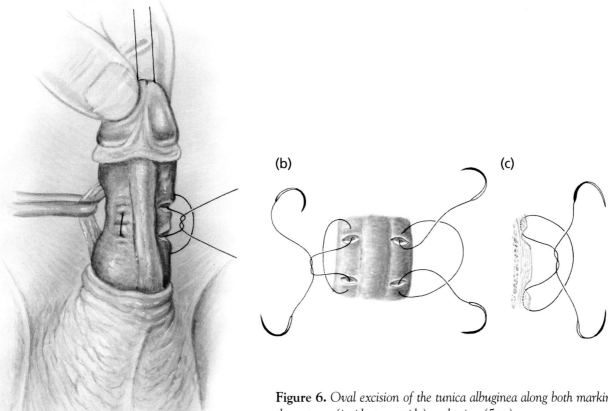

(b)

(c)

Figure 6. *Oval excision of the tunica albuginea along both markings, placement of the sutures (inside to outside) and tying (5 ×).*

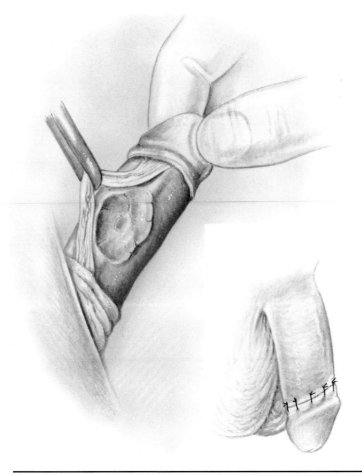

Figure 7. *The modified Nesbit procedure results in an additional extension.*

Figure 8. *Skin closure with interrupted sutures (catgut 4/0).*

Antegrade Scrotal Sclerotherapy for Varicocele

A.M. Mottrie, R.A. Bürger, R. Hohenfellner
Department of Urology,
University of Mainz School of Medicine,
Mainz, Germany

Comment

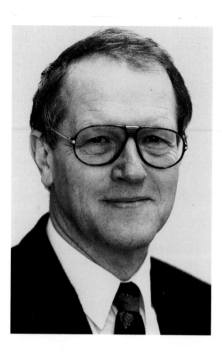

We have performed antegrade sclerotherapy of testicular varicoceles since 1984. We have done more than 2000 of these procedures and we know of many other institutions in which antegrade sclerosing of testicular varicoceles is also a routine procedure.

The technique of varicocele sclerosing is well described in this paper, and we wish only to add some of our experiences.

The described technique is of low cost, has few complications and can be performed on an outpatient basis. The indications can therefore be broad. (The implications of a varicocele and the necessity for treatment remain a subject of discussion. However, there is no doubt that a pathologic sperm count improves after successful treatment of a varicocele.)

The technique is easy for a urologist to learn, but should not be underestimated. Nevertheless, it usually takes only a few minutes to perform this technique (more in some special cases). During training in the technique, suitable patients should be chosen: young slim men with a long scrotal origin and varicocele of degree II or III are best. Preoperatively the spermatic cord should be well palpable. If local anesthesia is applied before the sterile covering, time can be saved. (Sedation is usually not necessary.) The scrotum should be raised.

The effect of all sclerosing drugs depends on injury of the endothelial cells of the intima. An abacterial inflammatory reaction leads to thrombosis of the vessel lumen. The thrombus becomes organized and so the vein is closed.

We use polidocanol. The maximal tolerable dose for men is 2 mg/kg body weight (for a 70 kg man, about 4.6 ml of 3% solution). We recommend 3 ml of a 3% solution for adults and single-sided sclerosing, and 2 ml 3% solution in double-sided sclerosing of testicular varicoceles. In children we have had good results with 3 ml 1% solution on each side.

The sclerosing drug closes refluxive veins because of its inflammatory effect over time, so that sperm counts improve for more than 6 months after sclerosing of the varicocele.

Complications are rare. If the procedure does not succeed (0.4–0.5%), local ligation and resection of the veins can be attempted using the Kocher procedure.

The most common complication is scrotal hematoma (1–2%), which can be prevented by local compression of the scrotum immediately after surgery. If preparation was difficult, a Penrose drain can be placed in the scrotum and should be removed within the next day. Prophylactic treatment with local cooling, heparin salve and oral antiphlogistics, e.g. diclofenac, is possible and is the treatment of choice for abacterial epididymitis. A severe complication is testicular atrophy, which we have seen only in single cases. It is important not to sclerose an artery, as this is usually accompanied by severe scrotal pain: washing out with 1–3% lidocaine solution and injection of 500 units of heparin may help. Ligation of a single artery is unimportant because the artery of the distal seminal cord is multiply branched. There is no incidence of hydroceles after the procedure. Residual or persistent disease has been seen in 0% of first degree, 9% of second degree and 11% of third degree varicoceles. In this case sclerosing can be repeated in the same way.

R. Tauber, Hamburg

Antegrade Scrotal Sclerotherapy for Varicocele

Introduction

A varicocele is an abnormal dilatation of the pampiniform venous plexus. Its association with topographic, histopathologic and functional derangements of the testis is well established. Varicoceles are found in 15% of the adult male population and in 39% of the infertile group.[1,2]

Possible pathophysiologic explanations include:[2]

- High testicular temperature

- Retrograde flow of a toxic substance

- Elevated venous pressure through malfunctioning venous valves or outflow obstruction at the right-angled entrance of the spermatic vein in the left renal vein

Possible histologic changes in testicular tissue include:[1,3]

- Endothelial proliferation of capillaries

- Desquamation of germinative epithelium

- Tubular fibrosis

- Degeneration of Sertoli cells and hyperplasia of Leydig cells

Indications[4]

- Varicocele in OAT syndrome

- Large varicocele in childhood

- Small varicocele in children with low testicular volume

- Recurrence and/or persistence after operative ligation or antegrade or retrograde sclerotherapy

Sclerotherapy is not indicated for:

- Varicocele with azoospermia

- Varicocele with normal sperm analysis

and is of limited value where there is:

- Collateral drainage to the pelvic veins

- Very large varicocele

Results[5-7]

Outpatient treatment (operation time 15–20 minutes) results in:

- Amelioration of sperm analysis in 76% of infertile men

- Paternity in 42%

- Freedom from recurrence/persistence in 91%

Sclerotherapy is technically possible in 83–99.5% of patients.

Instruments

- Standard instruments for interventions on external genitalia

- One vessel loop

- Cannula 24 Fr

- 3% polidocanol

- Local anesthetic (e.g. 1% xylocain)

- Nonionic contrast medium

- 3/0 Dexon 5 × 75 cm

- 4/0 catgut DS19 70 cm

Operative technique step by step (Figures 1–10)

- The procedure is performed under local anesthesia: 5–10 ml of 1% lidocaine is injected at the region of the external inguinal ring with additional infiltration at the scrotal incision site

- The spermatic cord with the scrotal skin is held between the thumb and index finger. An incision of the stretched scrotal skin over a length of 1–1.5 cm is then made one finger lateral and caudal to the base of the penis

- The spermatic cord is mobilized and looped

- After incision of the fascia of the spermatic cord, a vein is isolated from the pampiniform plexus (laterodorsal fatty tissue) and distally ligated

- A 24 Fr cannula is inserted proximally and secured with a single ligature. Injecting a few milliliters of isotonic fluid while inserting the cannula can be helpful

- Using C-arm fluoroscopy and injection of 3–5 ml of nonionic contrast medium (Omnipaque 300, Nycomed,

Birmingham, UK) into the vein, it is possible to delineate the anatomy of venous drainage. It is essential to show that the isolated vein is not draining into major pelvic veins

- The sclerosing agent is injected in an antegrade direction using an air block technique (1 ml of air, followed by 3 ml of the sclerosing agent). The patient is instructed to perform a Valsalva maneuver during injection

- Injection is done only once. The cannula is then removed and the vein ligated proximally. The fascia is closed, the spermatic cord reduced and the skin closed with two stitches using 3/0 catgut. Manual compression of the spermatic cord for about 3–5 minutes is performed for hemostasis.

Postoperative care

- Supportive underwear for 3–5 days
- Avoidance of physical stress for 1 week
- Control examination after 3–6 months: the sclerosing agent initially causes a vasculitis with progressive closure of the total venous lumen over a period of 3 months

References

1. Kass EJ, Belman AB. Reversal of testicular growth failure by varicocele ligation. *J Urol* **137** (1987) 475–6.
2. Thomas AJ, Geisinger MA. Current management of varicoceles. *Urol Clin North Am* **17** (1990) 893–907.
3. Hadziselimovic F, Herzog B, Liebundgut B, Jenny P, Buser M. Testicular and vascular changes in children and adults with varicocele. *J Urol* **142** (1989) 583–5.
4. Weidner W. Varikozele. In: Hautmann (ed.) *Therapie urologischer Erkrankungen*, chapter VIII. Stuttgart: Ferdinand Enke Verlag (1992) S. 210.
5. Tauber R, Johnsen N. Die antegrade skrotale Verödung zur Behandlung der Testisvarikozele. *Urologe A* **32** (1993) 320–6.
6. Tauber R, Johnsen N. Antegrade scrotal sclerotherapy for the treatment of varicocele: technique and late results. *J Urol* **151** (1994) 386–90.
7. Wechsel HW, Strohmaier WL, Bichler K-H. Die antegrade Sklerosierung. *TW Urol Nephrol* **5** (1993) 378–82.

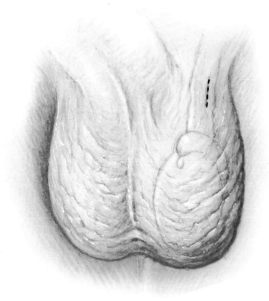

Figure 1. *Scrotal incision 2 cm lateral and caudal to the base of the penis.*

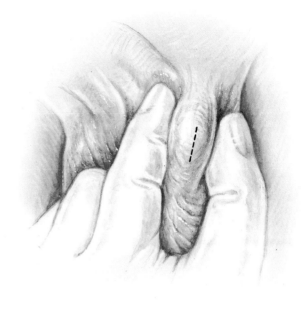

Figure 2. *The spermatic cord is held between the thumb and index finger. The scrotal incision is made over a length of 1–1.5 cm.*

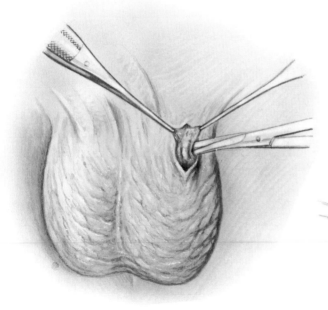

Figure 3. *Mobilization of the spermatic cord.*

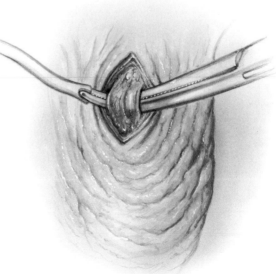

Figure 4. *The spermatic cord is looped and its fascia incised.*

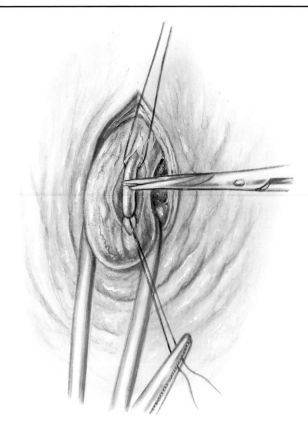

Figure 5. *A vein is located from the pampiniform plexus, ligated distally and incised proximally.*

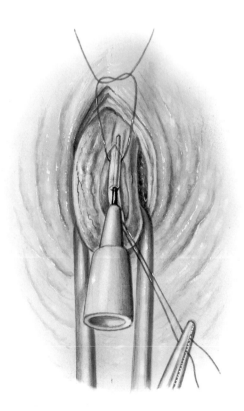

Figure 6. *Insertion and fixation of a 24 g cannula.*

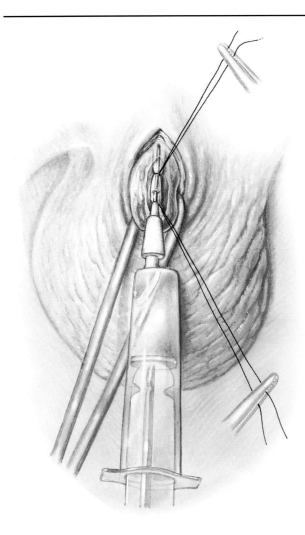

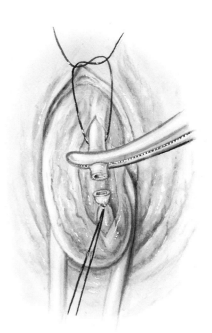

Figure 8. *The cannula is then removed and the vein ligated proximally.*

Figure 7. *1 ml of air, followed by 3 ml of the sclerosing agent, is injected while the patient is performing the Valsalva manoeuvre.*

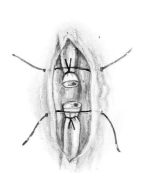

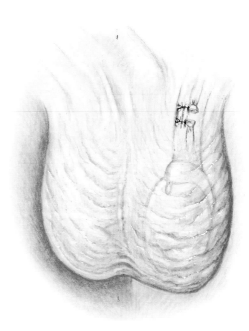

Figure 9. *The fascia of the spermatic cord is closed.*

Figure 10. *The skin is closed with two stitches of 3/0 catgut.*

Circumcision

R. Stein, F. Steinbach[a], R. Hohenfellner
Department of Urology,
University of Mainz School of Medicine,
Mainz, Germany
[a]University of Magdeburg,
Magdeburg, Germany

Introduction

At birth, there is a physiologic phimosis or inability to retract the foreskin in the majority of neonates because of natural adhesions between the prepuce and the glans. During the first 3–4 years of life, as the penis grows, epithelial smegma accumulates under the prepuce, gradually separating the foreskin from the glans.[1] A phimosis can be primary, or secondary due to inflammation or recurrent trauma.

There are a lot of techniques for circumcision; the operation using a scalpel is a safe procedure with excellent cosmetic results.[1–4]

Indications

- Phimosis causing ballooning of the foreskin
- Recurrent balanitis
- Paraphimosis
- Dyspareunia due to a tight frenulum or preputial ring (relative)
- Ritual circumcision
- Cosmetic reasons (extremely long foreskin)

Contraindications

- Hemorrhagic diathesis (relative)
- Suspicion of a carcinoma of the penis

Surgical risks

- In ritual or cosmetic circumcision, the patient should be informed that there is no medical indication for circumcision
- All the complications (see below) should be discussed

Special instruments and materials

- Bipolar electric forceps
- Feather knife or scalpel
- Catgut 4/0 and 5/0; in small children 6/0

Anesthesia

- Insufflation anesthesia or local anesthesia (the latter is not recommended for children)

- Caudal block

Operative technique step by step (Figures 1–7)

- Careful disinfection, retraction of the foreskin and removal of the smegma
- Disinfection of the glans penis and extension of the foreskin with two clamps at the 6 o'clock and 12 o'clock positions
- Marking of the incision line and incision proximal to the corona in a curved line to the frenulum
- Incision with either the scalpel or the feather knife, the cut being straight without interruptions
- Division of Scarpa's fascia (dartos fascia) with the knife and careful coagulation of the small vessels
- Moving of the clamps to the 3 o'clock and 9 o'clock positions and division of the foreskin at 12 o'clock, with the scissors, to the last 3–4 mm of the inner layer of the foreskin (in cases with severe adhesion, a sharp dissection between the prepuce and the glans may become necessary – but beware of carcinoma of the penis)
- Folding down of the foreskin and stretching of the inner layer of the foreskin; division of the skin 3–4 mm proximal to the corona, at the frenulum, like a V with the knife (a stay suture at the glans is not necessary)
- Careful coagulation to control bleeding (using bipolar cautery) and reconstruction of the frenulum with two or three interrupted sutures (bleeding from the frenular artery can be controlled with catgut sutures (4/0 or 5/0))
- Adaptation of the wound with interrupted sutures
- Dexpanthenol wound dressing

Surgical tricks

- For removal of the adhesion a bulb-headed probe and one or two drops of lidocaine or dexpanthenol are helpful
- Careful and sparing coagulation reduces the extent of postoperative edema

Postoperative care

- The first micturition after operation is usually painful for children. Some drops of lidocaine or a bath with camomile lotion may help

- Bathing with camomile lotion after the first day until wound healing is complete

- Fistula of the urethra (requiring urethroplasty)

- Stenosis of the meatus (requiring meatotomy)

Complications

- Postoperative bleeding (treated by compression or purse-string suture of the frenular artery)
- Local wound infection, sometimes leading to sepsis
- Severe edema or hematoma (treat with ethacridine lactate)
- Removal of too much skin (correction by mobilization of the dermis, or if necessary covering with a split skin graft)
- Removal of too little of the inner layer with unsatisfactory cosmetic results (corrected by resection)
- Injury of the dorsal nerves and vessels by coagulation

References

1. Nesbit TE, King LR. Zirkumzision. In: Hohenfellner, Thüroff, Schulte-Wissermann (eds) *Kinderurologie in Klinik und Praxis*, 1st edn. Stuttgart: Georg Thieme (1986) 522–7.
2. Broecker BH. Circumcision. In: Glenn JF. *Urologic Surgery*, 4th edn. Philadelphia: J.B. Lippincott (1991) 841–4.
3. Johnston JH. Phimosis. In: Eckstein, Hohenfellner, Williams (eds) *Surgical Pediatric Urology*, 1st edn. Stuttgart: Georg Thieme (1977) 414–5.
4. Kaplan GW. Circumcision complications. *Dial Ped Urol* 17 (1994) 6–8.

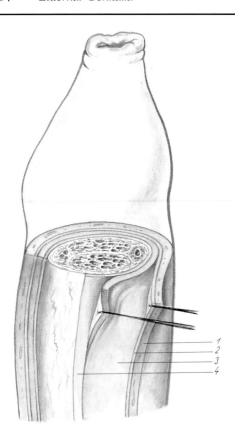

1
2
3
4

Figure 1. The superficial fascia, Scarpa's fascia and Buck's fascia. Between the fascias there is good space for preparation. The superficial vessels are in Scarpa's fascia (dartos fascia).

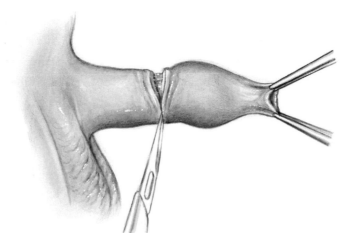

Figure 2. Extension of the prepuce with two clamps and division of the skin with a scalpel distal to the corona.

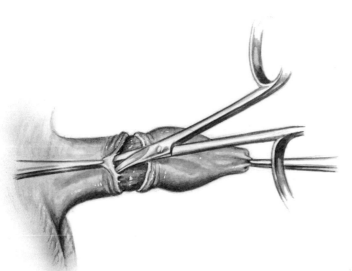

Figure 3. Optional mobilization of the dorsal skin and preparation of Scarpa's fascia.

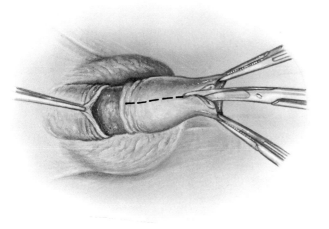

Figure 4. *Retraction of the prepuce with two clamps at 3 o'clock and 9 o'clock and incision of both layers at 12 o'clock.*

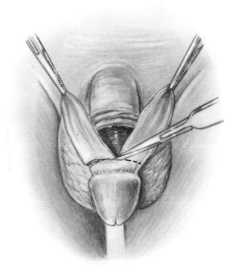

Figure 5. *Folding down of the foreskin and division 3–4 mm proximal to the corona.*

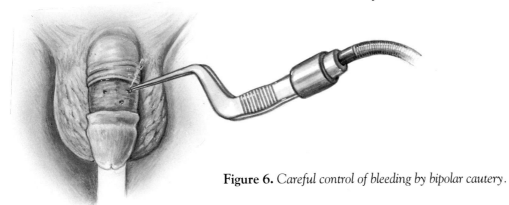

Figure 6. *Careful control of bleeding by bipolar cautery.*

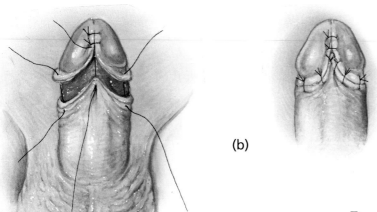

(b)

(a)

Figure 7. *Reconstruction of the frenulum by two or three purse-string sutures (ligation of the frenular artery) and adaptation of the wound with 5/0 or 6/0 catgut.*

Ileocecal Neovagina

R.A. Bürger, U. Witzsch, S. Schumacher,
J. Fichtner, J. Leissner, R. Hohenfellner
Department of Urology,
University of Mainz School of Medicine,
Mainz, Germany

Introduction

Vaginal reconstruction with skin flaps or peritoneum or vaginal replacements with sigmoid colon often end in shrinkage and extreme mucus secretion, which leads to odor and unsatisfactory results.[1-5] The advantages of a neovagina created from an ileocecal segment are:[6]

- Perfect vascularization of the ileocecal region
- Mobility of the ileocecal segment with a long vascular pedicle
- Rapid reduction of mucus secretion
- No tendency to shrink

Indications

- Traumatic or operative loss of the vagina
- Shrinkage after radiation
- Vaginal aplasia
- Sexual transformation

Preoperative diagnostics and care

- In congenital vaginal aplasia, ultrasonography and intravenous urography (look for urologic disorders, which are present in 10–20% of cases), and magnetic resonance imaging or laparoscopy for exact determination of genital disorders
- Intestinal cleaning with oral Fordtran's solution (6–8 liters)
- Perioperative antibiotics, e.g. cephalosporine or metronidazole

Complications

- Narrow introitus
- Temporary mucus secretion
- Prolapse of the neovagina

Instruments and materials

- Vaginal speculum
- Hand-crafted glass phantom (Laborbedarf, Nordheim, Germany)
- Monocryl 3/0 or 4/0 (Ethicon, Edinburgh, UK)

Operative technique step by step (Figures 1–13)

- This is an abdominal and vaginal technique. The patient is positioned supine with the legs placed on movable leg holders
- Mobilization of the ileocecal segment, ascending colon and right flexure. Disconnection of a 12–15 cm segment of the cecum and ascending colon
- Tension-free ileocolostomy with one-layer seromuscular single stitches (e.g. Monocryl 4/0), with a step-wise anti-mesenteric small bowel incision to match the diameters. Closure of the mesenteric slot with single stitches. If necessary, reconstruction of the ileocecal valve to avoid postoperative diarrhea[7]
- If possible, simultaneous vaginal incision (by a second team) between the external urethral and the posterior vaginal commissure. Blunt preparation toward the pouch of Douglas so that three fingers can be put into the canal. Sharp dissection of fibrotic tissue between the urethra and bladder on one side and the rectum on the other
- For regular insertion of the ileocolic artery, anticlockwise rotation up to 180° of the bowel segment. Tension-free transposition of the ascending colon, incision through the pelvic floor in front of the vulva
- For high insertion of the ileocolic artery (no turnaround possible) luxation of the cecal pole caudally through the preformed canal in front of the vulva. Closure of the aboral opening and transverse incision of the cecal pole
- Anastomosis between the vulva and the vaginal stump with single stitches (3/0 catgut) and fixation of the neovagina at the right psoas muscle. Extraperitonealization as far as possible

Surgical tricks

- If a mesenteric length of 2–3 cm is missing for luxation of the ileocecal segment in front of the vulva, a transverse incision of the peritoneum just above the vascular supply is helpful to prolong the mesenterium for tension-free anastomosis
- Heavy and extensive scar tissue at the introitus must be totally resected. For closing and widening, a transposition flap may be turned in

Postoperative care

- Insertion of a glass phantom two or three times a week up to the time of regular sexual intercourse

- Gentle phantom application with lidocaine
- Gastric tube for 3–5 days; alternatively, gastrostomy
- Parenteral nutrition up to the time of the first bowel movement
- No sexual intercourse for 4 weeks

References

1. Counseller VS. Congenital absence of the vagina. *JAMA* **136** (1948) 861–6.
2. Kindermann G. Die Sigmascheide: Erfahrungen in der Behandlung bei angeborenem Fehlen oder späterem Verlust der Vagina. *Geburtshilfe Frauenheilkd* **47** (1978) 650–3.
3. Knapstein P, Friedberg V. Plastische Eingriffe an Vulva und Vagina. *Gynäkologie* **14** (1981) 42–8.
4. Ratnam SS, Rauff M. Funktionserhaltende Operationen bei Vaginalatresie. *Gynäkologie* **13** (1980) 116–19.
5. Zängl A. Konstruktion der Vagina durch Sigmatransposition. *Langenbecks Arch Chir* **339** (1975) 413–16.
6. Bürger RA, Riedmiller H, Knapstein PG, Friedberg V, Hohenfellner R. Ileocecal vaginal construction. *Am J Obstet Gynecol* **161** (1989) 162–7.
7. Fisch M, Spies F, Hohenfellner R. Rekonstruktion der Ileozökalklappe. *Akt Urol* **23** (1992) Operative Techniken 6.13.

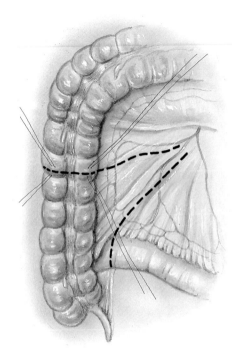

Figure 1. *Isolation of a 12–15 cm ileocecal segment for creation of the neovagina.*

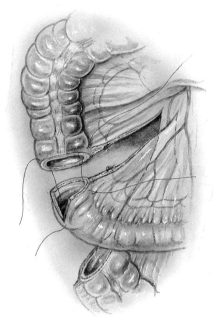

Figure 2. *Restoration of bowel continuity with an ileoascendostomy using one-layer seromuscular stitches (Monocryl 4/0).*

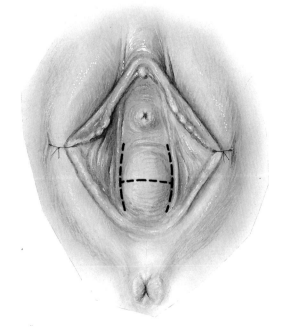

Figure 3. *H-shaped incision of the anterior vaginal wall.*

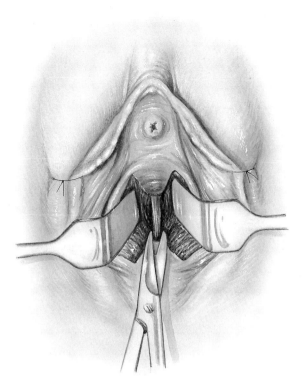

Figure 4. *Sharp and blunt preparation of the canal to the pouch of Douglas.*

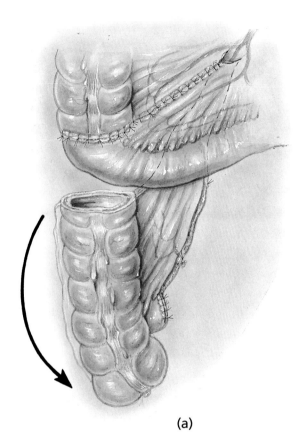

(a)

Figure 5. *(a,b) For normal location of the ileocolic artery anticlockwise rotation up to 180° and anastomosis with the vulva. (c) For high location of the ileocolic artery caudal transposition and opening of the cecal segment for anastomosis with the vulva.*

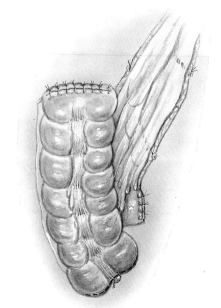

(c)

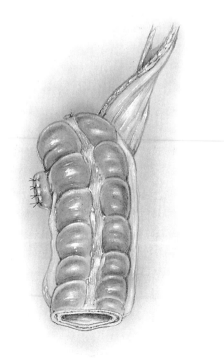

(b)

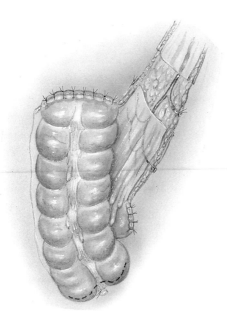

Figure 6. *For a short mesentery, transverse incision of the mesoserosa for 2–3 cm will gain length.*

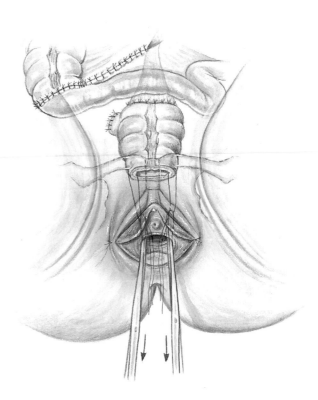

Figure 7. *Pull through of the neovagina through the pelvic floor.*

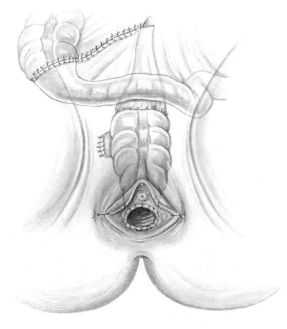

Figure 8. *Anastomosis of the neovagina to the vulva with single stitches (4/0 catgut).*

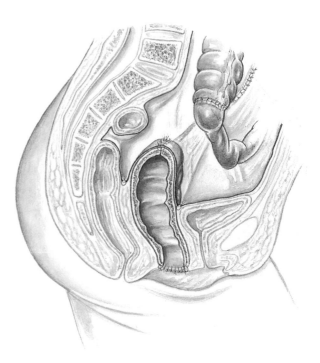

Figure 9. *Location of the neovagina in relation to the pelvic organs.*

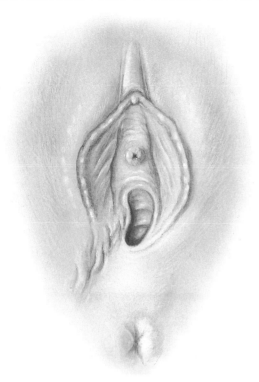

Figure 10. *Deep and wide scar for secondary healing of episiotomy with narrowing of the introitus.*

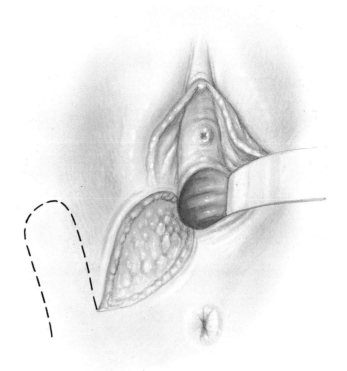

Figure 11. *After scar excision, widening of the narrowed introitus. A transpositional flap is marked.*

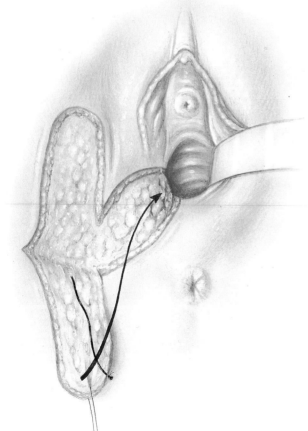

Figure 12. *Mobilization of the flap (be careful with the supplying vessels).*

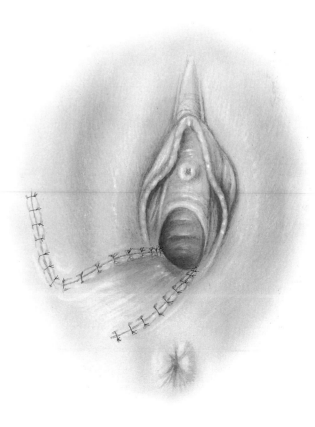

Figure 13. *Fixation of the flap and skin closure with 4/0 or 5/0 catgut.*

Vaginal Reconstruction Using the Defunctional Urinary Bladder (Bladder Neovagina)

R. Wammack, M. Fisch, R. Hohenfellner
Department of Urology,
University of Mainz School of Medicine,
Mainz, Germany

Introduction

Vaginal replacement or reconstruction is becoming a more important aspect during exenteration and urinary diversion surgery. Of the multitude of operative procedures available, techniques using free tissue transfer[1] or myocutaneous flaps[2] and vaginal reconstruction by means of bowel segments are established and well known.[3-5]

Often, the closed distal colonic segment (Hartmann stump) can be used for vaginal reconstruction while a continent urinary diversion using the ileocecal region prevents a second incontinent stoma. The ileocecal valve should be reconstructed in such cases, as the functional loss of bowel may result in intestinal malabsorption.[6]

Heavy irradiation may, however, make vaginal reconstruction using standard techniques very difficult. Patients having radiogenic rectovaginal or vesicovaginal fistulas or anal incontinence and a colostomy are difficult to manage in this respect. In patients with pronounced radiation damage, the defunctionalized urinary bladder may be used for vaginal reconstruction.

Indications

- Patient's and partner's desire for operative treatment of the cloaca and possibility of sexual intercourse

Instruments

- Standard instruments for bowel and bladder surgery
- Bent clamp
- Scott retractor
- Suture material: polyglycolic acid 4/0, chromic catgut 5/0

Operative technique step by step (Figures 1–7)

- Patient in the dorsosacral position
- Midline laparotomy (already performed for urinary diversion or colostomy)
- Insertion of a bladder catheter
- Opening of the bladder between two stay sutures from the abdominal approach
- Widening of the vesicovaginal fistula with forceps

- Incision of the anterior vaginal wall from the urethral meatus to the orifice of the vaginal fistula
- Incision of pelvic floor at the 3 and 9 o'clock positions using electrocautery
- Running sutures along the incised vaginal wall permits effective hemostasis

Surgical tricks

In the unlikely event that the newly created bladder neovagina is not sufficiently long, augmentation with bowel, preferentially using the Hartmann stump, is possible. Alternatively, a short isolated segment of detubularized ileum, anastomosed side-to-side, may be used (Figure 8).

If greater omentum is left, it should be used to cover the neovagina toward the abdominal cavity.

Postoperative care

- A glass phantom remains in the neovagina for 5 days and is intermittently placed in the introitus until regular sexual intercourse takes place
- Baths with chamomile solution are advisable

References

1. Farber M, Mitchell GW. Surgery for congenital absence of the vagina. *Obstet Gynecol* **51** (1978) 364–7.
2. Benson C, Soisson AP, Carlson J, Culbertson G, Hawley-Bowland C, Richards F. Neovaginal reconstruction with a rectus abdominis myocutaneous flap. *Obstet Gynecol* **81** (1994) 871–5.
3. Bürger R, Knapstein PG, Hohenfellner R. Die ileozökal-Neovagina. In: Schmidt W. (ed.) *Jahrbuch der Gynäkologie und Geburtshilfe* (1991) Zülpich: Biermann Verlag.
4. Novak E. Die Verwendung von Kolon bei der chirurgischen Behandlung der Vaginalagenesie. *Gynäkologie* **132** (1980) 122.
5. Wesley JR, Coran AG. Intestinal vaginoplasty for congenital absence of the vagina. *J Pediatr Surg* **27** (1994) 885–9.
6. Fisch M, Wammack R, Spies F *et al.* Ileocecal valve reconstruction during continent urinary diversion. *J Urol* **151** (1994) 861–5.

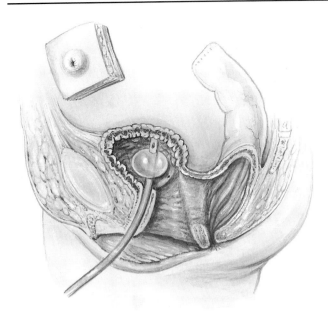

Figure 1. *Profound irradiation damage: irradiated Hartmann stump, and cloaca with rectovesicovaginal fistula.*

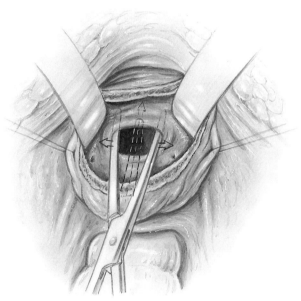

Figure 2. *Abdominal view of the opened small-capacity radiation-damaged bladder. Forceps widen the vesicovaginal fistula.*

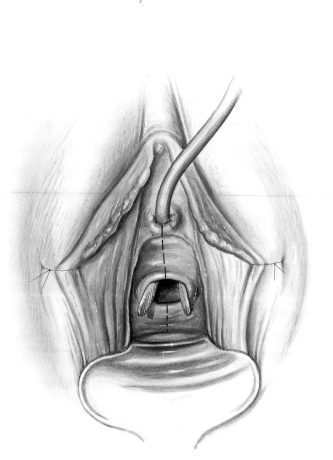

Figure 3. *Vaginal view showing the forceps as introduced from the abdominal approach. Incision of anterior vaginal wall along the dotted line.*

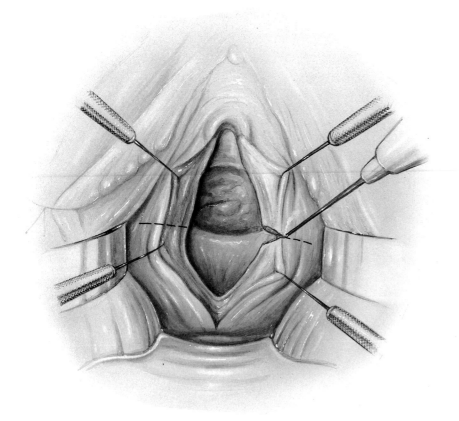

Figure 4. *Widening of the introitus by lateral incisions made by electrocautery at the 3 and 9 o'clock positions.*

Figure 5. *Running suture of the resection margins achieves hemostasis.*

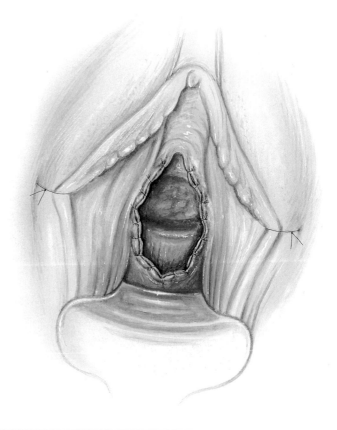

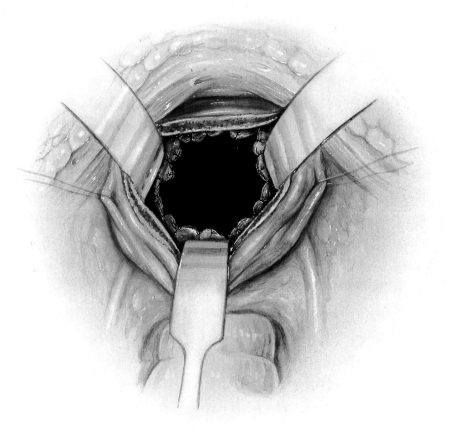

Figure 6. *Abdominal view of the neointroitus*

Figure 7. *The completed neovagina.*

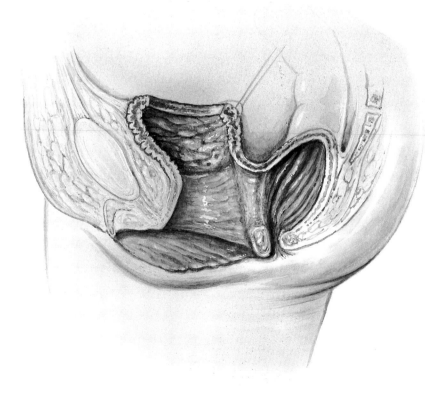

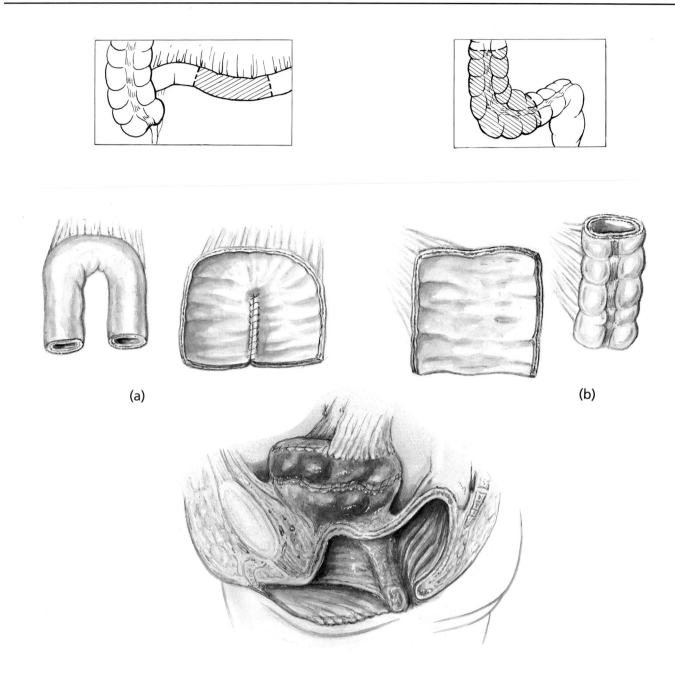

Figure 8. *Optional augmentation of the bladder neovagina. (a) Isolation of an ileal segment, antimesenteric opening and anastomosis of the medial and distal margins to form a pouch. (b) Alternatively a colonic segment may be isolated, detubularized and used as a patch.*

Reconstruction of the Male External Genitalia with a Penoid

G.H. Jordan, C.J. Devine
Devine Center for Genitourinary Reconstructive Surgery,
Sentara Norfolk General Hospital,
Norfolk, Virginia, USA

Comment

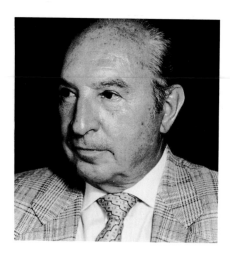

or with the AMS penile prosthesis or testicular prosthesis that are implanted 1 year later. Suprapubic urinary diversion was never necessary.

In many cases vaginal skin was used for construction of the glans. However, improved techniques for glans reconstruction, as presented by these authors, are desirable.

References

1. Chang TS, Hwang WY. Forearm flap in one-stage reconstruction of the penis. *Plast Reconstr Surg* **74** (1984) 251.
2. Meyer R, Daverio PJ, Duquesne J. One-stage phalloplasty in transsexuals. *Ann Plast Surg* **16** (1986) 6.
3. Meyer R, Daverio PJ. One-stage phalloplasty without sensory deprivation in female transsexuals. *World J Urol* **5** (1987) 9.

R. Meyer, Lausanne, Switzerland

The authors are to be congratulated on their fine chapter. Only free flaps can cover all the prerequisites in the reconstructive surgery of the penis. I also favor the forearm flap. Shortly after the publication of Chang and Hwang[1] the method was introduced by Daverio, Duquesne and myself for sexual transformation from female to male. Our modification has been published in 1986 and 1987.[2,3] The length of the forearm flap is approximately 12–14 cm, the width 13 cm. The flap is divided into a radial and an ulnar strip. The neourethra is formed out of the ulnar part and later anastomosed with the neourethra constructed from vaginal skin. The radial part (9 cm) forms the outer part of the penoid. The radial artery is anastomosed to the inferior epigastric artery, and the cephalic vein is brought to the saphenous vein. Some of the branches of the medial antebrachial cutaneous nerve are brought together with the genital branches of the left ilioinguinal and the iliohypogastric nerves. Genital sensibility is provided by anastomosis of the lateral antebrachial cutaneous nerve with the right perineal branches of the pudendal nerve. Simultaneous hysterectomy with subsequent vaginal closure allows the construction of a neoscrotum from vaginal and labial skin. We used to cover the forearm with split skin; however, in our last 10 cases we have used a full-thickness flap from the groin or the breast. To avoid fistulas and strictures, we now construct the neourethra from forearm skin (according to Chang) and not vaginal skin.

Biemer, who modified our method, often constructs a perineal opening (boutonnière) to avoid urethral problems; however, we have not encountered any problems at this site

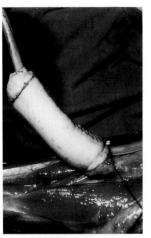
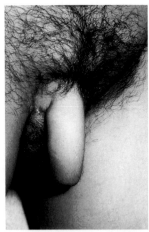

1,2

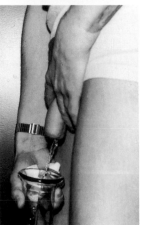
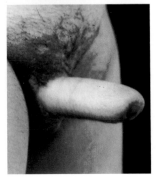

3,4

Figure 1. *Reconstruction of a phallus from a forearm flap.*
Figure 2. *Neophallus.*
Figure 3. *Voiding via the neophallus.*
Figure 4. *Erection with the AMS penile prosthesis.*

Reconstruction of the male external genitalia with a penoid

Introduction

Reconstruction of the penis after traumatic amputation has been performed since the end of the 1930s.[1,2] Many methods, including the use of fascia and muscle strips, the use of scrotal skin, and prosthesis implantation, have been developed.[3–9] On several occasions up to five consecutive operations were necessary.[9] Several-stage procedures implementing the 'tube within a tube' technique and its modifications soon became the therapy of choice.[3,4] The advent of microsurgery and the successful transfer of free transplants by means of microsurgical anastomoses have led to a considerable reduction in the number of operations performed. The use of vein-to-vein grafts has also proved to be of advantage.[11] The ideal reconstruction of a penoid is performed as a one-stage procedure using a free skin flap with an overlapping vascular and nerve pedicle.[12–17] Good tactile and erogenous sensibility, a urethra with the meatus located at the tip of the glans, the possibility of standing micturition, a good cosmetic result, and enough graft material for a future prosthesis implantation should be aimed at. These criteria are best fulfilled by using a skin flap from the forearm.[16] The overlapping function of the radial and ulnar arteries should guarantee sufficient vascularization. However, the need for several experienced surgeons and the surgical complexity are disadvantages: the surgical team at our institution consists of a urologic surgeon with experience in reconstructive surgery, a plastic surgeon and sometimes also a vascular surgeon.

The urethroplasty is the critical stage of the procedure, as in any other reconstruction of the phallus. If sufficient vascular supply at the time of reconstruction is uncertain, the gracilis muscle can be moved perineally as a well-vascularized flap.

A sufficient vascular and nerve supply to the penoid should be ensured before the prosthesis is implanted. The use of artificial materials bears a higher infection risk, and so we do not implant a prosthesis during the initial procedure.

Preoperative examination

- Allen test to check the collateral circulation between the radial and the ulnar arteries

- If this test fails to provide a definite result, angiography

Operative technique step by step

A flap of about 12 × 17 cm is taken from the arm that is not dominant (Figures 1 and 2). If the Allen test is positive, a vein interposition between the stumps of the radial artery is not required.

Cricket bat flap (Figures 3–8)

This is the preferred flap after traumatic penis amputation or amputation for malignancy, and in children[18] because of the easier dissection of the radial artery. It provides excellent venous drainage over the venae comitantes in addition to the cephalic and basilic veins and/or the superficial medial antebrachial vein. The nerve supply is provided by the antebrachial cutaneous lateral and medial nerves.

The neourethra is placed over the radial or ulnar artery. The flap width depends on age (adults, 3.5 cm; boys aged 6–7 years, *ca.* 2 cm); the length depends on the portion to be replaced.

Biemer's flap (Figure 9)

Here, the skin flap for construction of the neourethra is placed in the middle. The epithelium lining to the left and right adjacent sides is removed, and the lateral skin flaps are joined together to form a phallus with the urethra in the middle.[19] This technique is especially of advantage when the construction of a relatively long phallus is planned.

Dissection of the skin flap

- Placement of a tourniquet. Skin incision extending up to the fascia

- Incision of the fascia at the base of the flap over the radial artery. (The artery runs in a groove along the edge of the brachioradialis muscle, in the distal part running more superficially.) The superficial branch of the radial nerve arises from the depth of the muscle belly as well-running parallel to the artery. (Caution is necessary as the nerve is easily injured.)

- If the nerve is severed, it should be reanastomosed immediately. Paresthesia or painful neuroma may result

- Mobilization of the lateral antebrachial cutaneous nerve (which supplies the volar and distal radial area of the forearm) and the medial antebrachial cutaneous nerve (which divides in the anterior and ulnar branches)

- Mobilization of the radial artery and the accompanying veins. After mobilization has been completed, opening of the tourniquet and careful hemostasis

Neourethra

- De-epithelialization of the skin flap between the neourethra and the skin of the phallus shaft

- Two-layer closure of the neourethra over a silicone catheter with interrupted chromic catgut sutures, followed by a running suture with 5/0 or 6/0 PDS (Ethicon, Edinburgh, UK)

- Embedding of the neourethra in the middle of the flap and closure of the distal portion to form a penoid. The de-epithelialized portions thicken the distal phallus in the cricket bat flap and thus give it the appearance of a glans

- The proximal portion remains open so that, if necessary, the stumps of the corpora cavernosa can be inserted (after trauma or amputation)

Reconstruction of the glans

- Circular incision of the distal portion at the level of the corona

- A skin flap that has been removed from the genital area is built into a tube over a thin catheter

- Placement of this flap in the incision and skin closure

- In a second step after 3 weeks, opening of the skin over this flap (the different texture of this tissue and the different color of the implanted skin graft make the glans evident)

- A large phallus *ca.* 8–10 cm can be built with this technique

Dissection of the genital area

- The constructed phallus has to remain connected to its nerve and vessel supply until dissection of the genital area has been completed

- Dissection of the genital area is performed simultaneously by a second surgical team

Urethra

- In cases of transsexualism, stretching of the female urethra and extending it distally by using the front vaginal wall

Vessels

- Paramedian or midline incision, mobilization of the inferior epigastric artery and vein or the deep circumflex artery, and presentation of the vessels on their course to the origin

- Avoid traumatic injury by preserving the paravascular tissue. (A disadvantage of this is that it produces tension on the anastomosis and a high vascular resistance.) An alternative is a vein graft to the femoral artery

- Mobilization of the great saphenous vein

- End-to-side anastomosis of the distal end of the vein with the femoral artery above the branching of the deep artery. (This fistula remains until the final anastomosis with the skin graft is performed.)

- Mobilization of the contralateral great saphenous vein. A couple of its branches are spared. (The anastomosis is better with multiple veins in the skin graft.) Note that venous blood stasis in this high-pressure system can lead to failure

- The anastomosis with the femoral artery yields a high blood flow to the transplant, and so every visible vein should be connected to a vein branch (and, if it exists, also to the dorsal vein of the penis)

- The veins or vein grafts are passed medially through a tunnel from the inguinal incision

Nerves

- Mobilization of the dorsal nerves of the penis. If there is no dorsal nerve, anastomosis with the pudendal nerve or its dorsal branches

- If the nerve is too short, interposition of a free piece of the sural nerve

Transposition

- Division of the nerve, followed by division of the artery and finally division of the vein

Urethral anastomosis

- Urethral anastomosis to prevent later manipulation of the vessel anastomoses with consequent vessel spasms

- Interrupted sutures (chromic catgut), and a second layer of running suture (PDS 6/0). Urethral splint with a white silicone catheter

- The duration of ischemia does not influence the survival of the penoid

Vascular anastomosis

- Utilization of a surgical microscope

- Midline division of the loop of the arteriovenous fistula. Anastomosis of the vein graft with the radial artery using interrupted sutures (nylon or Prolene (Ethicon) 10/0)

- Anastomosis of the veins with the great saphenous vein. (Ideally all the veins are anastomosed with the spared branches of the great saphenous vein.)

- Inspection of vascular patency with a doppler

- The phallus is wrapped with warm towels after completion of the anastomoses

- Inspection for vascular spasms

Nerve anastomosis

- After completion of vascularization, anastomosis of the

lateral and medial antebrachial cutaneous nerves with the dissected nerves of the genital area (nylon or Prolene 10/0 or 11/0)

- Closure of the shaft skin

Care of the forearm

- Simultaneous closure of the forearm during the microscopic section of the procedure in the genital area

- A thick split-thickness skin graft from the upper leg is obtained and fixed with chromic catgut

- Dressing and cast immobilization of the forearm

Surgical tricks and complications

Fistulas are the main complication of the urethral anastomosis. Small fistulas almost always close spontaneously. In large fistulas the gracilis muscle can be used for cover. If the vascular supply is suspicious, covering with gracilis muscle from the non-dominant side follows. In cases of transsexualism, a bilateral stalked skin flap from the region above the clitoris is mobilized at the same time.

The phallus is shifted to the pubic bone crest by transposition to the base of the penoid. The urethral anastomosis is covered with the transposed muscle. Complications at this site are rare in male patients.

Postoperative care

- Careful examination of the phallus with a doppler, marking the sites with the strongest signals (in this way, detailed postoperative control is possible)

- Installation of a pH meter to monitor the acidosis of the transplant

- Strict bed rest for 2–3 days at a room temperature of 27–32 °C

- Hospitalization for 2–3 weeks

- Administration of 100 mg acetylsalicylic acid/day

- Suprapubic catheter for 2–3 weeks

- High-dose antibiotic coverage

- Prosthesis implantation in a second operation

References

1. Bogarz NA. Plastic restoration of the penis. *Sov Khir* **8** (1936) 303–7.
2. Frumpkin AP. Reconstruction of the male genitalia. *Am Rev Sov Med* **2** (1944) 14–21.
3. Gillies HD, Harrison RH. Congenital absence of the penis. *Br J Plast Surg* **1** (1948) 8–28.
4. Arneri V. Reconstruction of the male genitalia. In: J.M. Converse (ed.) *Reconstructive Plastic Surgery*, 2nd edn. Philadelphia: W.B. Saunders (1977) 3910–19.
5. Goodwin WE, Scott WW. Phalloplasty. *J Urol* **68** (1952) 903–8.
6. Puckett CL, Montie JE. Construction of male genitalia in the transsexual, using a tubed groin flap for the penis and a hydraulic inflation device. *Plast Reconstr Surg* **61** (1978) 523–30.
7. McGregor IA, Jackson IT. The groin flap. *Br J Plast Surg* **25** (1972) 3–16.
8. Orticochea M. New method of total reconstruction of the penis. *Br J Plast Surg* **25** (1972) 347–66.
9. Orticochea M. The musculo-cutaneous flap: a heroic substitute for the method of delay. *Br J Plast Surg* **25** (1972) 106–10.
10. Devine PC, Winslow BH, Jordan GH, Horton CE, Gilbert DA. Reconstructive phallic surgery. In: J.A. Libertino (ed.) *Pediatric and Adult Reconstructive Urologic Surgery*, 2nd edn. Baltimore: Williams and Wilkins (1987) 552–61.
11. Puckett CL, Reinisch TF, Montie JE. Free flap phalloplasty. *J Urol* **128** (1982) 294–9.
12. Daniel RK, Terzis J. Neurovascular free flaps. In: A. Deniller, B. Strauch (eds) *Symposium on Microsurgery*. St Louis, Missouri: (1976) 66–73.
13. McGraw JB, Furlow LT Jr. The dorsalis pedis arterialized flap: a clinical study. *Plast Reconstr Surg* **55** (1975) 177–85.
14. Taylor GI, Daniel RK. The anatomy of several free flap donor sites. *Plast Reconstr Surg* **56** (1975) 243–53.
15. Muhlbauer W, Herndl E, Stock W. The forearm flap. *Plast Reconstr Surg* **70** (1982) 336–42.
16. Chang TS, Huang WY. Forearm flap in one-stage reconstruction of the penis. *Plast Reconstr Surg* **74** (1986) 251–88.
17. Ponten B. The fascio-cutaneous flap: its use in soft tissue defects of the lower leg. *Br J Plast Surg* **34** (1981) 215.
18. Farrow GA, Boyd JB, Semple JL. Total reconstruction of the penis employing the 'cricket bat flap' single stage forearm free graft. *AUA Today* **3** (1990).
19. Biemer E. Penile construction by the radial arm flap. *Clin Plast Surg* **15** (1988) 425–30.

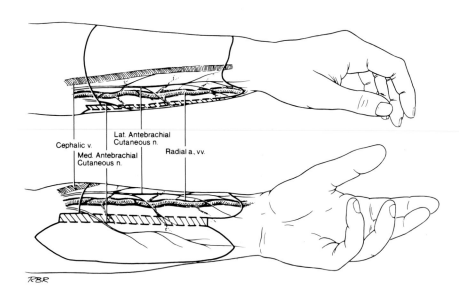

Figure 1. *Radial forearm flap. The ulnar portion becomes the neourethra, the middle portion is de-epithelialized, and the largest (radical) portion is turned into the shaft.*

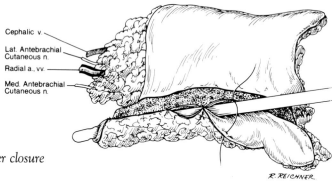

Figure 2. *Construction of the neourethra with two-layer closure (chromic catgut and PDS) follows after mobilization.*

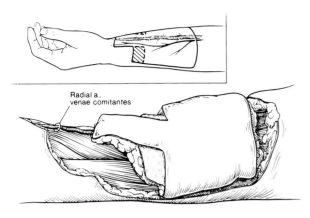

Radial a.,
venae comitantes

Figure 3. *The stalk is placed distally over the radial artery and turns later into the neourethra. De-epithelialization of the hatched area and mobilization of the flap. The radial artery has not been divided yet.*

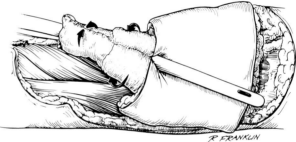

R FRANKLIN

Figure 4. *Placement of the silicone catheter and closure of the neourethra.*

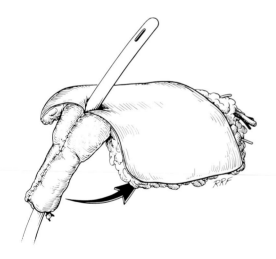

RRF

Figure 5. *Embedding of the neourethra into the proximal portion of the flap. The vessels are ligated shortly before reanastomosis.*

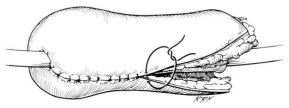

RRF

Figure 6. *Closure of the epidermis with interrupted sutures.*

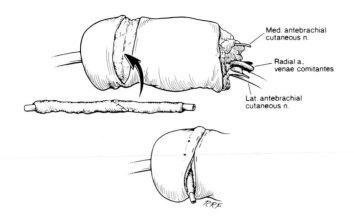

Figure 7. *Circular skin incision at the level of the corona and burying of the tubularized skin flap (taken from the genital area).*

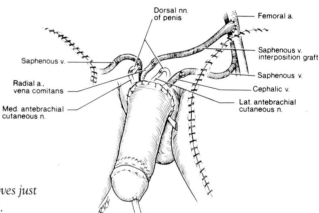

Figure 8. *Ligation and reanastomosis of the vessels and nerves just after completion of the vessel dissection in the genital area.*

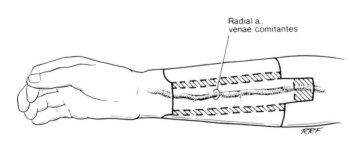

Figure 9. *The urethra is placed in the midline on top of the radial artery, an epithelialized flap is excised at both sides and the skin is closed laterally with two suture rows to form a phallus.*

Phalloplasty with an Extended Pedicled Groin Island Flap

S. Perović
*Department of Urology,
University of Belgrade, Serbia*

Comment

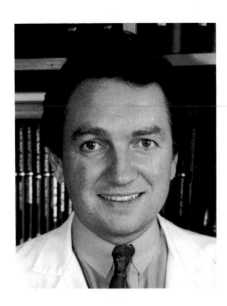

If a patient with a micropenis or amputation of the penis, or a female transsexual wants to have a phalloplasty, the following principles have to be considered:

- The shaft of the penis should be hairless and of a suitable calibre

- The location from which tissue is removed should have no deforming scars

- The urethra should be constructed in such a way that no stricture, fistula or hairs impair voiding

- Ideally a hardening should be possible (during which the risk of perforation is very high because of the low sensibility of the penoid)

- The erogenous innervation should be integrated

Without claim to completeness, the literature published since 1936 shows the different techniques used to meet these demands. Unfortunately, none of these techniques is able to achieve all the aims. The technique proposed by Perović has many advantages. Compared with the forearm and deltoid flaps, the scars at the site of tissue removal are less distinct. By dropping the microsurgical anastomosis of vessels the operating time is considerably decreased. (The sex-adapting operations with forearm or deltoid flaps take 10–16 hours, even in the hands of experienced reconstruction surgeons.) However, nerve injuries caused by compartmental syndrome are no

rarity, and a disadvantage of this technique, as Perović himself acknowledges, is the low sensibility of the neophallus. Whether this construction of the urethra is linked to a lower rate of stricture and fistula than other techniques remains to be proved by larger series. The absence of a prosthesis and the expected growth of hair on the penoid also show that this operation method cannot solve all problems.

In spite of all this criticism, the phalloplasty with an extended pedunculated island flap from the groin seems to be an acceptable alternative to the microsurgical procedures with free flaps. Nevertheless, one should not raise too much hope in patients: a minimally acceptable cosmetic and functional result is often reached only after multiple operations.

Bibliography

1. Bogoras N. Über die volle plastische Wiederherstellung eines zum Koitus fähigen Penis (penis plastica totalis). *Zentralbl Chir* **63** (1936) 1271.
2. Chang TS, Hwang WY. Forearm flap in one stage reconstruction of the penis. *Plast Reconstr Surg* **74** (1984) 251.
3. Gilbert DA, Horton CE, Terzis JK *et al*. New concepts in phallic reconstruction. *Ann Plast Surg* **18** (1987) 128.
4. Gillies H, Harrison R. Congenital absence of the penis. *Br J Plast Surg* **1** (1948) 8.
5. Goodwin WE, Scott WW. Phalloplasty. *J Urol* **68** (1952) 903.
6. Harashima T, Inoue T, Tanaka I *et al*. Reconstruction of penis with deltoid flap. *Br J Plast Surg* **43** (1990) 217–22.
7. Hester TR *et al*. One stage reconstruction of the penis. *Br J Plast Surg* **31** (1978) 279–85.
8. Kaplan I, Wesser D. A rapid method of constructing a functional, sensitive penis. *Br J Plast Surg* **24** (1971) 342.
9. Matti BA, Mathiews RN, Davies DM. Phalloplasty using the free radial forearm flap. *Br J Plast Surg* **41** (1988) 160–4.
10. Meyer R, Daverio PJ. One stage phalloplasty without sensory deprivation in female transsexuals. *World J Urol* **5** (1987) 9–13.
11. Orticochea M. A new method of total reconstruction of the penis. *Br J Plast Surg* **25** (1972) 347.
12. Puckett CL, Montie JE. Construction of male genitalia in the transsexual using a tubed groin flap for the penis and a hydraulic inflation device. *Plast Reconstr Surg* **61** (1978) 523.
13. Puckett CL, Reinisch JF, Montie JE. Free flap phalloplasty. *J Urol* **128** (1982) 294.

W. Stackl, Vienna, Austria

Phalloplasty with an Extended Pedicled Groin Island Flap

Introduction

Among the different techniques of phalloplasty, the microsurgical transplantation of free flaps is the most frequent used. In contrast we prefer an extended pedicled island flap of the groin.

Introduced in the 1970s and the 1980s, the island flap of the groin was first modified to allow a one-stage operation in 1984. In contrast to others we do not execute a direct preparation of vessels. The risk of damaging the vessels, particularly owing to the frequent anatomical variations encountered, is therefore decreased.

Advantages

- Largeness of the flap (depending on the frame of the patient)
- Richness of the lymphatic supply
- Simple technical performance (saving time)
- Low rate of complications
- Simple closure of the skin defect

Disadvantage

- Low sensibility of the neophallus

Indications

- Absence of the penis (in female transsexuals or due to congenital anomalies) or complete traumatic amputation of the penis: in these cases a complete phalloplasty is performed
- Very short penis or penis stump caused by incomplete amputation, or untreated or partially treated anomalies of the penis: in these cases augmentation phalloplasty is required

The technique is mainly performed in adults or adolescents, but in childhood (usually prepuberty) strong psychological reasons (in the children or their parents) are a special indication.

Contraindications

- Previous surgery or trauma combined with damage of vessels in the inguinal or iliacal region

Preoperative preparations

- Intensive massage and application of ointment to prevent scars and increase the elasticity of the skin and the dimensions of the flap (to facilitate closure)
- Utilization of a tissue expander, if the available skin is limited

Instruments

- Standard instruments for plastic reconstructive surgery of the genital region
- Synthetic reabsorbable suture material

Operative technique step by step

- Supine position of the patient with a pad under the posterior
- With a doppler, the femoral artery, the source and course of both branches of the superficial circumflex iliac artery and the superficial epigastric artery are identified and marked
- Measurement of the flap: about 22 cm length and 12 cm width. The base of the flap is positioned over the femoral artery, about 2 cm above the inguinal ligament
- When a wide flap is necessary, it is better to extend it cranially or laterally
- Lifting of the flap below the deep fascia, starting from the proximal part to the base
- Preparation of the flap to the medial border of the sartorius muscle (with care not to damage the vessel system), the superficial circumflex iliac artery and the superficial epigastric arteries
- De-epithelialization of the base of the flap (about 4–5 cm) up to the medial part (about 2 cm) (neourethra) with elongation of the peduncle to facilitate transposition of the flap in the region of the lower symphysis
- De-epithelialization of a skin strip (about 1 cm) between the medial and the lateral part of the flap
- Tubularization of the lateral part around a fenestrated silicone stent (neourethra)
- Tubularization of the medial part of the flap around the neourethra ('tube within a tube' technique)
- Subcutaneous tunneling between the region of transplantation and the origin of the tissue

- Drawing of the neophallus through the subcutaneous tunnel by rotating the peduncle from 90° to 180° without compressing the vascularization

- Mobilization and elongation of the original urethra and anastomosis with the neourethra. Mobilization, dorsal removal and incorporation of the clitoris in the neophallus and adaptation to the skin of the transplantation region in a female transsexual

- In cases of amputation of the penis or malformation of the penis, anastomosis of the neourethra with the original spatulated urethra and suturing of the skin of the neophallus with the stump of the corpora cavernosa

- Closure of the abdominal skin defect

- Formation of the neoglans by the modified Norfolk technique

Surgical tricks

- The size of the flap can be better estimated by flexion of the leg to 45° and by lightly pinching the skin with the fingers

- The success of the operation depends on the mobilization of the flap below the deep fascia (fasciocutaneous flap). Mobilization of the flap base at the caudal and medial border is performed by blunt preparation of the subcutaneous fat. The flap base is lifted off from lateral to medial. The lateral side is partially covered by the deep fascia of the thigh. The connection between the sartorius and tensor fasciae latae muscles is identified by palpation of a little groove between these two muscles (taking care to avoid damaging the deep branch of the superficial iliac circumflex artery)

- The tubularization of the flap is facilitated by careful removal of fat tissue (lipomectomy) in obese patients

- Closure of the abdominal skin defect is possible by flexion of the leg to 45° and skin mobilization

Postoperative care

- Antibiotic and antiphlogistic therapy until day 7

- Bedding of the patient in a semisupine position with flexion of the corresponding leg

- Bedding of the neophallus to the other side to avoid sharp twisting

- Rest in bed until day 3

- In simultaneous plasty of the urethra, suprapubic drainage of urine for 3 weeks with a transurethral catheter for 2 weeks

- Without simultaneous plasty of the urethra, transurethral catheter for 3–4 days

- Stenting of the neourethra for 6 weeks

Comments

- To reduce complications (stenosis, fistula, diverticula) it is better to perform the anastomosis of the original urethra with the neourethra in a second operation

- Plasty of the neoglans is performed in a second operation, normally when the healing process is complete

- In children, the neophallus has to be big enough to allow for somatic and genital growth

Bibliography

1. Chang TW, Hwang WY. Forearm flap in one-stage reconstruction of the penis. *Plast Reconstr Surg* **74** (1984) 251–8.
2. Gilbert DA, Jordan GH, Devine CJ Jr, Winslow BH, Schlossberg SM. Phallic construction in prepubertal and adolescent boys. *J Urol* **149** (1993) 1521–6.
3. Gilbert DA, Winslow BH, Gilbert DM, Jordan GH, Horton CE. Transsexual surgery in the genetic female. *Clin Plast Surg* **15** (1988) 471–87.
4. Guang CS, Jin JH. One-stage reconstruction of the penis with composite iliac crest and lateral groin skin flap. *Ann Plast Surg* **15** (1985) 519-28.
5. Guang CS, An GZ, Wei H, Ping D, Wei MS, Jie GM. Reconstruction of the external genitalia and repair of skin defects of the perineal region using three types of lateral groin flap. *Ann Plast Surg* **24** (1990) 328–34.
6. Hoopes JE. Surgical construction of the male external genitalia. *Clin Plast Surg* **1** (1974) 325–34.
7. He GL, Lin ZH, Liu Q, Yang XB, Zhang HL, Gao XS. One-stage penis reconstruction with abdominal fasciocutaneous flap based on the double arteries. *Chin Med J* **100** (1987) 255–8.
8. Lai CS, Chou CK, Yang CC, Lin SD. Immediate reconstruction of the penis with an iliac flap. *Br J Plast Surg* **43** (1990) 621–4.
9. Manktelow RT. Microvascular reconstruction. Berlin: Springer-Verlag (1986) 7–59.
10. Mukherjee GD. Use of groin and mid-thigh flap in reconstruction of penis with penile and perineal urethra and a dorsal skin-lined socket for a urethroplasty. *Ann Plast Surg* **6** (1986) 235–41.
11. Persoff MM. Groin flap phallus reconstruction with new method of urethroplasty. *Ann Plast Surg* **6** (1981) 132–7.
12. Puckett CL, Montie JE. Construction of male genitalia in the transsexual, using a tubed groin flap for the penis and a hydraulic inflation device. *Plast Reconstr Surg* **61** (1978) 523–30.

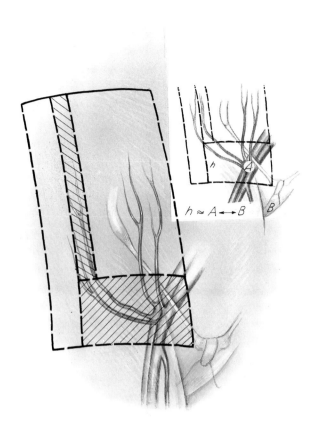

Figure 1. *Design and vascularization of the extended pedicled island flap, which consists of three parts: a lateral part, which is hairless and thin, about 2 cm wide and 22 cm long, to build the neourethra; a medial part, about 10 cm wide and 19–20 cm long, for the reconstruction of the stump of the neophallus; and a part (hatched), which is de-epithelialized.*

Figure 2. *Lifting of the flap base, which incorporates a part of the fascia of the sartorius muscle (preserving the superficial circumflex iliac artery). Variations of the source of the superficial circumflex iliac artery (SCIA) and the superficial epigastric artery (SEA) are frequent: both arteries may have a common source, and the superficial epigastric artery can be absent.*

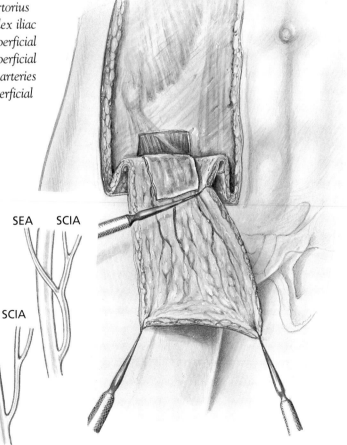

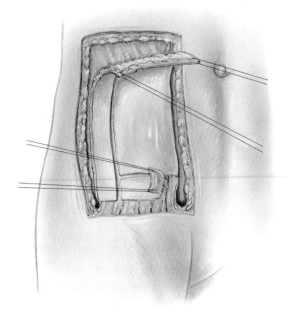

Figure 3. *De-epithelialization of the flap base and a 1 cm wide strip between the lateral and the medial parts. The lateral part of the base is not de-epithelialized because this allows an elongation to facilitate anastomosis of the neourethra. The distance between the lateral (neourethra) and the medial (neophallus) parts of the flap can be enlarged by careful blunt preparation.*

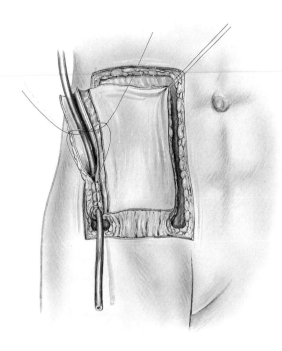

Figure 4. *Tubularization of the lateral part.*

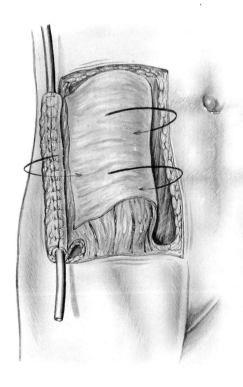

Figure 5. *'Tube within a tube' technique.*

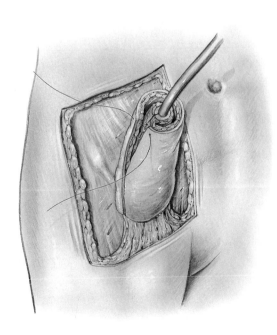

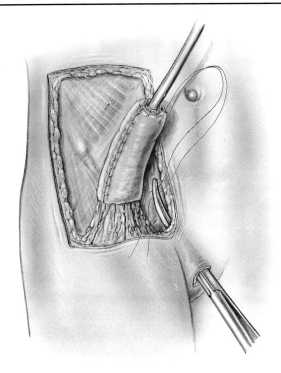

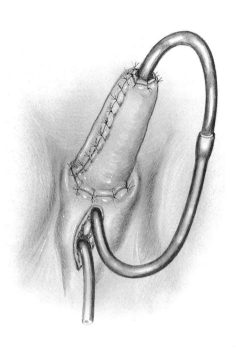

Figure 6. *The newly formed phallus is transposed to the transplantation region (the lower border of the symphysis). In female transsexuals the clitoris is mobilized and transposed dorsally.*

(b)

(c)

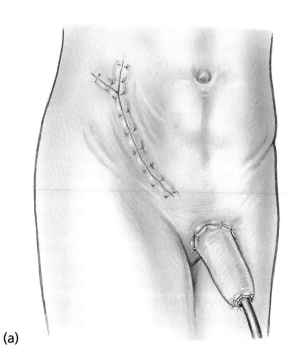

(a)

Figure 7. *The neophallus is fixed in the recipient region. The transplantation region can be skin (in female transsexuals), a short penis or a stump of a penis (a penile malformation or trauma to the penis). Anastomosis of the urethra is completed in the same or a second session. Direct closure of the wound where tissue has been removed.*

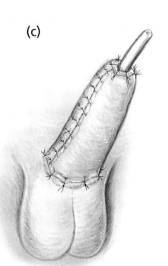

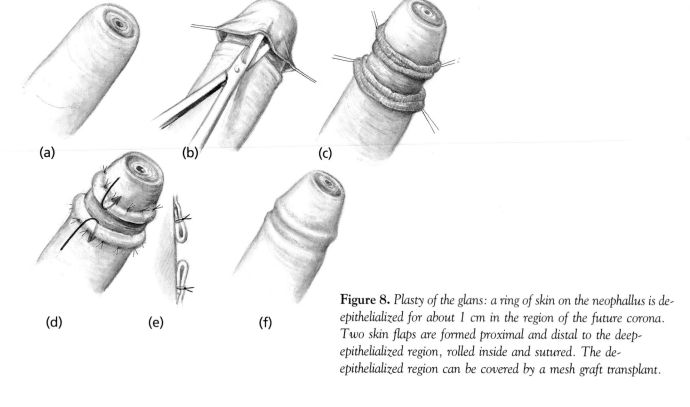

(a)   (b)   (c)

(d)   (e)   (f)

Figure 8. *Plasty of the glans: a ring of skin on the neophallus is de-epithelialized for about 1 cm in the region of the future corona. Two skin flaps are formed proximal and distal to the deep-epithelialized region, rolled inside and sutured. The de-epithelialized region can be covered by a mesh graft transplant.*

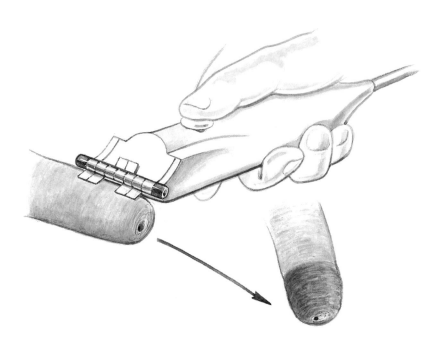

Figure 9. *Alternative plasty of the glans. The upper layer of the dermis can be removed from the distal end of the phallus with a dermatome.*

Hypospadias Repair with Buccal Mucosa Onlay Graft

J. Fichtner, A. Macedo, M. Fisch,
R. Bürger, R. Hohenfellner
Department of Urology,
University of Mainz School of Medicine,
Mainz, Germany

Introduction

With an incidence of 1 in 300 male newborns, hypospadias is the most frequent anomaly of the male genitalia. Over 300 surgical techniques for its correction have been described, and a standardized treatment strategy with low morbidity is badly needed. Our experience with buccal mucosa since our first publication[1] in 1992 seems to underline the advantages of this particular substitute material. We have observed a surprisingly low complication rate (12%) in a selected group of patients with complex hypospadias, most of them being hypospadias cripples with multiple unsuccessful previous operations. However, the final value of this technique can only be judged with a longer follow-up of at least 10 years.

The pattern of enthusiasm after the initial description of a new technique followed by disillusion has become particularly obvious with the Duckett tube:[2] initial low complication rates were followed by reports of significant morbidity, and the technique was abandoned in favor of the onlay.

Because of these significant complication rates, it becomes especially important to differentiate between functionally necessary procedures and those performed for esthetic reasons. Since techniques for correction of anomalies of meatal position are associated with significant complication rates and 70% of all hypospadias cases are performed for esthetic reasons only, counselling of the parents before they give their informed consent is particularly important.

Indications

- *Esthetic*: in glanular, coronal and subcoronal hypospadias without associated penile deviation, surgery may be delayed and the patient allowed to make a decision at a later time. (Meatotomy and circumcision only is also possible.)

- *Functionally necessary*: proximal hypospadias, and all forms with associated deviations or other functional deficit

Timing of surgery

Surgery should be performed between the 2nd and 4th years of life, with a possible reintervention 9 months later and completion before school age. (Hospital stay should be in mother–child units or outpatient.)

Pretreatment

A 6 week pretreatment of the penis with daily application of either 1% testosterone or dihydrotestosterone cream facilitates the reconstructive procedure, especially in the small penis with bad skin.

Instruments

- Microsurgical tools
- Magnifying glasses
- Tourniquets
- Sponges with 1 : 10 000 adrenaline
- Buccal submucosal injection (for hemostasis) of 1 : 100 000 adrenaline in saline
- Suprapubic catheter
- PVC Websinger stent, 10 Fr
- Nonadhesive wound dressing
- Suture material: 5/0–7/0 catgut or chromic catgut and nonresorbable sutures for the Nesbit plication

Conversion to a two-stage procedure

Residual deviation after complete chordectomy, together with a poorly vascularized and fragile urethral plate, necessitates division of the urethral plate, Nesbit plication, ventral skin closure and two-stage strategy.

Anesthesia

Intubation, caudal block. Nasal intubation facilitates dissection of the buccal mucosa.

Surgical technique step by step

A.

Esthetic indication: meatotomy and possible circumcision (Figures 1 and 2)
- Meatotomy with deep incision and lateral mucosal sutures and possible additional circumcision

Harvesting of the buccal mucosa (Figures 3–6)
- Harvesting of mucosa from the lower lip and, if necessary, the inner cheek. A sufficiently long graft can be harvested even for scrotal hypospadias. Dissection of the pure mucosa graft without damage to the oral musculature is facilitated by submucous injection of adrenaline 1 : 100 000 in saline. Shrinkage of approximately 25% has to be taken into account when outlining the graft.

- Careful thinning of the graft with dissecting off the submucous fatty tissue

- Coagulation of the wound in the lip or cheek and insertion of a sponge. A suture is not necessary in this very rapidly healing wound

B.

Functional indication: coronal to scrotal hypospadias with chordee but intact urethral plate for onlay (one-stage procedure) (Figures 7–18)

- Downstripping of the entire shaft skin together with Scarpa's fascia and corda and freeing of the dorsal bundle after circular skin incision 3 mm proximal to the corona

- Elevation of the urethra from the underlying tissue facilitated by placement of two vessel loops

- Dissection of the lateral bands to both sides of the urethral bed between the corpora cavernosa and extensive chordectomy

- Elevation of the glans wings and dissection until deep under the wings of the cord bands

- Artificial erection, When persisting deviation is present a modified Nesbit procedure with inverting sutures is performed

When a poorly vascularized thin and fragile urethral plate is noticed after these steps, a two-stage procedure is indicated: surgery should be completed by a ventral skin flap, with onlay 9–12 months later as described below

- Urethral reconstruction with onlay of the graft to the remaining urethral plate with the mucosal side to the urethra and running suture over a Websinger stent, which is inserted only as far as the bulbar urethra (for drainage or secretion without urine contamination) and fixation of the stent with a catgut suture at the urethral plate

- Adaptation of the glans wings to the distal neourethra

- Covering of the suture line with dorsally mobilized Scarpa's fascia and subcutaneous tissue

- Plastic reconstruction of the neomeatus, which is placed at the coronal level

C.

Functional indication: proximal hypospadias with chordee and insufficient urethral plate for onlay after chordectomy (second stage) (Figures 19–21)

- 9–12 months after the initial chordectomy and ventral skin flap, the second stage is performed with incision along the envisioned urethral plate and lateral dissection of the shaft skin

- The buccal mucosa onlay graft is sutured with running suture to the plate, positioning the meatus at the corona, and covered with Scarpa's fascia and subcutaneous tissue

Surgical tricks

Abandoning positioning the neomeatus at the tip of the glans avoids extensive glans dissection, with the possibility of impaired blood supply and meatal stenosis due to circular closure of the glans wings at the tip of the glans over the neomeatus. This results in a lower rate of meatal stenosis and consecutive fistula associated with this final step. In a cohort of adults with incidental hypospadias we have had no associated functional deficits. All of them voided in the standing position with a single stream.[3] The covering of the neourethra with three vascularized sheaths (Scarpa's fascia, superficial fascia and skin) is especially important.

Postoperative care

- Nonadhesive wound dressing for 7–10 days

- Stenting of the neourethra with a 10 Fr Websinger, which reaches only to the bulbar urethra for secretion drainage

- Urinary diversion with a suprapubic tube for 3 weeks and removal after an intact urethra and residual-free voiding has been demonstrated on voiding cystourethrography

- Antibiotic prophylaxis until the suprapubic tube is removed

Ten things to aim for

- Functional indication

- Surgery between 2 and 4 years of age

- 6 weeks prior treatment with testosterone cream

- One-stage procedure if possible

- Use of buccal mucosa

- Onlay technique

- Use of rapidly resorbable suture material

- Well-vascularized covering sheaths

- Stent for 10 days, cystostomy for 3 weeks

- Nonadhesive wound dressings

Ten things to avoid

- Esthetic indication
- Surgery too early
- Enforcement of a one-stage procedure
- Meatal positioning near the tip of the glans
- Use of hairy skin
- Slowly resorbable sutures
- Repeated dilatation of the meatal stenosis
- Voiding before 3 weeks
- Removal of wound dressings before 7 days
- Stent removal before 10 days

References

1. Bürger R, Müller SC, Hohenfellner R. Buccal mucosa graft: a preliminary report. *J Urol* **147** (1992) 662–4.
2. Onckett JW Jr. Transverse preputial island flap technique for repair of severe hypospadias. *Urol Clin N Amer* **7** (1980) 423.
3. Fichtner J, Filipas D, Mottrie AM, Voges GE, Hohenfellner R. Analysis of meatal location in 500 men: wide variation questions need for meatal advancement in all pediatric anterior hypospadias cases. *J Urol* **154** (1995) 833–4.

1. Esthetic indication: Meatotomy and circumcision

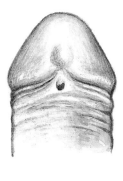 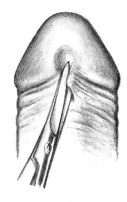

Figure 1. *Meatotomy with a deep incision between the hypospadiac meatus and blind-ending groove.*

Figure 2. *Everting sutures of the mucosa.*

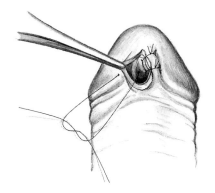 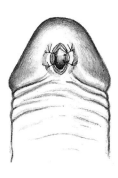

Harvesting of buccal mucosa

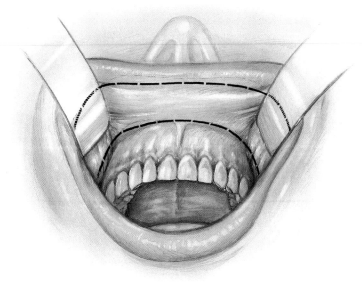

Figure 3. *Outlining of the graft from the lip and possibly the inner cheek.*

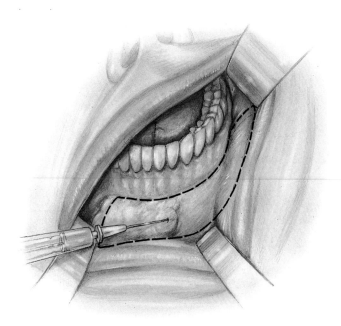

Figure 4. *Submucous injection (1 : 100 000 adrenaline) facilitates dissection of the graft.*

Figure 5. *Sharp dissection of the graft with careful avoidance of the underlying musculature.*

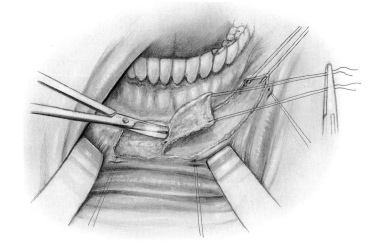

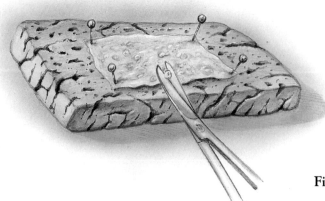

Figure 6. *Thinning of the graft and resection of the fatty tissue.*

2. Functional indication: Coronal-penile hypospadias with deviation but sufficient urethral plate for onlay => one stage

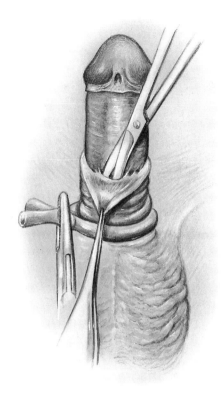

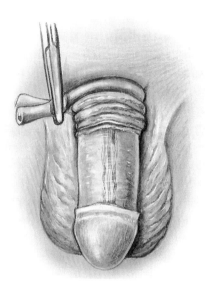

Figure 7. *Stripping down of the shaft skin together with Scarpa's fascia after coronal incision.*

Figure 8. *Dorsally freed bundle.*

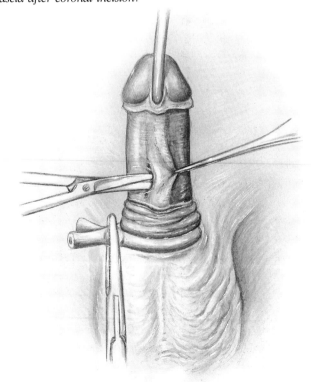

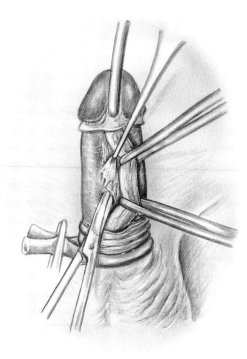

Figure 9. *Lifting of the urethra off the underlying tissue (Mollard).*

Figure 10. *Sharp dissection of the lateral cord bands to both sides of the urethral bed after placement of two vessel loops.*

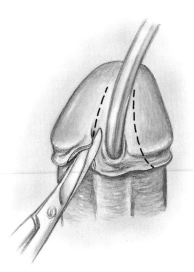

Figure 11. *Line of incision for mobilization of the glans wings.*

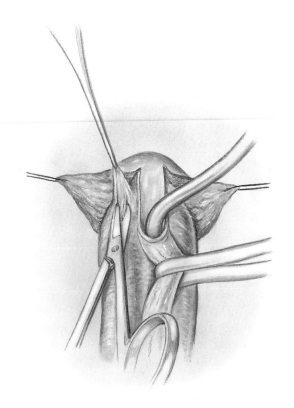

Figure 12. *Dissection deep under the wings for removal of the cord.*

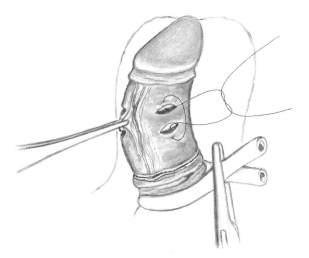

Figure 13. *Residual deviation requires a modified dorsal inverting Nesbit plication.*

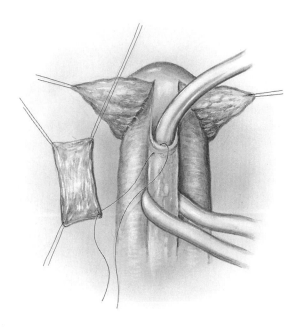

Figure 14. *Suturing of the buccal mucosal graft (mucosa side to the urethra).*

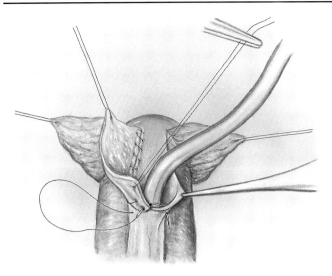

Figure 15. *Running suture of the graft.*

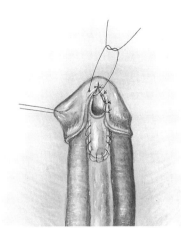

Figure 16. *Adaptation of the glans wings to the neourethra. Do not leave the tourniquet for longer than 20 minutes.*

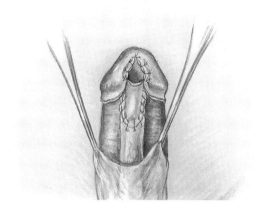

Figure 17. *Covering of the urethra with mobilized Scarpa's fascia.*

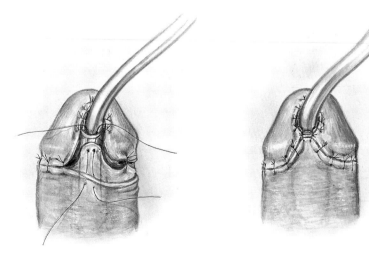

Figure 18. *Plastic reconstruction of the coronal neomeatus.*

3. Functional indication: proximal hypospadias with chorda but insufficient urethral plate for onlay => two-stage

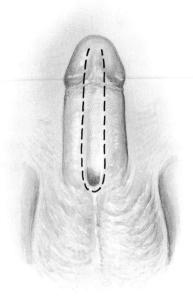

Figure 19. *Incision along the outlined urethral plate.*

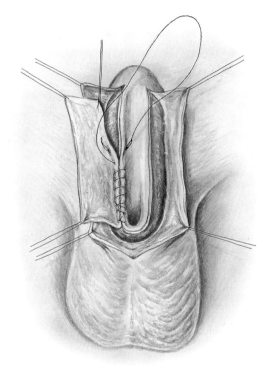

Figure 20. *Suturing of the onlay graft to the plate after lateral dissection of the penile shaft skin.*

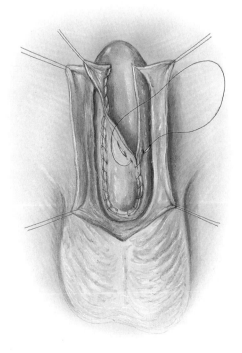

Figure 21. *Running suture of the onlay graft with three-layer closure of covering sheaths over the neourethra (Scarpa's fascia, superficial fascia and skin).*

Construction of a Scrotum from Prepuce

J.E. Wright
Paediatric Surgeon,
116 Everton Street,
Hamilton NSW 2303, Australia

Comment

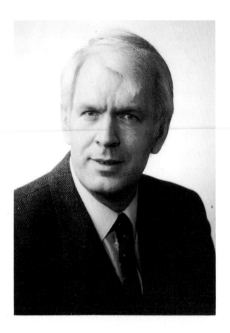

The male genitalia are formed between the 6th and 13th weeks of gestation from the genital tubercle. Malformations of the scrotum are observed in severe forms of hypospadias as scrotum bifidum or penoscrotal transformation. The absence of one half of the scrotum or the ectopic formation of a part of the scrotum is rare; however, in these cases the existing scrotum can be used in reconstruction. The reasons for scrotal anomalies are not well understood. One theory is that during the period of relative oligohydramnios the pressure on a developing extremity causes the malformation, but this seems too mechanical.

In female-to-male transsexuals the labia majora are used for the construction of a scrotum. After loss of the scrotal skin due to gangrenous diseases like Fournier syndrome or extensive cancer surgery, tissue expander can be used to enlarge the remaining skin, myocutaneous skin flaps or split skin for a mesh graft plasty. There are few publications concerning the absence of a scrotum, and the operative techniques normally used offer no solution for this problem. The technique presented by Wright is impressive because of the construction of the scrotum and the placing of both testes in the neoscrotum in one session. The cosmetic result 13 months after the operation, presented in the original publications in 1993, are satisfactory.

The author considers it important that the skin used to construct the scrotum should have androgen receptors because adequate development and enlargement after puberty are not guaranteed by the use of the skin. Methods to determine the presence of androgen receptors in the fibroblast of the prepuce have been available for some years, so that it is now possible to investigate this further. However, I think that it is more important to bring the testis down into the correct position at the age of presentation (16 months). This is debatable if the perineal testis is more or less orthotopic but the other testis is inguinal, as this position of the testis would make the chance for fertility higher.

This operative technique extends the methods of plastic surgery available to pediatric urologists. In my opinion this is the method of choice in children with no scrotum but with sufficient prepuce if it is not needed for reconstruction of the urethra.

R.-H. Ringert, Göttingen, Germany

Construction of a scrotum from prepuce

Introduction

Congenital absence of the scrotum is rare. It was first described, together with a technique for construction of a scrotum from prepuce, in 1993 in the *Journal of Pediatric Surgery*.[1] The condition is obviously associated with undescended testes, which may be in the groin or in the perineum.

It is important that a scrotum be constructed so that testes can be inserted in this 'cooling chamber' to allow them to develop adequately and for spermatogenesis to take place after puberty. It is important that the scrotum be constructed from skin with androgen receptors so that it will develop adequately and enlarge after puberty. The appropriate skin is the prepuce.

I have developed a technique to achieve this, which has proved successful in one patient.

Operative technique step by step (Figures 1–8)

- Under general and caudal anesthesia, the patient is placed supine with the legs apart

- The prepuce is retracted, with preliminary dilatation if necessary. All available preputial skin must be preserved. A circumferential incision is made around the inner layer of the prepuce keeping it distal with a short coronal cuff on the dorsal surface but more proximal with a large coronal cuff ventrally. The prepuce is then unfolded, preserving its blood supply, to form a single tubular flap

- A midline incision is made in the perineum from the most proximal aspect of this circumcizing incision, following the raphe of the perineum. This incision opens up the tube of preputial skin to become a large flap

- The perineal incision is undermined and through it testes are mobilized. If necessary, supplementary inguinal incisions can be performed to achieve adequate cord length. The testes are then delivered into the perineum

- A dorsal buttonhole incision is made in the preputial flap as far proximal as possible while still allowing enough skin to cover the dorsal surface of the penile shaft

- This Beck–Ombredanne flap[2] is then swung over the glans to cover the perineum

- The mobilized testes are accommodated within this flap, which is sutured to the margins of the perineal incision with fine absorbable sutures (polyglycolic acid or polyglactin)

- A septum can be created between the two testes by suturing the skin of this flap or its subcutaneous tissue to the fascia of the perineum in the midline

- Skin edges are united using fine absorbable sutures such as 6/0 polyglycolic acid or polyglactin. No dressing is necessary

Postoperative care

There is considerable postoperative swelling, and close supervision is required to ensure that there is no infection and that the blood supply to the skin edges is adequate.

It takes many months for the bruising and swelling to settle down, but the final result is a scrotum which is barely distinguishable from a normal one.

References

1. Wright JE. Congenital absence of the scrotum: case report and description of an original technique of constructing a scrotum. *J Ped Surg* **28** (1993) 264–6.
2. Beck C. Hypospadias and its treatment. *Surg Gynecol Obstet* **24** (1917) 511–32.

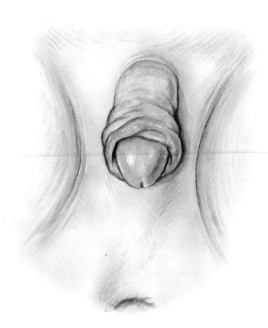

Figure 1. *Congenital absence of the scrotum.*

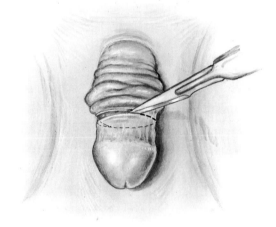

Figure 2. *Circumferential incision around the inner layer of the prepuce, keeping distal with a short coronal cuff on the dorsal surface and more proximal with a large coronal cuff ventrally.*

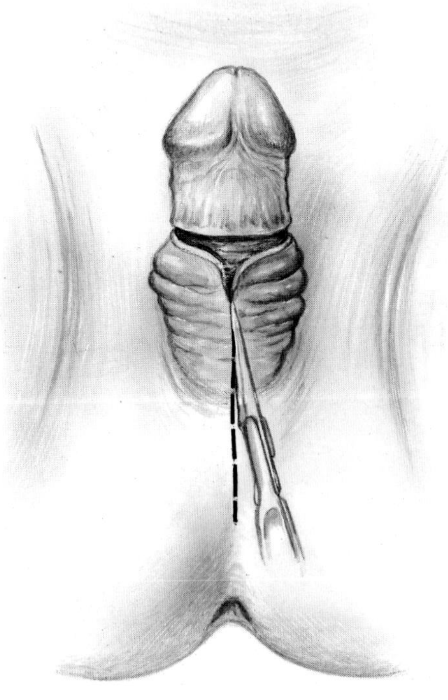

Figure 3. *Midline incision from the most proximal incision following the raphe of the perineum.*

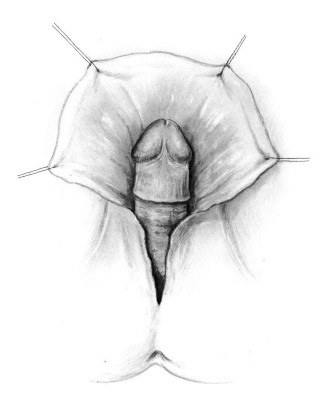

Figure 4. *Unfolding of the prepuce (blood supply).*

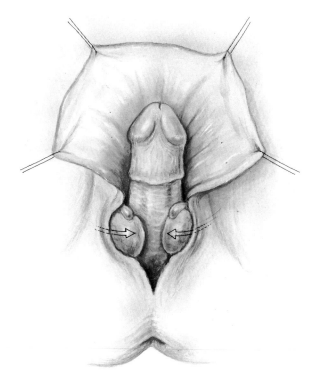

Figure 5. *Mobilization of the testis and fixation in the scrotum.*

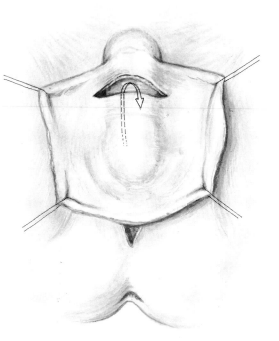

Figure 6. *'Button-hole' incision in the preputial flap.*

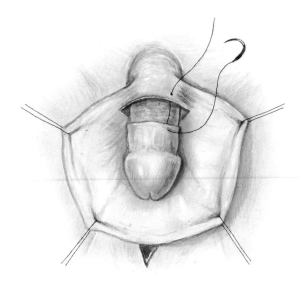

Figure 7. *The Beck–Ombredanne flap is swung over the glans; adaptation of the skin.*

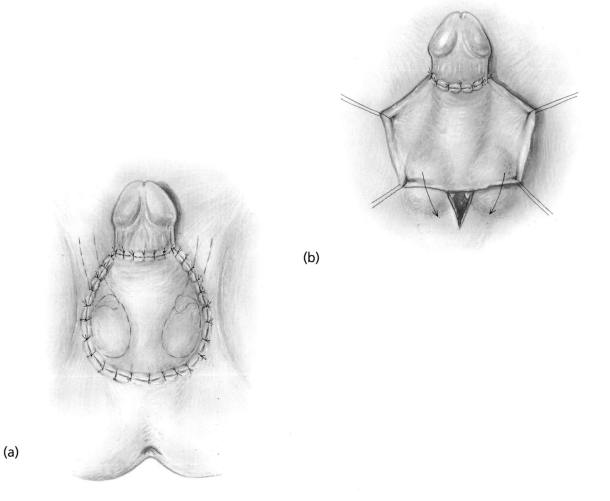

(b)

(a)

Figure 8. *Fixation of the prepuce with interrupted sutures.*

Special Techniques

VI

Operative Therapy of the Nutcracker Phenomenon

F. Steinbach[b], R. Stein, M. Hohenfellner[a]
J.W. Thüroff[a], R. Hohenfellner
Department of Urology,
University of Mainz School of Medicine,
Mainz, Germany, and
[a]*Department of Urology, Klinikum Barmen,*
University of Witten/Herdecke School of Medicine,
Wuppertal, Germany
[b]*University of Magdeburg,*
Magdeburg, Germany

Comment

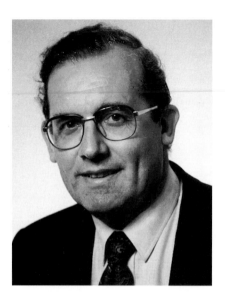

The diagnosis in patients with hematuria represents a complex problem. In most cases the diagnosis is made by routine examinations. However, if this is not possible, rare causes such as malformations of the vessels and systemic vascular disease should be kept in mind. In these patients more extensive investigations are necessary. Computed tomography, magnetic resonance imaging, angiography, pharmacoangiography and, in selected cases, phlebography are helpful.

The anterior 'nutcracker' syndrome has to be included in the differential diagnosis. In this condition, the left renal vein is compressed between the aorta and the superior mesenteric artery. The effect of compression is increased in patients with a deep renal bed due to extension of the left renal vein. A relatively deep renal bed is found in patients with extensive lumbar lordosis causing ventralization of the aorta.

In one of our patients with nutcracker syndrome, operated on in 1983, the hemoglobin level was decreased to 5.8 g/dl. Computed tomography was helpful in diagnosis. In addition to a dilated left renal vein, a declination of the vessel was seen at the level of the aorta. After injection of contrast medium, multiple small enrichments of contrast medium were found at the region of the left renal sinus and the lower pole of the kidney. Intravenous urography demonstrated a notching of these collateral vessels. In cases with this notching phenomenon, phlebography should be performed.

Pressure measurements in the left renal vein show a large interindividual variation. The larger the collateral circulation, the lower the pressure gradient between the inferior vena cava and the left renal vein. In our patient the difference was 6 cmH$_2$O. The left renal vein was located 1 cm above the renal artery and was dilated and extended up to the renal hilus.

In cases with a real nutcracker phenomenon the intrarenal venous blood flow cannot be normalized by ligation of the collateral vessels only: the pressure gradient is raised by this procedure. The best operative strategy would be to bring the renal vein more caudal. In our patient, intraoperative pyeloscopy revealed the bleeding in the region of the fornices so familiar from the literature. Because the ischemic period was short, we did not cool the kidney. After transposition of the renal vein, the vessel was no longer dilated or extended. For preservation of the vessel anastomosis we performed a nephropexy at the anterior abdominal wall.

Seven years after the operation, the patient is free of symptoms, has no periods of hematuria and is normal on intravenous urography and renography.

Bibliography

1. Coolsaet BLRA. Ureteric pathology in relation to right and left gonadal veins. *Urology* **12** (1978) 40–9.
2. Steinbach F, Stöckle M, Hohenfellner M, Schweden F, Riedmiller H, Hohenfellner R. Vaskulär bedingte Hämaturie. *Akt Urol* **20** (1989) 326–31.
3. Stewart BH, Reiman G. Left renal venous hypertension: 'nutcracker' syndrome. *Urology* **20** (1982) 365–9.
4. Weiner SN, Bernstein RG, Morehouse H, Golden RA. Hematuria secondary to left peripelvic and gonadal vein varices. *Urology* **22** (1983) 81–4.
5. Wendel RG, Crawford ED, Hehmann KN. 'Nutcracker' phenomen: an unusual cause for renal varicosities with hematuria. *J Urol* **123** (1980) 761–3.

A.A. Daenekindt, Eindhoven, The Netherlands

Operative Therapy of the Nutcracker Phenomenon

Introduction

The anterior 'nutcracker' or superior mesenteric artery phenomenon was first described as a cause of sinistral hematuria in 1972 by De Schepper.[1] The left renal vein is compressed between the superior mesenteric artery and the aorta; the subsequent increase in pressure in the renal vein leads to the development of collateral veins in the form of peripelvic and periureteral varices. Bleeding, particularly in the calix region, caused recurrent microhematuria and macrohematuria. In addition, this is conducive to the development of a sinistral varicocele or ovarian venectasia, with unilateral renal vein thrombosis and flank pain.

Similar symptoms can be observed in the posterior nutcracker phenomenon, where the course of the left renal vein is retroaortal.

The aim of operative therapy is reduction of pressure in the renal vein and thus an unhindered venous flow out of the left kidney. This is achieved by caudal transposition of the left renal vein.

Preoperative diagnostics

It is essential to prove the existence of compression of the left renal vein, as well as to exclude other causes of hematuria such as urologic diseases (especially malignancy) and the rarer vascular abnormalities and systemic diseases with vascular involvement.[2] Cystoscopy shows bleeding from the left ureteral orifice. The basic urologic examinations consisting of physical and laboratory examinations, sonography of the retroperitoneum and excretory urography (IVU) usually do not meet these two objectives.

The IVU may be completely normal or, in the renal pelvic and ureteral region, may show contrast media in recesses (the 'notching' phenomenon), caused by peripelvic and ureteral varices.

On ultrasonography, a significantly dilated left renal vein and an acute angle between the aorta and the superior mesenteric artery may indicate a compression phenomenon.

To confirm the diagnosis, it is necessary to use a combination of several diagnostic procedures:

- *Cystoscopy.* Proof of bleeding from the left orifice

- *Retrograde pyelography.* Even during a minimal retrograde filling, prompt contrast media passage into the smallest

peripheral veins indicates the pyelovenous shunt

- *Selective phlebography of the left renal vein with simultaneous measurement of pressure.* Besides the peripelvic varices, which lead to hematuria through spontaneous rupture, a sharp interruption of the contrast medium visualization of the renal vein near the crossing of the upper mesenteric artery is typical

  The intravascular pressure central and peripheral to the compression point should be determined with the patient in the supine and standing positions. Whereas only slight degrees of change in the pressure are apparent in the supine patient, these almost always increase significantly in the standing position

  A borderline between normal and pathologic pressures cannot be defined exactly because of individual variation. The normal difference in pressures ranges between 1 and 5 cmH$_2$O, but can also be more than this.[3] The pathologic readings for the patients examined here ranged between 12 and 14 cmH$_2$O.

- *Computed tomography or magnetic resonance imaging.* A significantly dilated left renal vein compressed between the aorta and the superior mesenteric artery may indicate the nutcracker phenomenon

Indications

In most cases the nutcracker phenomenon can be managed conservatively by giving plasminogen inactivators. A surgical procedure, however, is indicated if there is recurrent macrohematuria sufficient to affect blood hemoglobin levels and flank pain caused by the passing of blood clots.

Special instruments

- Bulldog clamps
- Satinsky clamps
- Ice-bags
- Satinsky scissors
- Polyglyconate suture material (4/0)
- 2500 units heparin in 40 ml 0.9% sodium chloride solution
- Slush ice

Operative technique step by step (Figures 1–7)

In the nutcracker phenomenon, the surgical objective is caudal transposition of the left renal vein. The vascular junction of the superior mesenteric artery and the aorta is not corrected.

- The patient is placed in a hyperextended supine position, and the abdomen is opened from the sternum to 5 cm above the symphysis

- The small intestine is shifted to the right and the dorsal peritoneum is incised lengthwise over the aorta

- Complete exposure of the confluence of the left renal vein and the vena cava inferior is achieved by mobilization of the duodenum and incision of Treitz's ligament

- To mobilize the left renal vein, it is necessary to ligate the suprarenal vein and the ovarian or testicular vein as well as the lumbar veins, which enter dorsally

- Intravenous application of 20 mg of furosemide and cooling of the kidney with ice-bags

- The left renal artery is clamped and the renal vein cut above a Satinsky clamp leaving a narrow caval cuff

- 2500 units of heparin in 40 ml of sodium chloride solution are injected into the lumen of the vein to prevent the formation of blood clots

- The left renal vein is shifted caudally 4–6 cm; if the inferior mesenteric artery proves to be a limiting factor it can be ligated

- A caval window is formed on the lateral side of the inferior vena cava by excising an oval patch corresponding to the caliber of the renal vein

- Two lateral corner sutures are placed, and the posterior and anterior anastomoses are made with running sutures

- The kidney circulation is restored and the ice-bag removed, and the defect in the vena cava wall is closed with a running suture

- The ischemic period for the kidney is approximately 15–20 minutes; therefore intraoperative perfusion of the kidney is not necessary

Postoperative care

- To prevent a thrombosis in the area of the vascular anastomosis, the prothrombin time should be stabilized at over 50 seconds by means of constant infusions of heparin for a period of 4 days

- The kidney circulation can be improved by administering dopamine (2–4 µg/kg per min for 4 days)

Surgical tricks

Macrohematuria can persist for several weeks after the operation before the pyelovenous shunt closes. If there is heavy bleeding, the pyeloureteral junction can be plugged with a balloon catheter pushed retrogradely into the renal pelvis. Simultaneously tranexamic acid (3 × 0.25 g/day) and antibiotics are then administered. After 3 days the balloon catheter is removed and the medication stopped.

Final examination

To document kidney function a MAG 3 clearance (mercaptoacetyltriglycerol) test should be performed before the patient is discharged.

References

1. De Schepper A. 'Nutcracker'-phenomenon of the renal vein causing left renal vein pathology. *J Belg Rad* **55** (1972) 507–9.
2. Steinbach F, Stöckle M, Hohenfellner M, Schweden F, Riedmiller H, Hohenfellner R. Vaskulär bedingte Hämaturie. *Akt Urol* **20** (1989) 326–31.
3. Beinart CK, Sniderman W, Tamura S, Vaughan ED, Sos TA. Left renal vein to inferior vena cava pressure relationship in humans. *J Urol* **127** (1982) 1070–1.

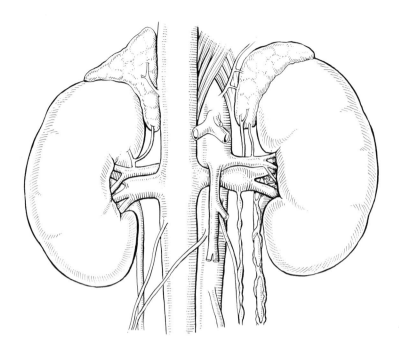

Figure 1. *Compression of the left renal vein in the angle between the superior mesenteric artery and the aorta leads to an increase in pressure in the renal vein with consecutive development of peripelvic and periureteral varices.*

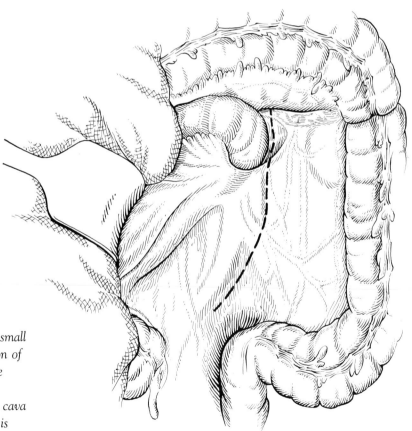

Figure 2. *Transposition of the small intestine to the right and incision of the dorsal peritoneum above the aorta and the mesenteric root. Complete exposure of the vena cava and the renal vascular pedicle is achieved after incision of Treitz's ligament and mobilization of the duodenum.*

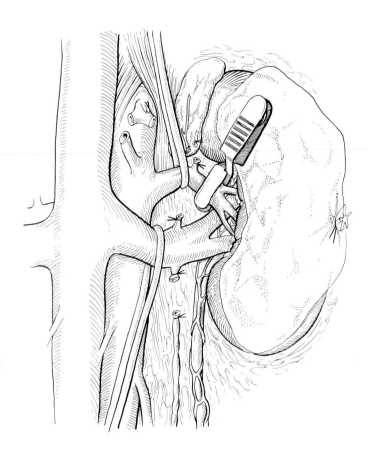

Figure 3. Mobilization of the renal vessels by ligating the suprarenal artery and vein, the testicular or ovarian vein and, if necessary, the lumbar veins entering dorsally. After external cooling of the kidney, clamping of the renal artery using a bulldog clamp.

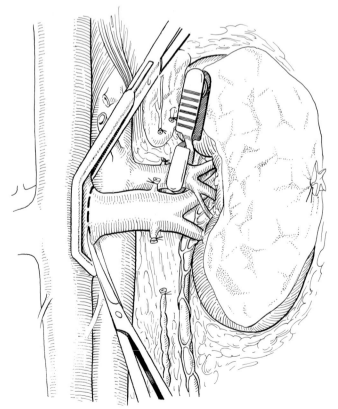

Figure 4. Incision of the renal vein with Satinsky scissors, leaving a narrow vena caval cuff. Injection of 2500 units of heparin into the lumen of the vein to prevent clot formation.

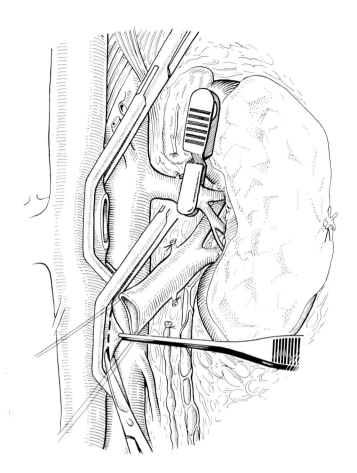

Figure 5. Construction of a vena caval window approximately 4–6 cm caudal to the former entrance.

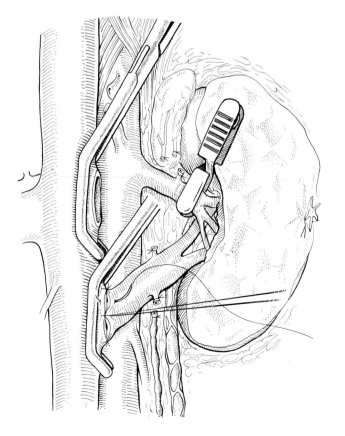

Figure 6. By mobilizing the kidney ventrally and medially, the vascular anastomosis is performed. After placing corner sutures, the posterior and anterior anastomosis is made using an atraumatic running suture (4/0). To avoid suturing the posterior wall, the interrupted suture in the middle of the anterior wall is pulled slightly.

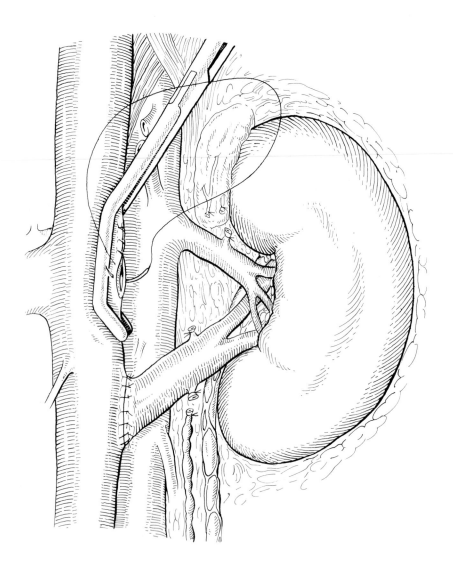

Figure 7. *Restoration of the venal circulation and closure of the vena caval defect with an atraumatic running suture (4/0) after termination of ischemia.*

Transverse Colonic Conduit

M. Fisch, R. Hohenfellner
Department of Urology,
University of Mainz School of Medicine,
Mainz, Germany

Comment

The different forms and techniques of bladder substitution and continent diversion dominate discussion of urinary diversion. Nevertheless, the introduction of a technique with a wet stoma is no anachronism: a transverse colonic conduit is indicated if one of the newer techniques is not practicable because of complications or if a classic ileal of sigmoid colonic conduit is technically impossible.

For the anastomosis of irradiated bowels or ureters, there are as many publications showing no problems as there are warning of enormous postoperative complications, but the number of unreported complicated operations is surely higher. Reliable intraoperative assessment of radiation damage is not possible, and the transverse colonic conduit avoids this risk by anastomosis of undamaged segments (Figure 1).

Some cases in female patients with extended fistulas developing in the small pelvis seem to be technically inoperable, especially following radiotherapy or previous unsuccessful operations leaving nephrostomas on both sides or ureterocutaneostomies as the (unacceptable) final treatment. In these cases the transverse colonic conduit (especially the pyelotransversopyeolocutaneostoma) is useful because it does not depend on extensively damaged ureters. Efficient arterial blood supply by the middle colic artery makes the necessary removal of a long bowel segment in these cases unproblematic (Figures 2 and 3).

The surgeon inexperienced in abdominal surgery will be afraid of the first steps: removing the omentum to cranial, cutting the gastrocolic ligament and opening the omental

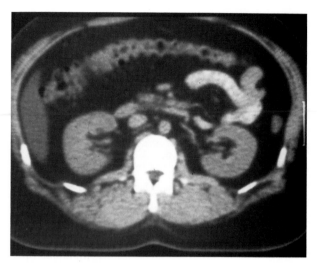

Figure 3

bursa, and if necessary extended mobilization of both colonic flexures to yield a tension-free bowel anastomosis. Calling a surgeon experienced in resection of the transverse colon is then recommended. The refluxive or antirefluxive ureter implantation and the pyelotranversostomy are approved and easy to perform with practice. The specific rate of complications of the transverse colonic conduit (anastomosis insufficiency and stenosis) is less than that in colonic surgery and low compared with other classic urinary drainage operations because healthy bowel is used.

P. Alken, Mannheim, Germany

Figure 1

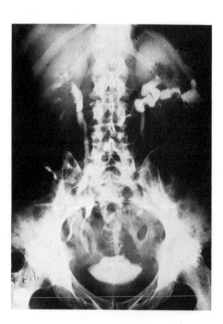

Figure 2

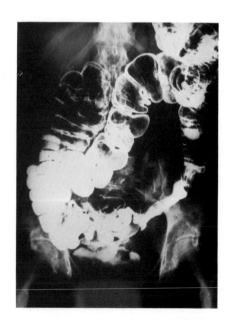

Transverse Colonic Conduit

Introduction

Since the first publication[1] in 1969, the transverse colonic conduit has been used more and more in patients with urologic or gynecologic malignancy who are receiving radiotherapy.[2-5] Its cranial position lies outside the irradiation field, which is of utmost importance for a segment to be used for urinary diversion. The long mesentery allows individual adaptation, and the transverse colon offers the possibility of antirefluxive as well as refluxive ureteral implantation[6-9] and is less prone to stoma stenosis than ileum.

Direct anastomosis of the conduit to the renal pelvis (pyelotransversopyelocutaneostomy) is an option in patients with total damage of the ureters by radiation or retroperitoneal fibrosis and in patients with recurrent urothelial tumor in a single kidney.[10]

Indications

- Urinary diversion in patients with urologic or gynecologic malignancy and radiation damage to the bowel and distal ureters

- Incontinence in patients with radiogenic cystitis

- Complex vesicovaginal and rectovesicovaginal fistula

- Unsuccessful primary urinary diversion requiring conversion[11]

Preoperative investigations and preparation

- Intravenous urography (to eliminate upper urinary tract disease), bowel enema with water-soluble contrast medium (to eliminate diverticula and polyposis)

- Intestinal irrigation with Ringer's lactate solution (8–10 liters) via a gastric tube or oral intake of 5–7 liters of Fordtran's solution; checking of electrolytic levels

- Deciding the position of the stoma in the epigastric region; attaching a stoma plate and bag, and check with the patient in a sitting, lying and standing position

Instruments and suture material

- Basic set for kidney surgery with additional instruments for intra-abdominal surgery

- Ring retractor

- Basin containing prepared iodine solution (for disinfection)

- Polyglyconic acid 4/0 for closure of the conduit, intestinal anastomosis to re-establish bowel continuity, and stoma

- Polyglyconic acid 5/0 for refluxive ureteral implantation

- Chromic catgut 5/0 and 6/0 for antirefluxive ureteral implantation

- Silk 4/0 for stay sutures (bowel)

- Catgut 4/0 for stay sutures (bowel mucosa), and fixation of ureteral stents

Operative technique step by step

- Insertion of a gastric tube (alternatively gastrostomy), a rectal tube and a central venous catheter

- Median laparotomy

- Identification of the ureters at the crossing over the iliac vessels and dissection in a cranial direction

- Mobilization of the right and left colonic flexures

- Resection of the radiogenically damaged ureters; a stay suture is placed at the end of the ureter

- Selection of a transverse segment approximately 15 cm in length, respecting the course of the vessels (Figure 1)

- Incision of the mesentery lateral to the supplying artery; the arcades are divided between mosquito clamps and ligated

- Dissection of the fat from the seromuscular layer of the bowel in the area where the segment will be cut; coagulation of bleeding vessels

- Isolation of the segment and cleaning by moist sponges

- Bowel continuity is re-established by a one-layer seromuscular suture using polyglyconic acid 4/0 (Figure 2)

- Closure of the mesenteric slit with a running suture

- According to the final position of the conduit, the left or right ureter is pulled through behind the mesentery to the other side (Figure 3)

- Ureteral implantation (see below)

- Fixation suture of the conduit

- Stoma formation (see below)

- Insertion of two silicone drainage tubes, one in the area of the conduit, the second down to the deepest point of the pelvis

- Wound closure

Ureteral implantation

Antirefluxive open-ended technique according to Goodwin and Hohenfellner[12] (Figure 4)
- The conduit is longitudinally opened over a length of approximately 4 cm starting from the end chosen for ureteral implantation (preferably the oral end)
- Four stay sutures (catgut 4/0) are placed to facilitate ureteral implantation
- A submucosal tunnel is dissected, starting from the end of the conduit (tunnel length 3–4 cm)
- An incision is made in the bowel mucosa at the end of the tunnel
- For implantation of the second ureter a second tunnel is prepared beside and parallel to the first
- The distal part of both ureters is carefully freed of fat and surrounding tissue, respecting the blood supply
- The ureters are pulled through the submucous tunnel
- The ureters are spatulated and resected to an adequate length
- The ureters are anchored by sutures at the 5 and 7 o'clock positions, through the seromuscular layer of the bowel and all layers of the ureter (chromic catgut 5/0)
- The anastomosis is completed by mucomucous single sutures (chromic catgut 6/0)
- To secure the ureterals a 6 Fr ureteral stent is inserted into each ureter and fixed to the bowel mucosa (catgut 4/0)
- The stents are led out through the aboral end of the conduit
- The oral end of the conduit and the incision line in the area of the teniae coli are closed with single seromuscular sutures (polyglyconic acid 4/0)

Refluxive ureteral implantation according to Wallace[9] (Figures 5 and 6)
- Both ureters are resected to an adequate length and spatulated over a distance of 3 cm
- A stay suture is placed at the 6 o'clock position and a ureteral stent inserted
- The first suture for anastomosis of the medial margins of

the ureters is placed at the 12 o'clock position and tightened later
- The anastomosis is performed by a running suture (polyglyconic acid 5/0)
- The ureteral stents are fixed to the ureteral mucosa (catgut 4/0) and subsequently brought out through the conduit
- The ureteral plate is anastomosed to the oral end of the conduit by two running sutures (polyglyconic acid 5/0)

Formation of the stoma (Figure 7)
- A circular area of the skin (approximately 3 cm in diameter) is excised and a cross-like incision made in the abdominal fascia
- The aboral end of the conduit is freed of fat and epiploic appendages
- The conduit is pulled through the fascia and the skin opening together with the ureteral stents by means of two Allis clamps
- The seromuscular layer of the conduit is fixed to the abdominal fascia by circular single stitches (polyglyconic acid 3/0)
- The oral end of the conduit is anastomosed to the skin by circular single stitches (polyglyconic acid 5/0), everting the stoma

Pyelotransversopyelocutaneostomy (Figures 8–15)
- The cecum and root of the mesentery are mobilized and Treitz's ligament dissected
- The right and left colonic flexure are freed
- The greater omentum is dissected from the transverse colon and the omental bursa opened
- The bowel is exteriorized
- The ureters are cut at the ureteropelvic junction
- The renal pelvis is spatulated longitudinally
- A 25–30 cm segment of transverse colon is isolated with an adequate blood supply
- A ureteral stent is placed in a calyx of the right kidney and fixed inside the renal pelvis (catgut 4/0)
- The right renal pelvis is anastomosed end-to-end to the aboral end of the conduit by two running sutures (polyglyconic acid 5/0)
- The ureteral stent is led out through the conduit before the anastomosis is completed

- The conduit is approximated to the left renal pelvis without tension
- A stent is inserted into the left kidney and fixed. (It is led out through the conduit later.)
- For anastomosis of the renal pelvis to the conduit, the wall of the conduit is incised at the teniae coli over an adequate length
- End-to-side anastomosis of the renal pelvis and the conduit is achieved by two running sutures (polyglyconic acid 5/0)

Surgical tricks

Transilluminating the mesentery by a cold light source reveals the vessels and facilitates selection of the segment as well as preparation of the mesenteric slits. When the conduit is positioned on the right side and the left ureter is relatively short, the ureter can be implanted antidromically to the right ureter (like the crossed hands of a ballerina). This is applicable for the Goodwin–Hohenfellner technique as well as the Wallace technique.

The colonic conduit can be peristaltic or antiperistaltic, so that the stoma may be positioned in the right or the left upper abdominal quadrant. For anisoperistaltic application, extensive mobilization of Treitz's ligament and the descending part of the duodenum becomes necessary; otherwise, compression of the duodenum by the conduit may result.

Postoperative care

- Antibiotics for 5 days
- Parenteral nutrition, gradually reduced after bowel contractions appear
- Removal of the gastric tube starting from day 3 (after clamping)
- Removal of the rectal tube starting from day 3
- Removal of the central venous catheter when parenteral nutrition is stopped and the patient is eating
- Loosening of the ureteral stents starting from day 9, and removal starting from day 10 (one stent after the other)

References

1. Nelson JH. *Atlas of Radical Pelvic Surgery*. New York: Appleton–Century–Crofts (1969) 181–91.
2. Altwein JE, Hohenfellner R. Use of the colon as a conduit for urinary diversion. *Surg Gynecol Obstet* **140** (1975) 33–8.
3. Morales P, Golimbu M. Colonic urinary diversion: 10 years of experience. *J Urol* **113** (1975) 302–7.
4. Schmidt JD, Buchsbaum H-J, Jacobo EC. Transverse colon conduit for supravesical urinary tract diversion. *Urology* **6** (1976) 543–6.
5. Schmidt JD, Buchsbaum H-J, Nachtsheim DA. Long-term follow-up: further experience with and modifications of the transverse colon-conduit in urinary tract diversion. *Br J Urol* **57** (1985) 284–8.
6. Camey M, Le Duc A. L'entéro-cystoplastie après cystoprostatectomie totale pour cancer de vessie: indications, technique opératoir, surveillance et résultats sur quatrevingt sept cas. *Ann Urol* **13** (1979) 114–23.
7. Leadbetter WF, Clarke BG. Five years experience with ureteroenterostomy by the 'combined' technique. *J Urol* **73** (1954) 67–82.
8. Mogg RA. Urinary diversion using the colonic conduit. *Br J Urol* **39** (1967) 687–92.
9. Wallace DM. Ureteric diversion using a conduit: a simplified technique. *Br J Urol* **38** (1966) 522–7.
10. Lindell O, Lehtonen T. Rezidivierende urotheliale Tumoren in Einzelnieren mit Anschluss eines Kolonsegmentes an das Nierenbecken. *Akt Urol* **19** (1988) 130–3.
11. Alken P, Jacobi GH, Thüroff J, Walz P, Hohenfellner R. Transversumkonduit. Berichte über das 7 klinische Wochenende der Urologischen, Universitätskliniken Mainz. Bern: Braun–Melsungen (1984) 157–71.
12. Hohenfellner R, Wulff HD. Zur Harnableitung mittels ausgeschalteter Dickdarmsegmente. *Akt Urol* **1** (1970) 18–27.

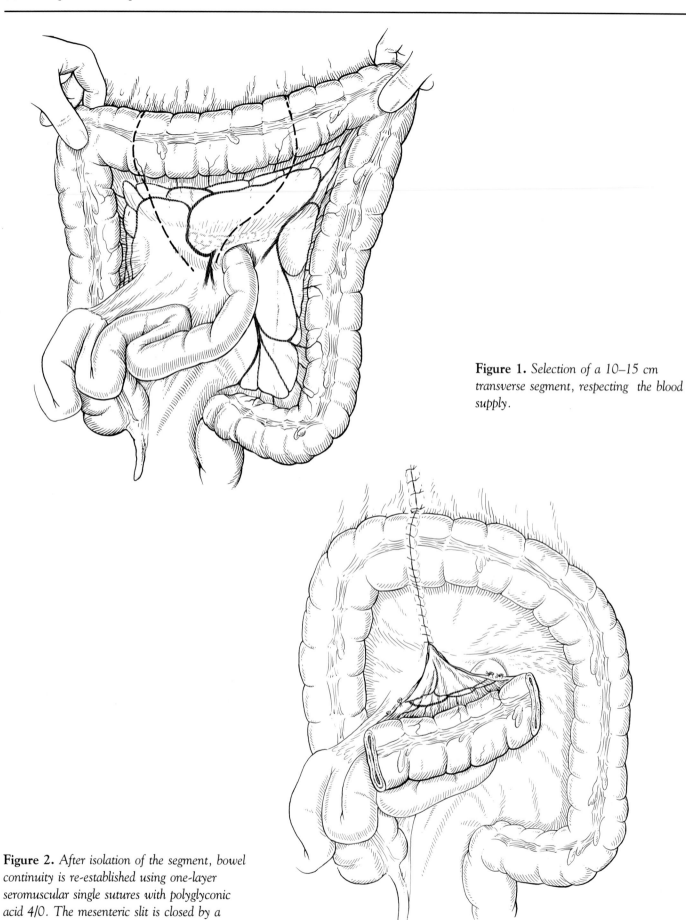

Figure 1. Selection of a 10–15 cm transverse segment, respecting the blood supply.

Figure 2. After isolation of the segment, bowel continuity is re-established using one-layer seromuscular single sutures with polyglyconic acid 4/0. The mesenteric slit is closed by a running suture (polyglyconic acid 5/0).

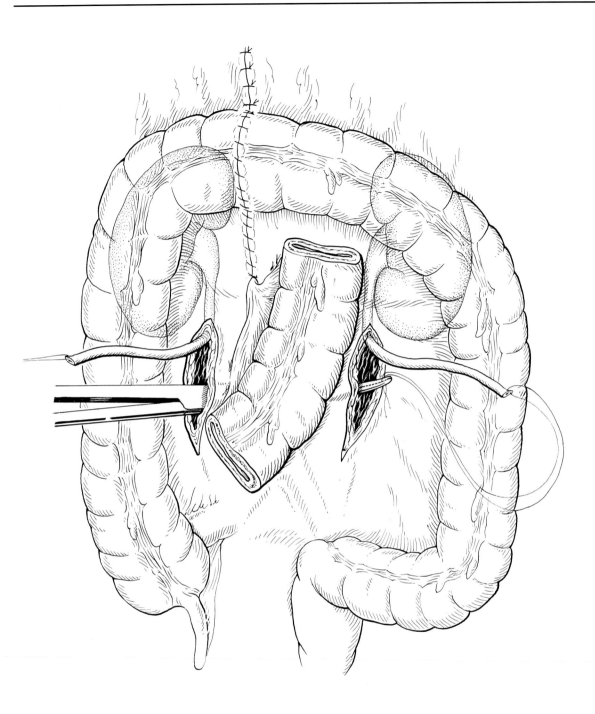

Figure 3. *When it is planned to position the conduit on the right side, the left ureter has to be brought to the right side behind the mesentery.*

Antirefluxive implantation

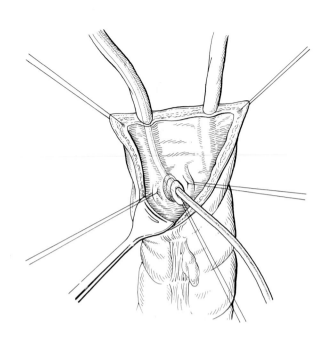

Figure 4. (a) Opening of the conduit in the area of the teniae coli over a length of approximately 4 cm, starting from the end chosen for ureteral implantation. To facilitate ureteral implantation four stay sutures are placed (catgut 4/0). A submucous tunnel is dissected starting at the end of the conduit (tunnel length 3–4 cm), and the bowel mucosa is incised at the end of the tunnel and the ureter pulled through.

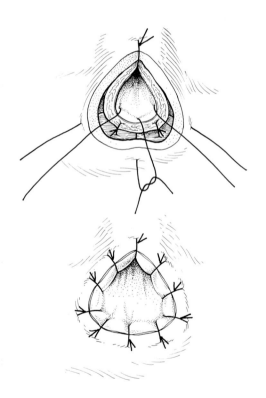

Figure 4. (b) Two anchor sutures placed at the 5 and 7 o'clock positions fix the seromuscular layer of the bowel and all layers of the ureter (chromic catgut 5/0). The anastomosis is completed by mucomucous single sutures (chromic catgut 6/0).

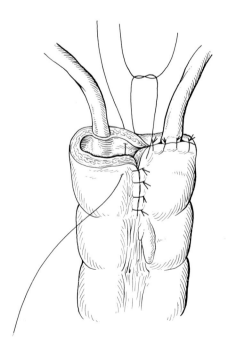

Figure 4. (c) After the contralateral ureter is implanted, the ureterointestinal anastomosis is secured by two ureteral stents (6 Fr), which are led out through the aboral end of the conduit. The conduit is closed by single seromuscular sutures (polyglyconic acid 4/0).

Refluxive implantation ('Wallace')

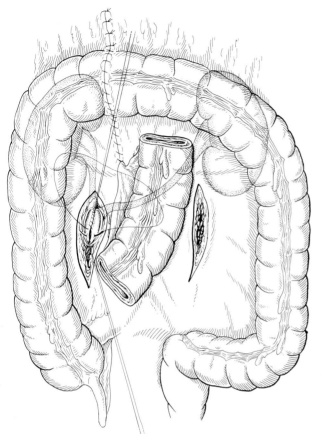

Figure 5. (*a*) *Resection of both ureters to an adequate length, with spatulation over a distance of 3 cm. A stay suture is placed at the 6 o'clock position, and the medial margins of the ureters are anastomosed starting cranially with a running suture (polyglyconic acid 5/0).*

Figure 5. (*b*) *Anastomosis of the ureteral plate to the oral end of the conduit. First, the back wall is anastomosed with a running suture (polyglyconic acid 5/0). Two stay sutures (cranial and caudal) facilitate suturing.*

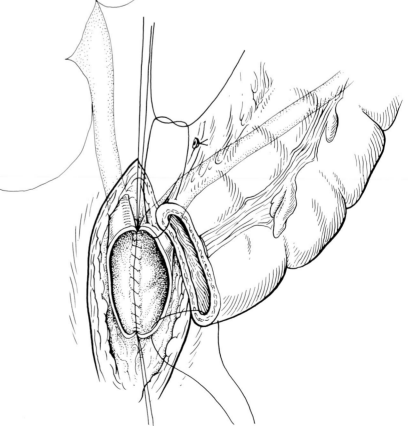

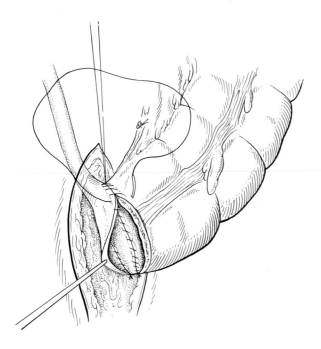

Figure 5. (*c*) *Two ureteral stents are inserted, fixed to the ureteral mucosa (catgut 4/0) and brought out through the conduit. The anastomosis to the anterior wall of the conduit is completed with a running suture (polyglyconic acid 5/0).*

Figure 5. (*d*) *The completed anastomosis. By lateral fixation, the conduit is placed in a retroperitoneal position.*

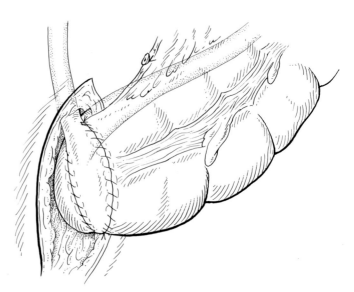

(b)

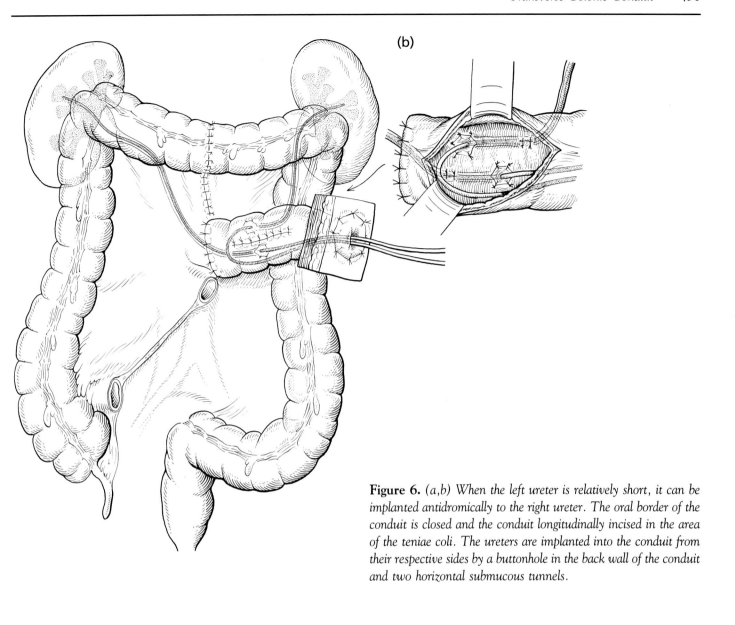

Figure 6. *(a,b) When the left ureter is relatively short, it can be implanted antidromically to the right ureter. The oral border of the conduit is closed and the conduit longitudinally incised in the area of the teniae coli. The ureters are implanted into the conduit from their respective sides by a buttonhole in the back wall of the conduit and two horizontal submucous tunnels.*

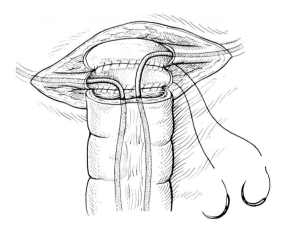

Figure 6. *(c) The antidromic implantation is also suitable for the Wallace technique, but the conduit has to be rotated 90° clockwise.*

Stoma formation

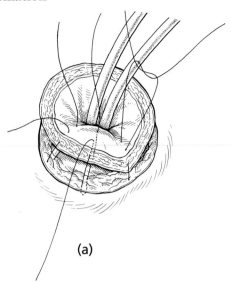

(a)

Figure 7. *(a,b) Excision of a circular area of skin (approximately 3 cm in diameter) and cross-like incision of abdominal fascia. The conduit is pulled through together with the ureteral stents. Fixation of the seromuscular layer of the conduit to the abdominal fascia by circular single stitches (polyglyconic acid 3/0).*

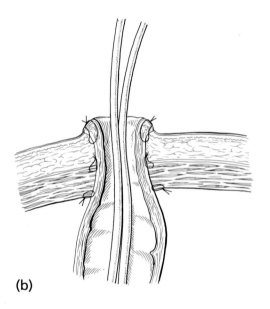

(b)

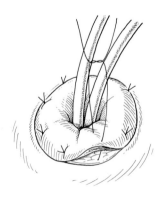

Figure 7. *(c) Anastomosis of conduit to the skin by circular single stitches (polyglyconic acid 5/0), everting the stoma.*

Pyelotransverso–Pyelocutaneostomy

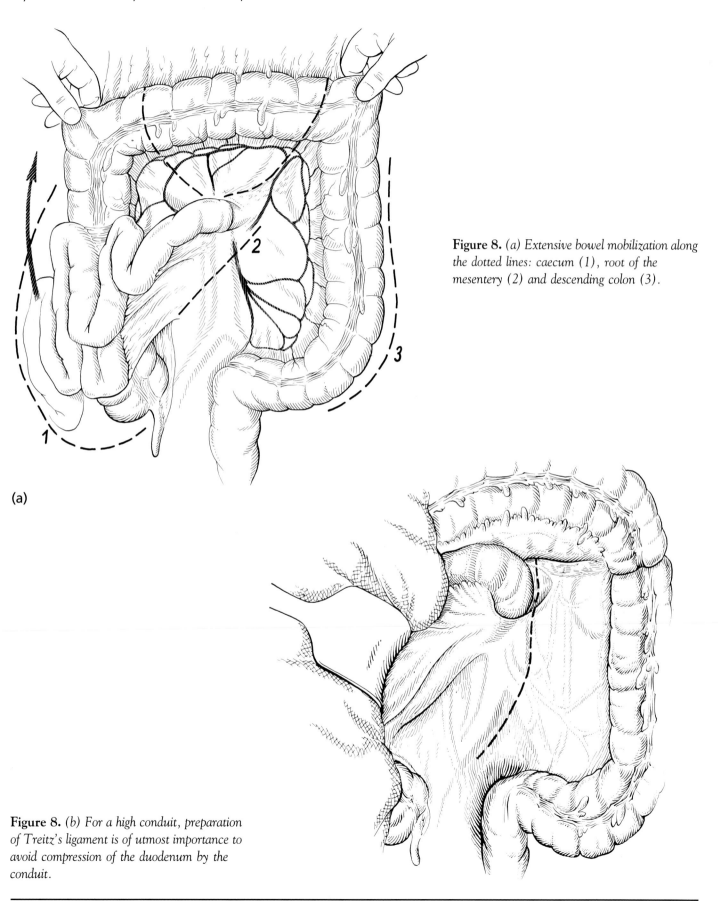

Figure 8. *(a) Extensive bowel mobilization along the dotted lines: caecum (1), root of the mesentery (2) and descending colon (3).*

(a)

Figure 8. *(b) For a high conduit, preparation of Treitz's ligament is of utmost importance to avoid compression of the duodenum by the conduit.*

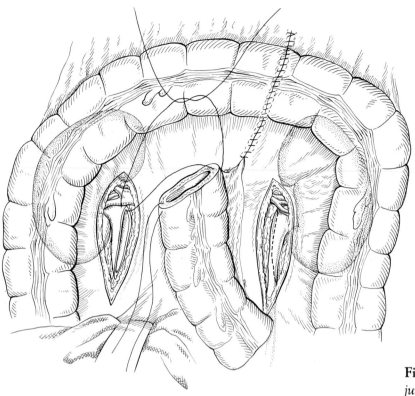

Figure 9. *The ureters are cut at the ureteropelvic junction. The renal pelvis is longitudinally spatulated and anastomosed end-to-end to the conduit with two running sutures (polyglyconic acid 5/0).*

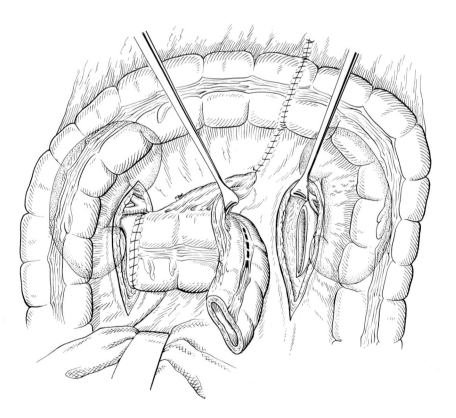

Figure 10. *Completed anastomosis of right pelvis. For anastomosis of the left renal pelvis, the wall of the conduit is incised at the teniae coli (dotted line).*

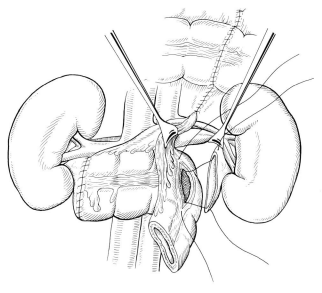

Figure 11. *Two stay sutures facilitate end-to-side anastomosis of the left renal pelvis to the conduit.*

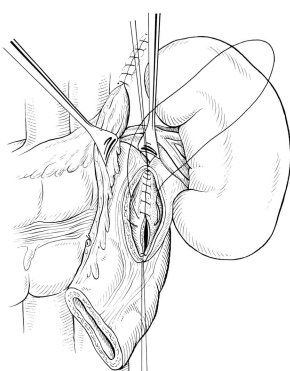

Figure 12. *Anastomosis of the back wall.*

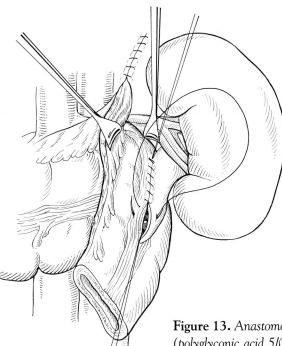

Figure 13. *Anastomosis of the anterior wall with a running suture (polyglyconic acid 5/0).*

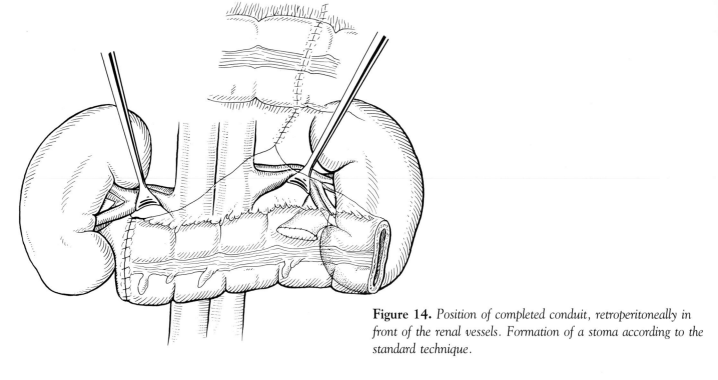

Figure 14. *Position of completed conduit, retroperitoneally in front of the renal vessels. Formation of a stoma according to the standard technique.*

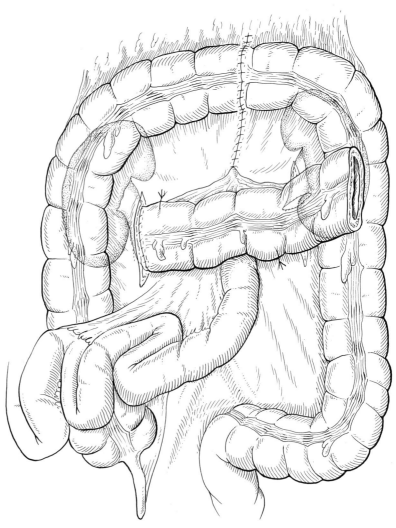

Figure 15. *Position of conduit in relation to other bowel sections: cranial to the duodenojejunic flexure and anterior to the descending colon.*

Rectus Muscle Flaps for Small Pelvis Coverage after Extensive Surgery

P. Kempf, B. Weyland
*Department of Surgery,
Rüsselsheim Hospital,
Rüsselsheim,*

Comment

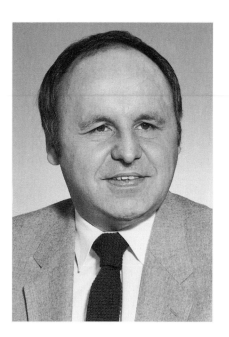

The small bowel has only limited toleration for radiation after partial or complete pelvic exenteration. High-dose (curative) radiotherapy, which is often applied using an external beam and afterloading technique, exceeds the radiation tolerance of small bowel. Any additional disease of the small bowel, benign or malignant, augments the side-effects of the radiation therapy, and in many patients leads to early termination of treatment. Therefore, radiotherapists often ask surgeons to locate and fix the small bowel outside the field of irradiation.

The author of this chapter points out that this often fails for lack of an adequate operating technique, especially in elderly patients. He presents a technique for use in addition to the existing techniques. Radiographs show that the small bowel is located far from the radiation field in the pelvis. In particular, the sacral and prostate areas are free for high-dose radiation therapy. For nonradiotherapy specialists, the relation between this technique and afterloading therapy is unclear, but this does not alter the quality of the technique. Unfortunately, only a small number of patients have so far been treated with this technique. A longer follow-up of more patients is needed to show whether this technique will affect the surgeon's work and lead to a higher number of patients being treated with an adequate dose of radiation.

B. Kober, Darmstadt, Germany

Rectus Muscle Flaps for Small Pelvis Coverage after Extensive Surgery

Introduction

Neoadjuvant radiotherapy of malignant neoplasms of the small pelvis is a standard method of local control.[1,2] Exact planning of the radiotherapy cycles and consideration of the topographic relations of the pelvic floor are necessary to avoid accidental irradiation of the small bowel. In contrast, adjuvant radiotherapy of residual tumor or local recurrences still presents problems. After total pelvic evisceration,[3] the small bowel falls automatically in the new dead space and lies therefore in any subsequent irradiation field. Severe damage can develop because of the extreme sensitivity of small bowel to radiation,[4] with negative effects on the quality of life of the patient.

Several coverage procedures have been described to protect the small bowel when adjuvant radiotherapy is planned. Popular methods are mobilization of the omentum in the small pelvis,[5,6] and sartorius muscle or gracilis muscle plasty.[7,8] However, these techniques are not free of problems. Patients with cancer are often cachectic and do not have sufficient omentum for mobilization and, in some cases omentum has to be removed as part of the radical oncologic operation. Gracilis or sartorius muscle plasty did not show the expected success when introduced into surgical practice. The muscle mass and size as well as the poor vascularization and distant location of these muscles from the small pelvis are unresolved problems. One alternative is the use of a flap of the latissimus dorsi muscle with microsurgical anastomosis to the vessels in the small pelvis, but the difficulty of this operation limits its usefulness.[9]

A simple and easy-to-perform technique for complete coverage of the small pelvis is to cover it by a flap of rectus abdominis muscle.[10–15] Vascularization is guaranteed by two arteries and two veins with extensive anastomosis between the upper and lower circles. Accidental or planned section of either of these two vascular systems does not therefore present a problem. Additionally, the size and location of this muscle are ideal for complete coverage of the small pelvis.

Operative technique (Figure 1–12)

- Midline longitudinal incision along the linea alba. The rectus abdominis muscle should be intact except in cases of previous transverse upper abdominal incisions (gallbladder or pancreas operations), Pfannestiel incision or McBurney incision

- After the tumor resection procedure, a longitudinal opening is made in the rectus abdominis muscle sheath

- The muscle is dissected proximal to the level of the first or second tendineal insertion with preservation of the vascularization. The muscle is removed from the aponeurosis with careful preparation of the vascular pedicle (inferior epigastric artery and vein) and control of the vascularization

- A small incision in the peritoneum permits positioning of the whole muscle in the abdominal cavity

- Atraumatic enlargement of the muscle avoids vessel lesions with subsequent vascular damages

- Fixation of the muscle at the pelvic wall with Vicryl (Ethicon, Edinburgh, UK) or chromic catgut suture

- Closure of the abdominal wall, and placement of a redon drain in the rectus abdominis sheath

Results, risks and surgical tricks

The indications for this technique are limited. We have performed this technique in only nine patients, seven of whom were female. The larger female pelvis is an important factor in the feasibility of the procedure.

This technique should be performed in careful aseptic conditions and the basic steps of hernia repair must be well known by the surgeon. The voided rectus abdominis sheath should be drained over several days by the use of a redon drain.

Adequate aseptic preparation of the bowel, before and during the operation avoids the occurrence of abscesses, as reported in the first case.[16]

The anterior abdominal wall was stable in all cases with no observation of relaxation. One female patient is free of symptoms 18 months after completion of radiotherapy.

Radiotherapy should start 14 days and in no case later than 6 weeks after the operation. At the end of the radiotherapy cycles, the afterloading tubes are removed. These represent a possible source of infection, especially after abdominoperineal rectum amputation.

References

1. Gerard A, Loygne J, Liegoise A, Kempf P. EORTC clinical trial for the treatment of rectal cancer using surgery, radiotherapy and chemotherapy. In: *Progress and Perspectives in the Treatment of Gastrointestinal Tumors.* Oxford: Pergamon Press (1981).

2. Kutzner J, Brückner R, Kempf P. Präoperative Strahlentherapie bei Rektumkarzinom. *Strahlentherapie* **160** (1984) 239–8.

3. Kutzner J *et al.* Interstitial remote controlled ^{192}Ir HDR afterloading therapy. Third International Afterloading Buchler Users' Meeting, 30–31 August 1990, Örebrö, Sweden.

4. Lenner V. Therapie von Strahlenfrüh- und -spätschäden des Darmes. *Dtsch Med. Wochenschr* **105** (1980) 912–14.

5. John H, Buchmann P. Verbesserung der perinealen Wundheilung nach Rektumamputation durch dei Omentumplombe. *Helv Chir Acta* **55** (1988) 673–7.

6. Russ JE, Smoron GL, Gagnon JD. Omental transposition flap in colorectal carcinoma: adjunctive use in prevention and treatment of radiation complications. *Int J Radiat Oncol Biol Phys* **10** (1984) 55–62.

7. Palmer JA, Vernon CP, Cummings BJ, Moffat FL. Gracilis myocutaneous flap for reconstructing perineal defects resulting from radiation and radical surgery. *Can J Surg* **26** (1983) 510–12.

8. De Ranier J, Crouet H, Andre M, Ollivier JM, Desdoits JM, Bouvet A, Souloy J. Les lambeaux de droit interne dans la courverture des pertes de substance périnéale en chirurgie carcinologique. *Presse Med* **14** (1985) 1967–9.

9. Kraybill WG, Reinsch J, Pucket CL, Bricker EM. Pelvic abscess following preoperative radiation and abdominoperineal resection: management with a free-flap. *J Surg Oncol* 25 (1984) 18–20.

10. Giampapa V, Keller A, Shaw WW. Pelvic floor reconstruction using the rectus abdominis muscle flap. *Ann Plast Surg* **13** (1984) 56–9.

11. Knapstein PG, Friedberg V. *Plastische Chirurgie in der Gynäkologie*. Stuttgart: Thieme Verlag (1987) 119–26.

12. Kroll SS, Pollock R, Jessup JM, Ota D. Transpelvic rectus abdominis flap reconstruction of defects following abdominal–perineal resection. *Am Surg* **55** (1989) 632–7.

13. Robertson CN, Riefkohl R, Webster GD. Use of the rectus abdominis muscle flap in urological reconstructive procedures. *J Urol* **135** (1986) 963–5.

14. Shukla HS, Hughes LE. The rectus abdominis flap for perineal wounds. *Ann R Coll Surg Engl* **66** (1984) 337–9.

15. Tobin GR, Day TG. Vaginal and pelvic reconstruction with distally based rectus abdominis myocutaneous flap. *Plast Reconstr Surg* **81** (1988) 62–79.

16. Kempf P *et al.* Zur Keimreduktion des Dickdarmes durch intraoperative Darmspülung. (in preparation).

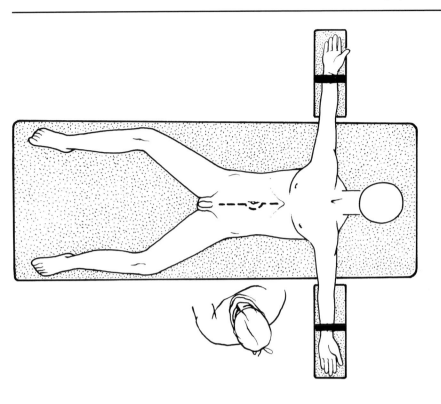

Figure 1. *Positioning of the patient.*

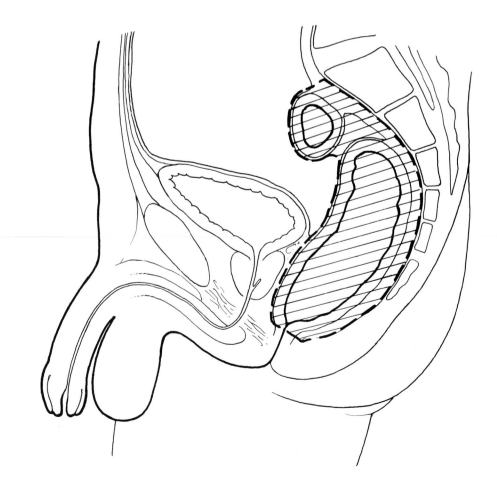

Figure 2. *Lateral view of the male pelvis. Dotted area marks the resected rectum.*

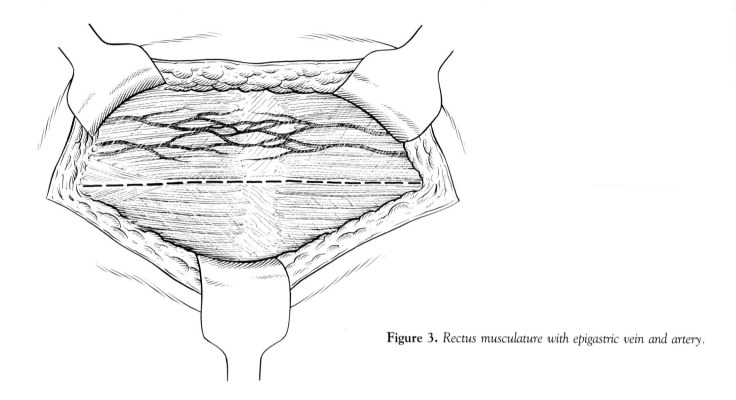

Figure 3. *Rectus musculature with epigastric vein and artery.*

Figure 4. *Dotted line marks resection lines for exenteration.*

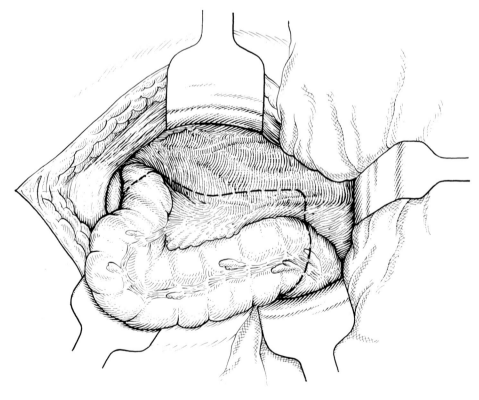

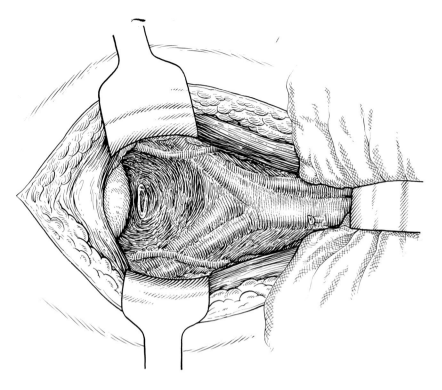

Figure 5. *The pelvis after exenteration.*

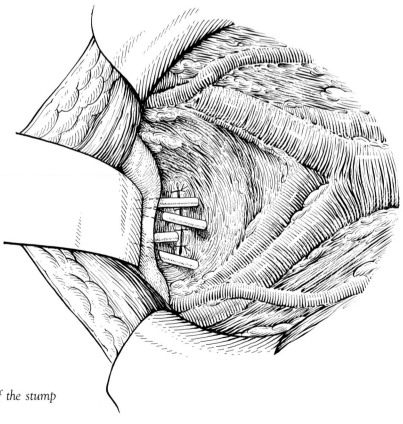

Figure 6. *After removal of the rectum or closing of the stump (Hartmann), afterloading-tubes are inserted.*

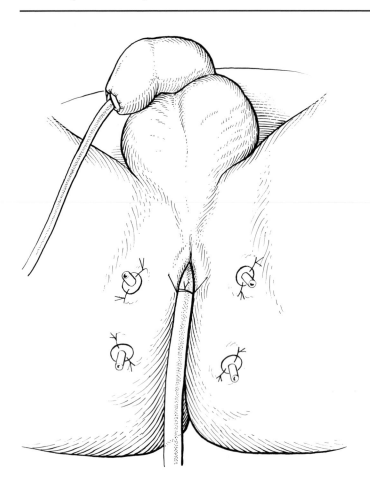

Figure 7. *Perineal view with drainage tube and afterloading tubes.*

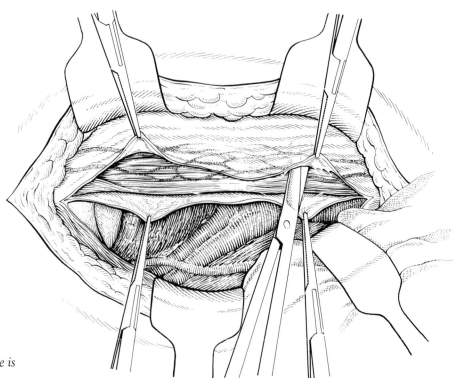

Figure 8. *Usually the right rectus muscle is used for coverage.*

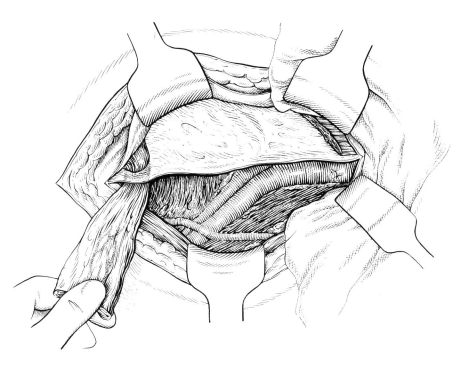

Figure 9. *The muscle is divided and brought in the abdomen.*

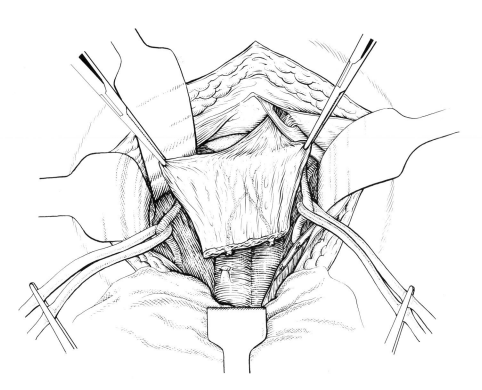

Figure 10. *Views from above, the muscle flap is large enough to cover aorta and v. cava.*

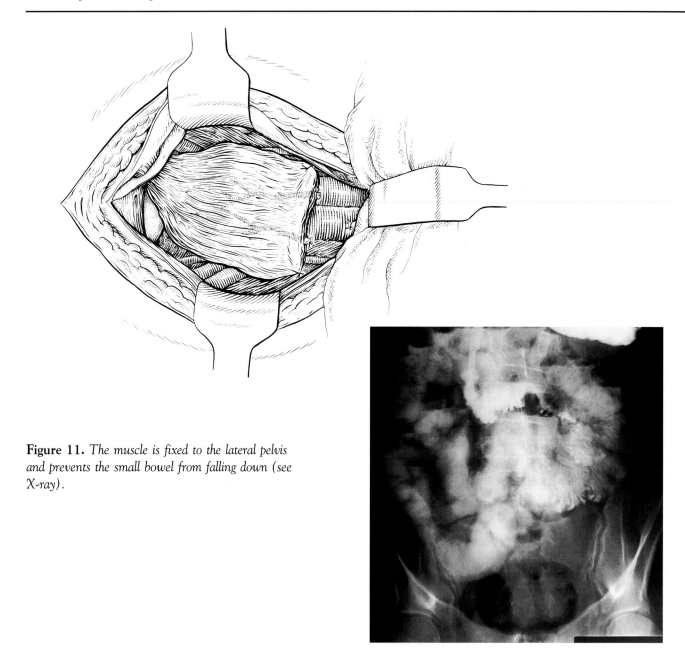

Figure 11. *The muscle is fixed to the lateral pelvis and prevents the small bowel from falling down (see X-ray).*

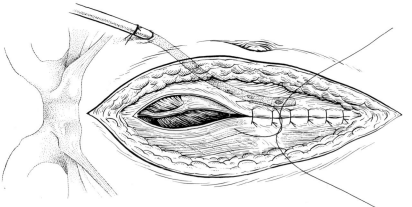

Figure 12. A drainage tube is placed.

The Sigma Rectum Pouch (Mainz Pouch II): A Modification of Ureterosigmoidostomy

M. Fisch, R. Hohenfellner
Department of Urology,
University of Mainz School of Medicine,
Mainz, Germany

Comment

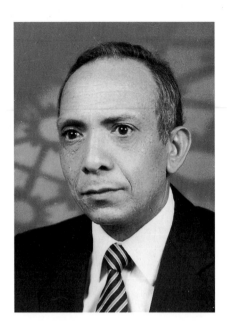

Evacuation of the rectal contents is the result of two mechanisms: an increase in the intra-abdominal pressure and peristaltic contractions extending along the entire length of the colon. Following ureterosigmoidostomy, voiding will be effected by a high-pressure system. There are two potential problems: reflux and nocturnal incontinence.

Several attempts have been proposed to modify the large bowel and create a low-pressure system:

- Mauclaire's rectal bladder with a terminal colostomy

- Excision of the teniae coli of the sigmoid colon

- Patching with a sheet of ileum

This chapter provides an innovative alternative: detubulization of the sigmoid in a fashion similar to Park's S pouch utilized for the ileum. The technique is distinctly simpler than the previously proposed procedures and, in my opinion, is a step in the right direction for optimization of ureterosigmoidostomy. I believe that the procedure should be further refined by the addition of an adjuvant step or procedure to reduce the surface area of the colon exposed for reabsorption of the urine contents.

Mohamed A. Ghoneim, Mansoura, Egypt

The Sigma Rectum Pouch (Mainz Pouch II): A Modification of Ureterosigmoidostomy

Introduction

The main drawbacks of classic ureterosigmoidostomy are:

- High intraluminal pressures caused by circular bowel contractions during peristalsis towards the anus, with a subsequent negative influence on continence and on the upper urinary tract
- Risk of ureteral implantation into the 'false' loop, especially when the sigmoid colon is extremely mobile[1]
- Risk of damage to the blood supply of the mesentery by fixation of the sigma after ureteral implantation

The sigma rectum pouch provides better results than the classic ureterosigmoidostomy, and has replaced it as a primary diversion. In addition, the sigma rectum pouch is amenable to revision after failure of classic ureterosigmoidostomy.

Detubularization and side-to-side anastomosis ensure low pressure and eliminate high-pressure contractions, thereby providing better protection of the upper urinary tract, and better continence rates are achieved. The operative technique is simple and reproducible, and the functional results comparable to those obtained using the more complex technique of the augmented rectal bladder.[2]

Indications

- Primary urinary diversion in patients with a competent anal sphincter (as demonstrated by water tap enema and rectodynamics)
- Revision of ureteral implantation after ureterosigmoidostomy

Contraindications

- Incompetent anal sphincter
- Irradiation of the pelvis
- Sigmoid diverticula
- Creatinine >1.5 mg%

Preoperative preparation

- *Bowel preparation*: oral administration of 4–7 liters of Fordtran's solution on the day before the operation, or 8–10 liters of Ringer's lactate solution via a gastric tube
- *Antibiotics*: metronidazole in combination with a cephalosporine is given at the beginning of the operation

Instruments and suture materials

- Standard instruments as for classic ureterosigmoidostomy
- Pouch wall: chromic catgut 5/0 (mucosa), polyglyconic acid 4/0 (seromuscular layer)
- Ureteral implantation: chromic catgut 5/0 and 6/0

Operative technique step by step (Figures 1–11)

- The patient is supine with the pelvis slightly elevated on a folded sheet
- Median laparotomy
- Incision of the peritoneum lateral to the descending colon and identification of the left ureter
- Incision lateral to the ascending colon and identification of the right ureter
- Dissection of both ureters up to the lower pole of the kidney, avoiding the longitudinal vessels running inside Waldeyer's sheath
- Dissection in the caudal direction down to the ureterovesical junction
- Cutting of the ureters as distal as possible, and placement of a stay suture at the 6 o'clock position
- Ligation of the ureteral stumps
- Pull-through of the left ureter behind the mesentery (above the inferior mesenteric artery)
- Identification of the junction between the sigmoid colon and the rectum
- Opening of the intestine at the teniae libera, starting from the rectosigmoid junction, over a total length of 20–24 cm distal and proximal to this point
- Placement of two stay sutures at the summit of the rectosigmoid to give the split intestine the shape of an inverted U
- Side-to-side anastomosis of the medial margins of the U by a two-layer running suture using 4/0 polyglyconic acid for the seromuscular layer and 4/0 chromic catgut for the mucosa

- For ureteral implantation, placing of four mucosal stay sutures right and left of the medial running suture

- Excision of the mucosa and the seromuscular layer to create a wide buttonhole between the two cranial stay sutures for the entrance of the ureter into the pouch

- Dissection of a submucous tunnel starting from this incision over a length of 2–2.5 cm

- Incision of the mucosa at its distal end and pull through of the ureter

- Resection of the ureter to an adequate length

- Completion of the implantation by placing two anchor sutures at the 5 and 7 o'clock positions and several single-stitch mucomucous sutures

- Closure of the cranial mucosal incision by a running suture with chromic catcut 6/0

- Implantation of the contralateral ureter

- Insertion of two 8 Fr ureteral stents, which are led out with the rectal tube, to secure the ureteral implantation

- Fixation of the pouch to the anterior longitudinal cord of the promontory in the area of the proximal end of the medial running suture by two Bassini sutures

- Closure of the anterior pouch wall by two-layer sutures (5/0 polyglyconic acid for the seromuscular and 4/0 chromic catgut for the mucosal layer); alternatively, seromuscular single stitches can be used

- Closure of the peritoneal incisions

- Covering of the anastomotic site of the pouch by omentum

- Insertion of a gastric tube (or gastrostomy) and a rectal tube, and a central venous catheter for parenteral nutrition

Surgical tricks

- When the anastomosis reaches deep down to the rectum, it is easier to suture the pouch starting caudally, as the deepest point of the anastomosis is the most critical part and can be reached more easily at the beginning of the anastomosis

- To facilitate fixation of the pouch to the promontory, one sutured end of the dorsal running suture can be pulled through dorsally outside of the pouch and tied with the fixation suture placed in the anterior cord of the promontory

- A Bassini needle facilitates placement of the fixation suture into the anterior cord

- During ureteral implantation extensive spatulation of the ureters is of utmost importance to avoid a cuff-like protrusion of the ureteral borders

- To avoid hematoma of the submucosal tunnel, the mucosa over the tunnel can be carefully incised at different points

Postoperative care

- The patient receives intravenous hyperalimentation for approximately 7 days

- The gastrostomy tube is clamped around day 5 and removed between days 7 and 9

- The bowel tube is left in place until days 3–5

- The ureteral splints are removed around day 8

- Intravenous urography is performed on day 15

Figures

The study of an 18-year-old woman served as an example for the drawing of the pictures. She has a congenital single kidney and presented with dilatation due to implantation stenosis after ureterosigmoidostomy (status post anterior exenteration and urinary diversion for an embryological carcinoma of the vagina). Therefore only one ureter is shown in the figures. Due to dilatation, ureteral implantation was performed using the open end technique.

References

1. Walz PH, Alken P. Der Einfluss anastomischer Normvarianten des Sigmas auf die Spätergebnisse der Ureterosigmoidostomie. *Akt Urol* **111** (1980) 161–8.
2. Kock NG, Ghoneim A, Lyche KG, Mahran MR. Urinary diversion to the augmented and valved rectum: preliminary results with a novel surgical procedure. *J Urol* **140** (1988) 1375–9.

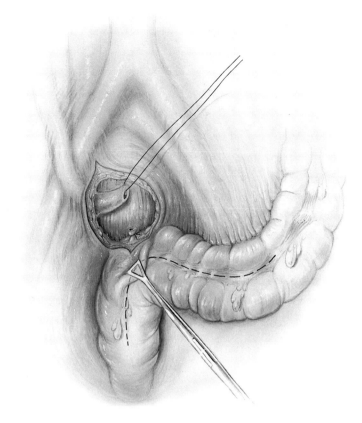

Figure 1. *The ureter is transected from the exterior aspect. Stay suture at the 12 o'clock position.*

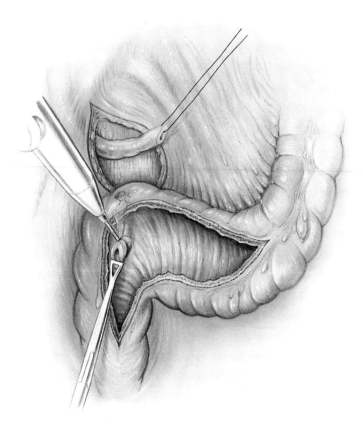

Figure 2. *Opening of the rectosigmoid at the taenia libera starting from the recto-sigmoid junction over a total length of 20 to 24 cm distal and proximal of this point. The previous ureteral implantation site is totally excised.*

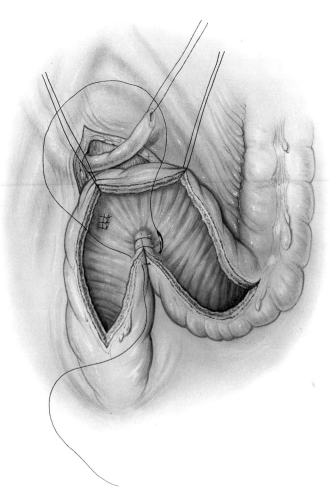

Figure 3. *Closure of the ureteral excision site by single polyglyconic acid sutures. Placing two stay-sutures at the summit of the rectosigmoid gives the split intestine the shape of an inverted U. Side-to-side anastomosis of the medial margins of the U is by two-layer running sutures using 4/0 polyglyconic acid for the sero-muscular layer and 4/0 chromic catgut for the mucosa.*

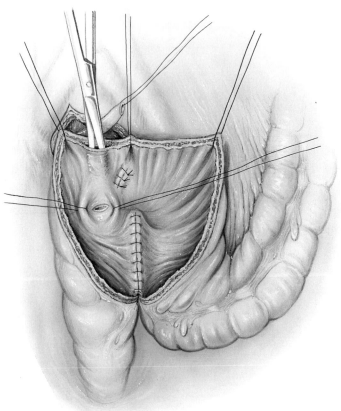

Figure 4. *A wide and 2–2.5 cm long submucosal tunnel is created starting at the cranial aspect of the pouch (open end technique). Four stay sutures facilitate preparation. Incision of the mucosa at the distant end of the tunnel.*

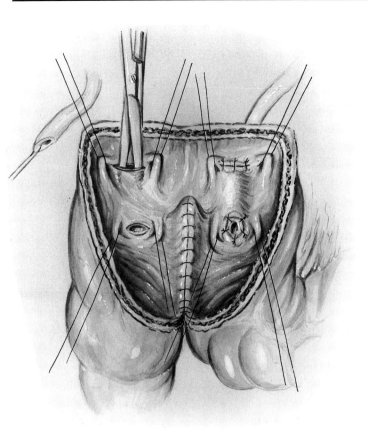

Figure 5. *Ureteral implantation according to Goodwin-Hohenfellner: creation of a wide buttonhole as an entrance of the ureter into the pouch and preparation of a submucous tunnel (2–2.5 cm in length). Incision of the mucosa is at its distant end; the ureter is pulled through. Ureteral implantation is by two anchor sutures at the 5 and 7 o'clock positions and single-stitch muco-mucous sutures. Closure of the cranial mucosal incision is by a running suture with chromic catgut 6/0.*

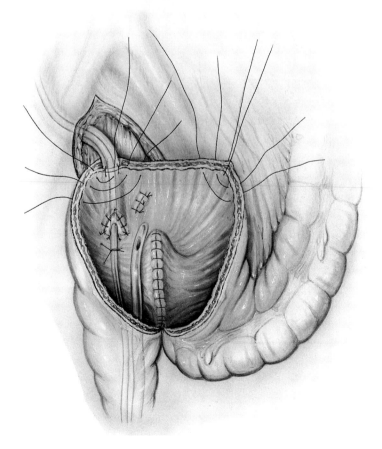

Figure 6. *After placement of an 8 French ureteral stent, which is led out with the rectal tube, closure of the pouch is started with single stitches at the corners.*

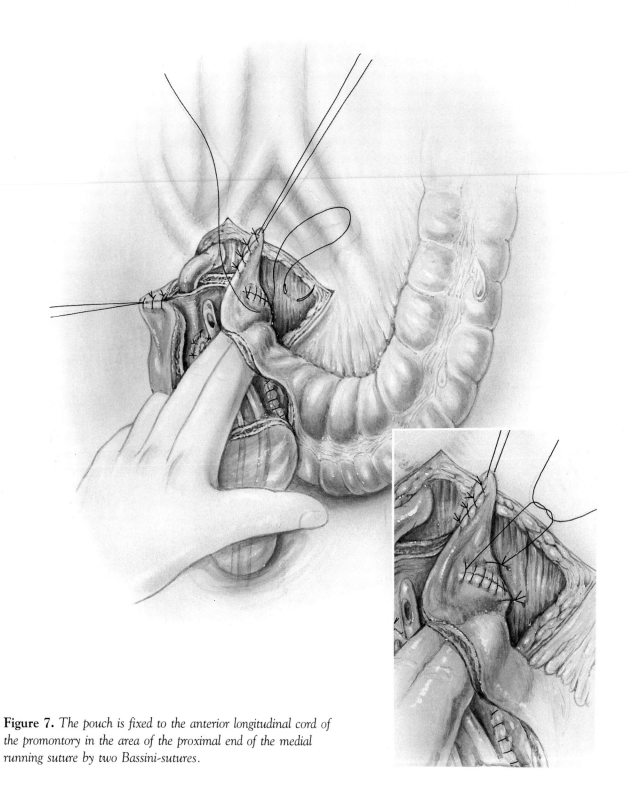

Figure 7. *The pouch is fixed to the anterior longitudinal cord of the promontory in the area of the proximal end of the medial running suture by two Bassini-sutures.*

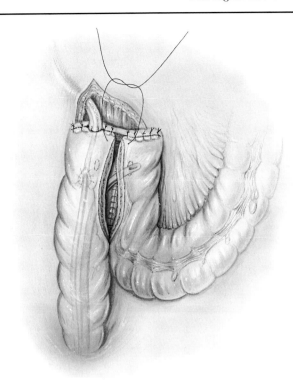

Figure 8. *Closure of the anterior pouch wall by seromuscular single stitches with polyglyconic acid 4/0.*

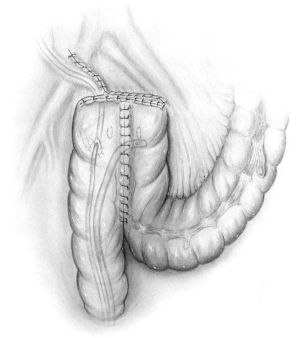

Figure 9. *Closure of the peritoneal incisions.*

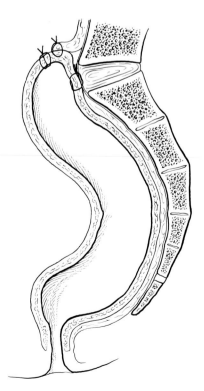

Figure 10. *Lateral view shows position of the fixation stitches.*

Continent Ileal Neobladder (Vesica Ileale Padovana, VIP)

F. Pagano, W. Artibani
Department of Urology,
Padua University Medical School,
Padua, Italy

Comment

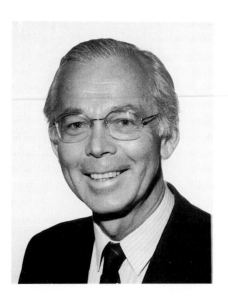

The authors offer radical cystectomy to patients with infiltrating bladder tumor without visceral or lymphatic metastasis. Of their 32 patients, 15 also received adjuvant chemotherapy. It would be interesting to compare the course of the disease in these patients with that in the patients who did not receive chemotherapy.

The bladder replacement described here is similar to Tasker's technique. We have also performed this procedure. Its advantages include the intact ileocecal region and the short length of the isolated ileum segment, which both help to reduce the incidence of metabolic disorders.

The results reported by the authors are as expected for this form of neobladder: good continence during the day, with a risk of urinary incontinence at night. The larger the bladder volume, the better the short-term results. Long-term results are still pending. It is important to pay attention to the residual urine after free micturition on control examinations.

Ureteroileal implantation bears some technical risks. It is most important to avoid the formation of a stenosis: implantation in a mucosal groove (Le Duc–Camey) achieves this, if the surgeon takes care to:

- Dissect the ureters with preservation of their distal vasculature

- Avoid kinking or torsion of the ureter

- Create a sufficiently large passage through the intestinal wall

A. Le Duc, Paris, France

Continent Ileal Neobladder

Introduction

After radical cystectomy, the continent ileal neobladder presents an ideal procedure for the construction of a detubularized reservoir very similar to the original bladder.

Indications

- Invasive malignancy restricted to the bladder in males

- Proof of a tumor-free prostatic urethra (preoperative biopsy), as well as inconspicuous pelvic lymph nodes (staging lymphadenectomy) is obligatory

Operative technique step by step (Figures 1–4)

- For protection of the distal urethral sphincter, the membranous urethra needs to be divided as close as possible to the prostatic apex, as in a radical prostatectomy. A 'nerve-sparing' cystoprostatectomy can be performed only in selected cases[1]

- To form the ileal neobladder, a 40–60 cm ileum segment with its aboral end reaching 15–20 cm proximal to the ileocecal valve is resected, and intestinal continuity is re-established with an end-to-end anastomosis

- The ileus segment has to be opened strictly antimesenterically with the electrocautery knife. A funnel to the urethral anastomosis is then constructed by placing 5 cm running anterior and posterior sutures

- A medially directed U-shaped twist in the proximal intestinal loop, with side-to-side anastomosis of the opposite borders, builds the bladder back wall and roof. This intestinal layer is then attached to the aboral intestinal parts by placing interrupted sutures or a running polyglycolic acid suture (3/0 Dexon, Davis and Geck, Gosport, UK). In this way, an oval-shaped reservoir is formed

- The urethrointestinal anastomosis is placed at the lowest point of the reservoir with six chromic catgut sutures. However, the anastomosis opening can also be placed at the lower end of the anterior funnel suture if the mesenterium is too short with limited mobility of the

neobladder. Thus, an additional distance of about 2 cm can be gained

- Ureteroileal anastomoses are performed at both sides according to Le Duc's technique.[2] The ureters are drained with 6 Fr stents, which are pulled through the front wall of the reservoir. A transurethral 22 Fr Foley catheter is used for prolonged neobladder drainage

The operation takes about an hour longer than the ileum conduit procedure.

Postoperative care

- The ureteral stents are removed 7–8 days later

- Retrograde cystography of the reservoir is performed after 2–3 weeks

- The Foley catheter can be removed if no extravasation is visible

- The patient has to learn to void urine regularly, by pressing his abdominal muscles while relaxing the pelvic floor. Micturition should leave no residual urine. A training program aiming at this should be started. The videourodynamic biofeedback method has proved helpful in this training

- Intravenous urography and videourodynamic tests should be performed after 3, 6 and 12 months

- Urethroscopy is performed once a year

Results

The first VIP procedure was performed in September of 1987 in a 55-year-old patient. Thereafter 32 patients (average 56 years) underwent the operation. All patients had locally invasive bladder carcinoma. In 15 cases adjuvant chemotherapy was needed.

One patient died, shortly after the operation, from a lung embolism. Two died 8 and 12 months after the procedure, one from a heart attack and one as a consequence of the tumor disease, respectively. Two other patients suffered urethral anastomosis insufficiency, which healed spontaneously. A ureteroileal stenosis formed in three cases, and an anastomosis narrowing in another three. Metabolic disorders and intestinal malfunction were not observed.

The most important clinical and urodynamic results are listed in Table 1.

Table 1. Clinical and urodynamic results after VIP bladder replacement in 19 patients with a follow-up of at least 6 months

	No. of patients
Day continence	
Complete	17
Minimal stress incontinence	2
Night continence	
Complete (sleeping time 6–7 hours)	16
Mild incontinence	2
Incontinence	1
Residual urine	0

VIP capacity: 400–650 ml
Basal neobladder tone 3–5 cmH₂O
Full bladder pressure: 10–30 average 17) cmH₂O
Maximal urine flow: up to 26 ml/s

References

1. Shlegel PN, Walsh PC. Neuroanatomical approach to radical cystoprostatectomy with preservation of sexual function. *J Urol* **138** (1987) 1402–6.
2. Le Duc A, Camey M. Un procédé d'implantation ureteroileale anti-reflux dans l'implantation ureteroileale anti-reflux dans l'enterocistoplastie. *J Urol (Paris)* **85** (1979) 449–54.
3. Pagano F. Artibani W, Ligato P, Piazza R, Garbeglio A, Passerini G. Vesica Ileale Padovana: a technique for total bladder replacement. *Eur Urol* (in press).
4. Walsh PC. Radical retropubic prostatectomy. In: Walsh PC, Gittes RF, Perlmutter AD, Stamey TA (eds) *Campbell's Urology*, 5th edn, vol 3. Philadelphia: W.B. Saunders (1986) 2769–71.

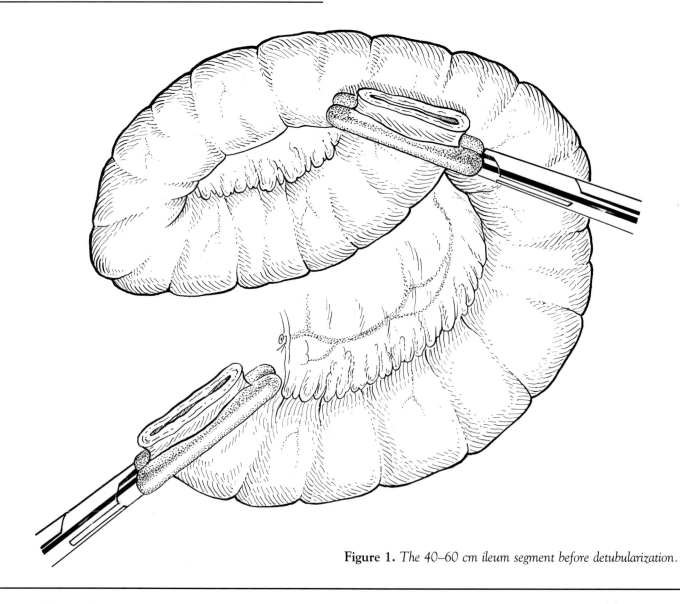

Figure 1. *The 40–60 cm ileum segment before detubularization.*

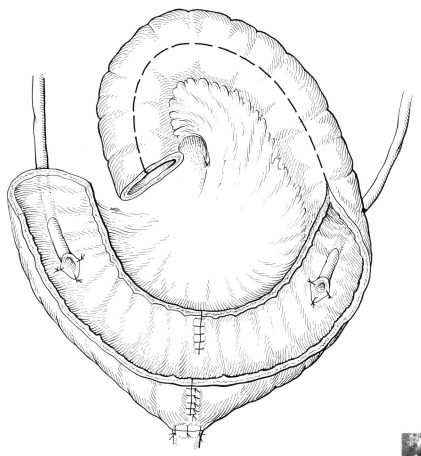

Figure 2. *Antimesenterial detubularization, construction of the bladder funnel by anteriorly and posteriorly placed sutures, and implantation of the ureters following Le Duc's technique.*

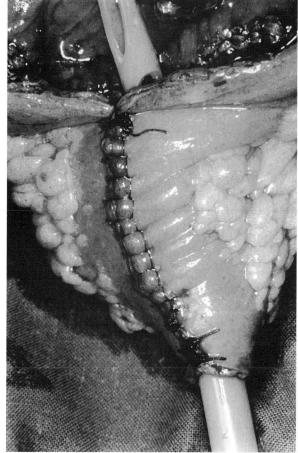

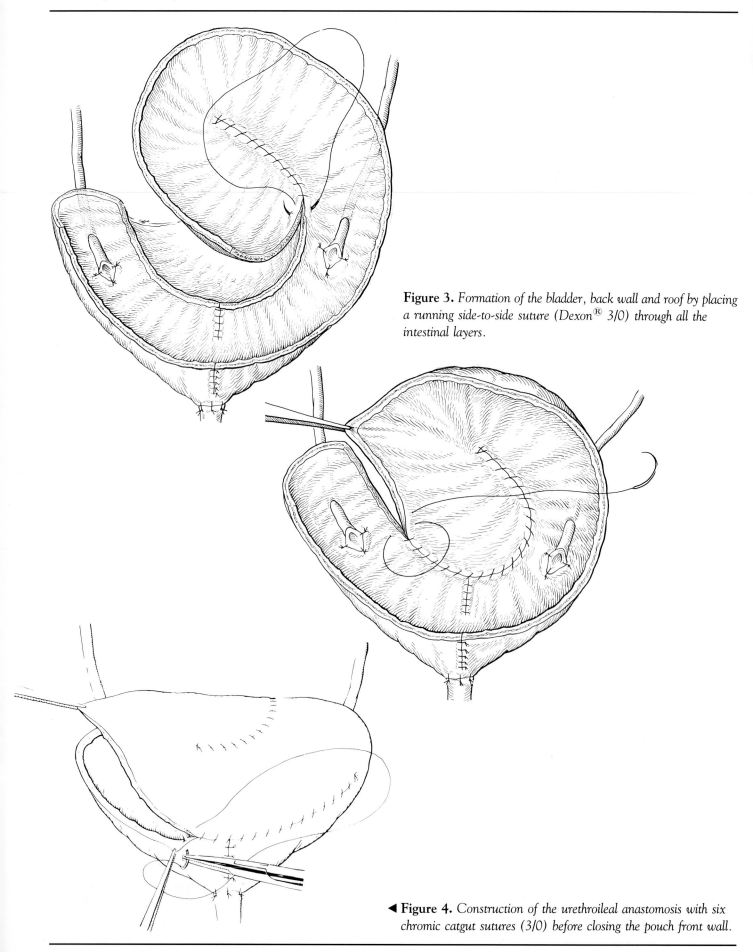

Figure 3. *Formation of the bladder, back wall and roof by placing a running side-to-side suture (Dexon® 3/0) through all the intestinal layers.*

◀ **Figure 4.** *Construction of the urethroileal anastomosis with six chromic catgut sutures (3/0) before closing the pouch front wall.*

Basic Principles of Stoma Care

M. Soeder, R. Hohenfellner
Department of Urology,
University of Mainz School of Medicine,
Mainz, Germany

Introduction

Cystectomy and the need for urinary diversion imply far-reaching therapeutic measures in modern urology. The ileum and the colon conduits are 'classic' forms of urinary diversion, which are associated with a 'moist stoma'. In the past years these standard procedures have increasingly been replaced by continent neobladders in suitable patients. One example, the Mainz pouch, allows voiding by means of intermittent self-catheterization through the navel. Urinary continence and the hidden navel stoma improve the patient's 'body image', thus improving the quality of life. This chapter concentrates mainly on care of the moist stoma.

Preoperative marking of the stoma (Figures 1 and 2)

Preoperative marking of the stoma should be carried out in every patient, regardless of the planned type of urinary diversion. It is part of the psychological preparation of the patient for the coming procedure, and it helps to define the ideal opening position of the stoma.

For uncomplicated postoperative care, the stoma should not be located right next to the umbilicus, the iliac crest, the rib border or the waist. Skin folds or scars very near the conduit site can also present difficulties in stoma care. The anatomically correct location for the stoma is in the region of the rectus abdominus muscle, where the patient has a direct view of it.

The patient should sit upright, stand, and lean forward with the upper body to allow the best possible location for the stomal opening to be decided. Only these body positions allow the detection of problem zones, i.e. skin folds. Materials needed for the marking of the stomal opening include a ruled marking disk and a waterproof marking pen or methylene blue for intracutaneous injection. Postoperative control is accomplished by adapting the complete stomal system to the marked conduit position. The patient can thus become acquainted with the expected situation.

Postoperative care

A stomal reservoir system should be adapted to the prominent stomal opening in the operating room. A sterile system that allows for a reservoir change without exerting pressure on the patient is to be used on this occasion. The stoma and the surrounding skin have to be inspected regularly to detect early complications – conduit necrosis or parastomal.

The continuous drainage of slime and urine will be ensured only if the reservoir base outlet hangs at the side of the patient's body. The outlet needs to be connected with a special collecting unit for fluid assessment. The definitive stomal reservoir system should be adapted after the ureteral stents have been removed, 10–12 days after the operation.

Stomal care at home

Patients should be sufficiently familiar with the stoma to take care of themselves before they are discharged from the hospital. It is also advisable to teach the patients' relatives about managing the stoma. Patients should choose the desired definitive stomal system themselves after they have been thoroughly advised. The use of a mirror to view the stoma has proved to be very useful, especially in obese patients.

Cleanliness is of utmost importance in taking care of the stoma. A raised conduit opening facilitates the nursing of the stoma, as the surrounding skin can be completely isolated with the stomal reservoir system.

The stoma size should be measured regularly during the first 3 months after the completed urinary diversion. This is important because, during this period, the conduit opening tends to shrink. For a perfect fit of the adhesive plate, the patient should use a template of the form and size of the stoma. This guarantees optimal skin protection.

There are many arguments for the daily changing of the reservoir unit:

- The warm humid milieu of the plastic reservoir allows for considerable bacterial growth

- Odour increases with time

- Precipitation of crystals may cause bleeding by friction against the skin

An increased fluid supply cannot prevent these side-effects. The disadvantage of one-piece reservoir units (Figure 3), in which the reservoir bag cannot be detached from the adhesive plate, is skin irritation due to the daily system change. On the other hand, two-piece units allow daily changing of the reservoir bag leaving the adhesive plate in place. Skin-friendly adhesives can be left in place for a couple of days.

Complications (Figures 4–8)

- Skin folds and grooves can be leveled out with adhesive paste (e.g. Stomahesive; Convatec, Munich)

- A stomal opening located at skin level requires compensation with the use of a belt, or with a support ring, so that the adhesive plate can adopt a convex position

- Skin irritation and maceration are mostly due to maladjustment or deficient maintenance of the system. As a consequence the parastomal skin is unprotected against urine. The cause of the problem needs to be corrected; that is, the parastomal skin needs to be perfectly sealed. If this is achieved but there is no improvement, a dermatologist should prescribe therapy with fat-free water-soluble tinctures or ointments; if necessary, the reservoir system can be changed to a different type

- Conduit stenosis or retractions needs surgical stoma correction

- Herniation and prolapse can be corrected surgically with a new stoma if the patient is in good surgical condition; otherwise, conservative treatment with a supporting bandage is offered

Urine control measurements (Figure 9)

Patients are often given unnecessary prolonged antibiotic therapy because of erroneous bacteriologic results. An important source of error is the method of removal of urine from the reservoir bag: a meaningful microbiologic examination result can only be achieved by a special technique using a double-lumen catheter (e.g. Tele-Cath, Pfrimmer Medicare).

Conclusions

A patient who has been thoroughly informed about stomal care can deal with the urinary diversion and return to normal everyday and professional life. Personnel engaged in stoma therapy should convey to patients the certainty that they will not be left alone with their worries and problems outside the clinic.

An accompanying videotape, *The Essentials of Stomal Care*, can be requested from Convatec.

Acknowledgements

This chapter was completed with the friendly assistance of Convatec (Munich).

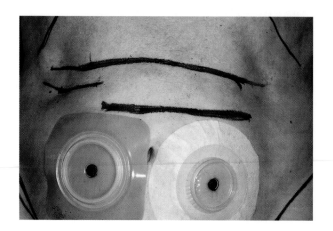

Figure 1. *Preoperative marking of the future stoma site. It should be performed in the standing, sitting and inclined patient for optimal positioning.*

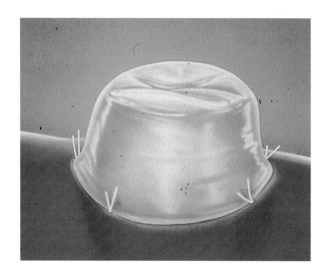

(a)

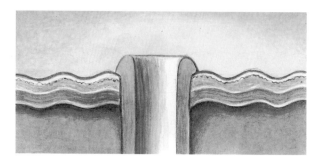

(b)

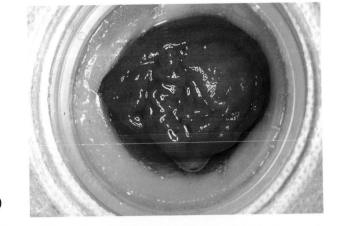

Figure 2. *Optimal raised stomal position. Eventual parastomal skin folds can be leveled out using a flexible basal adhesive plate (e.g. Convatec).*

(c)

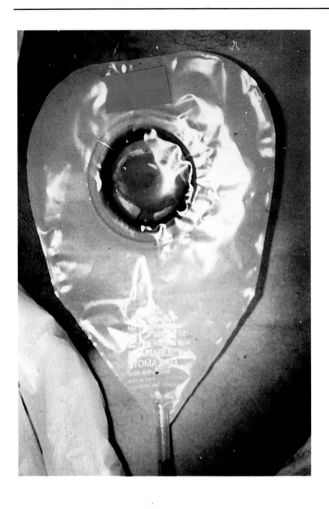

Figure 3. *Obsolete one-piece stomal kit. Skin protection, through a Karaya ring, fails to cover the parastomal skin.*

Figure 4. *Harvesting of a urine culture.*

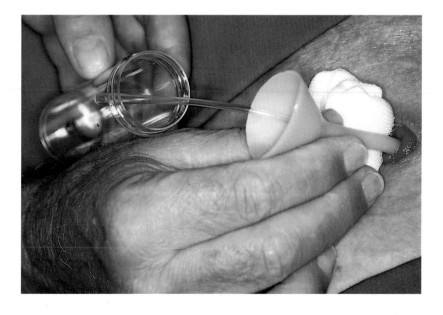

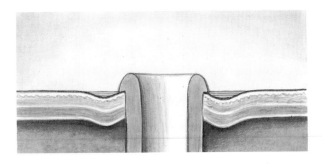

Figure 5. *Compensation for small parastomal skin folds with protective paste (e.g. Stomahesive).*

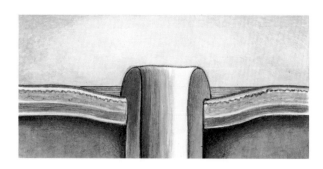

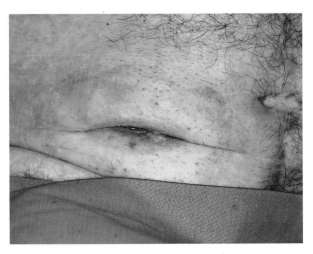

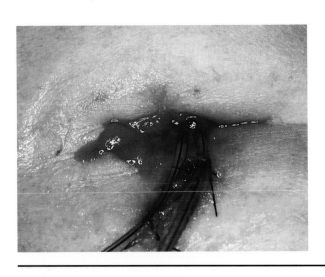

◀ **Figure 6.** *Pronounced differences in the level of the parastomal area (conduit opening at skin level and marked weight gain with consequent stomal retraction) can be compensated for with skin paste, a belt and a pressure system.*

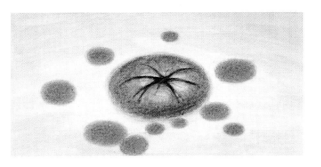

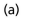

Figure 7. *Small areas of skin irritation caused by inadequate care can be managed with adhesive paste.*

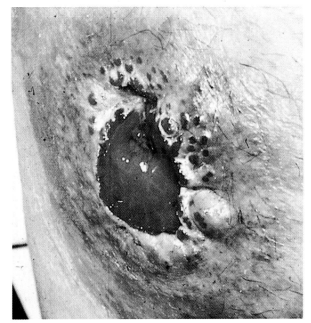

Figure 8. *(a) Hyperkeratosis with cutaneous defects caused by a disproportionately large basal plate for the central hole. (b) Marked skin irritations due to prolaps and inadequate care. (c) Extensive skin irritation can be managed with a protective plate covering the whole defective area.*

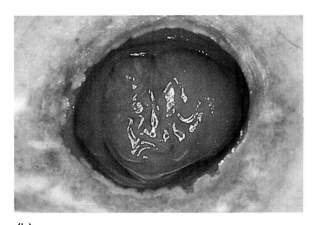

(b)

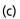

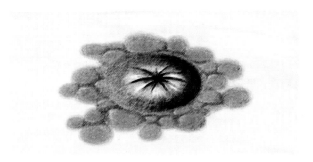

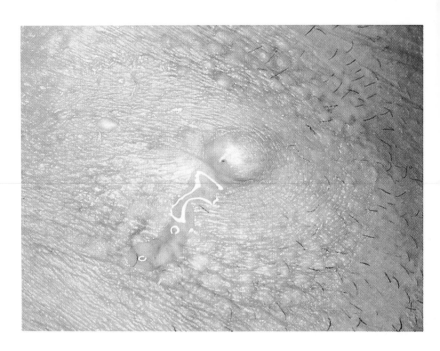

Figure 9 (a) and (b). *Stomal stenosis and unsuccessful stoma results, here in combination with multiple abdominal wall hernias needing surgical correction.*

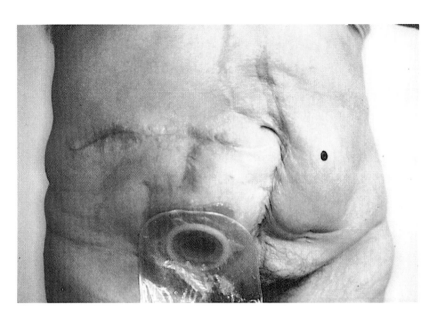

Retroperitoneal Lymphadenectomy: Surgical Approach to the Retrocrural Lymph Nodes

W. Höltl, S. Aharinejad[a]
Department of Urology,
Kaiser Franz Josef Hospital of the City of Vienna,
Vienna, Austria
[a]*Department of Anatomy I,*
University of Vienna,
Vienna, Austria

Introduction

As the management of advanced testicular neoplasms has improved, the need to remove clinically detectable residual disease persisting after chemotherapy has increased. Although the retroperitoneal lymph nodes are routinely dissected, the retrocrural nodes are not. Retrocrural lymph node dissection is needed in only 5–10% of patients requiring excision of residual disease after chemotherapy. Thus the technique has largely been neglected in textbooks on surgery.

Residual disease usually consists of necrotic or mature teratoma tissue. Vital malignant tumor tissue is rarely seen. Mature teratomas are known to have a slow but definite progressive growth potential (growing teratoma syndrome). Consequently, their surgical removal is inevitable. Their malignant potential is still poorly understood.

Anatomy

For planning the thoracoabdominal procedure, a full understanding of the blood vessels and nerves supplying the diaphragm is needed. The diaphragm is supplied by four arteries:

- The pericardiacophrenic artery, which accompanies the phrenic nerve caudally
- The musculophrenic artery which, like the former, originates from the internal thoracic artery
- The superior phrenic artery from the thoracic aorta
- The (abdominal) inferior phrenic artery, which arises from the abdominal aorta and uses the aortic hiatus for its passage through the diaphragm

When planning the diaphragmatic incision it is important to know that the diaphragm will not suffer any perfusion deficits if the left inferior phrenic artery is cut. This vessel is the first branch that the abdominal aorta gives off above the celiac trunk. It courses posteriorly and superiorly along the crus of the diaphragm and supplies the lumbar diaphragm on the abdominal side.

Indications

- Residual disease after chemotherapy for testicular tumors

Instruments

No instruments other than those for thoracotomy are needed.

Operative technique step by step

- Place the 30° right lateral position with the left side up (Figure 1)

- Make a left thoracoabdominal incision beginning at the seventh intercostal space in the anterior axillary line, and continue pararectally to the level of the umbilicus (Figure 2)
- Enter the abdominal and thoracic cavities (Figure 3)
- Incise the diaphragm as far lateral as possible, taking care to avoid the phrenic nerve which enters the diaphragm at the pericardial apex (Figure 4)
- Place a rib retractor
- Incise the parietal peritoneum lateral to the colon, to the esophageal aperture skirting the spleen superiorly (Figure 5)
- Pull the left colonic flexure medially and downward together with the spleen and the tail of the pancreas; expose the upper pole of kidney and the left adrenal
- Isolate the superior suprarenal artery (from the left phrenic artery) and the medial suprarenal artery (from the aorta); ligate them with 3/0 Vicryl (Ethicon, Edinburgh, UK) and cut them. Isolate them and cut the accompanying veins in the same manner
- Push the adrenal and the upper kidney pole downwards and laterally
- Pass a DeBakey or rectangular dissecting clamp underneath the crus of the diaphragm (Figure 6)
- Isolate and ligate the left phrenic artery and cut it again as it enters the diaphragm on its passage into the retroperitoneal space
- Split the diaphragm to the level of the esophageal hiatus
- Tape the superior mesenteric artery and celiac trunk behind the crura in patients with extensive tumor masses (Figure 7). Make sure to spare the artery of Adamkiewicz. An unpaired vessel, it arises at variable levels from the posterior wall of the aorta to the anastomosis between the aorta and the anterior spinal artery. Its injury may cause spinal lesion! Identify the azygos vein behind the para-aortic retrocrural lymph node group. To avoid injuring it, start dissecting the lymph nodes at the upper end of the tumor and work downwards
- No drain is necessary in the retrocrural space
- Close the diaphragmatic incision with running 3/0 Vicryl suture to ensure intraperitoneal lymphatic drainage
- Put a chest drain in (for 2–3 days) and close the incision as usual
- No drain is necessary in the abdominal cavity

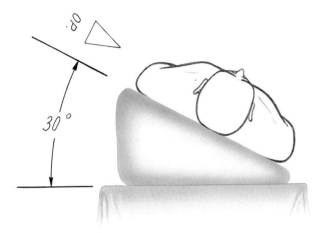

Figure 1. *Position of the patient.*

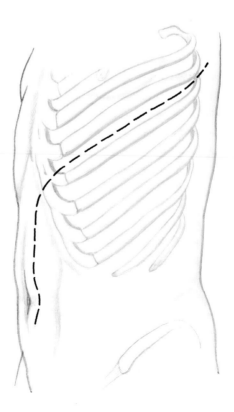

Figure 2. *Left thoracoabdominal incision.*

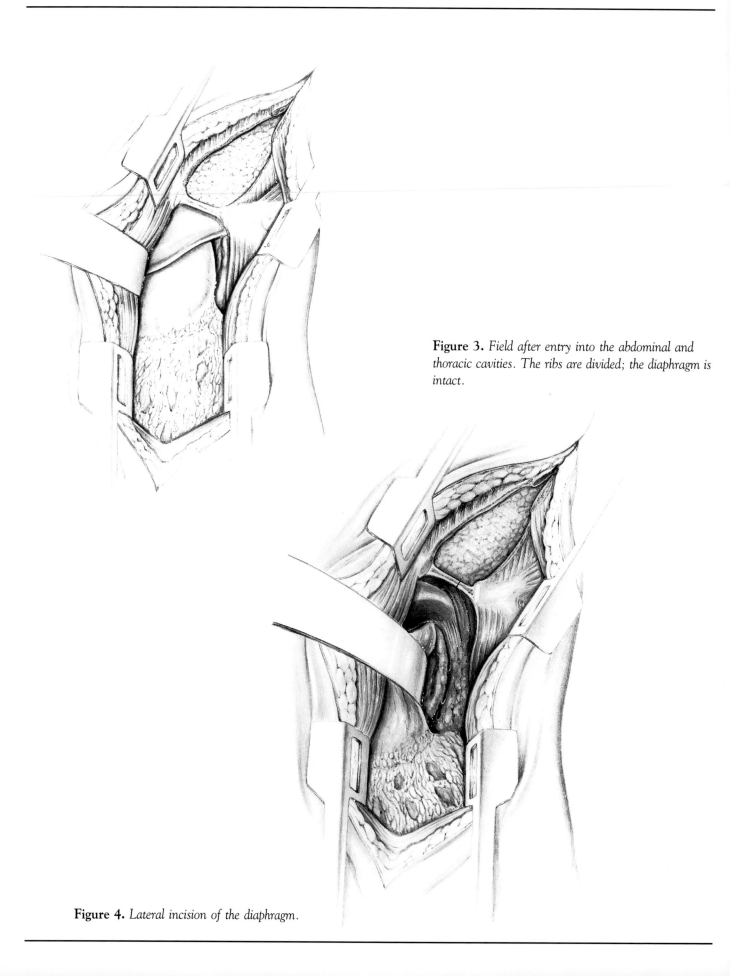

Figure 3. *Field after entry into the abdominal and thoracic cavities. The ribs are divided; the diaphragm is intact.*

Figure 4. *Lateral incision of the diaphragm.*

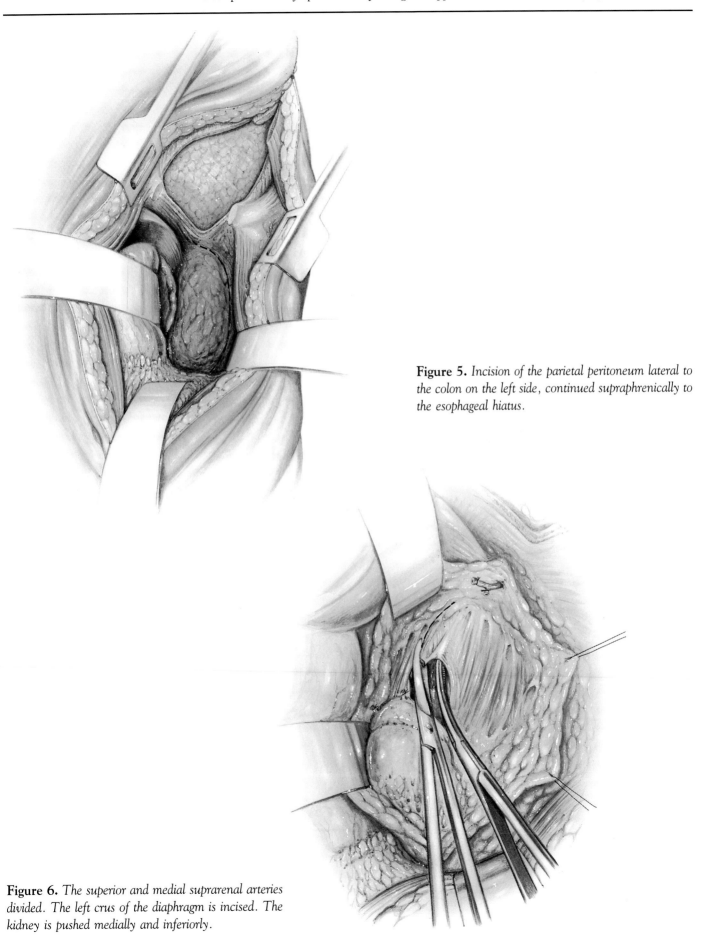

Figure 5. *Incision of the parietal peritoneum lateral to the colon on the left side, continued supraphrenically to the esophageal hiatus.*

Figure 6. *The superior and medial suprarenal arteries divided. The left crus of the diaphragm is incised. The kidney is pushed medially and inferiorly.*

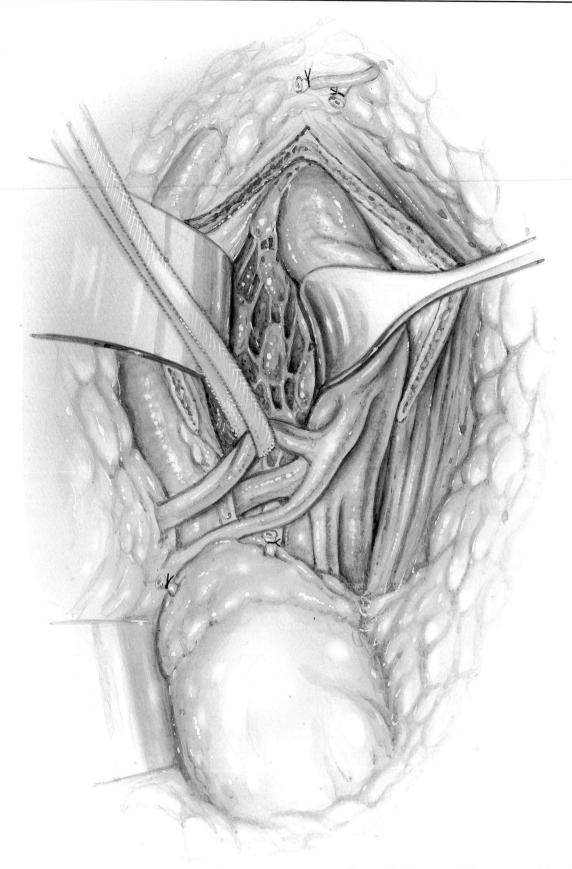

Figure 7. *Exposure of the retrocrural lymph nodes after isolation of the celiac trunk and superior mesenteric artery.*

The Mainz Pouch Procedure (Mixed Ileum and Cecum) for Bladder Augmentation, Bladder Replacement and Continent Diversion

R. Hohenfellner, M. Fisch,
R. Stein, J.W. Thüroff[a]
Department of Urology,
University of Mainz School of Medicine,
Mainz, Germany
[a]Department of Urology,
University of Witten/Herdecke Medical School,
Wuppertal, Germany

Comment

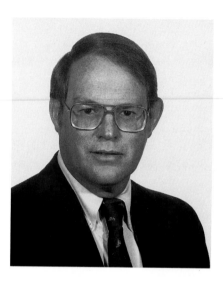

The authors are to be congratulated on their report of the uses of the mixed ileum and cecum augmentation procedure. The use of a composite (ileum and cecum) pouch adheres to the important principles of urinary tract reconstruction. Detubularization of the bowel segments not only increases the volume of the pouch using a given length of bowel, but also decreases the intraluminal pressure by increasing the radius of the bowel segments. These principles apply regardless of whether one is constructing a bladder augmentation, a continent cutaneous reservoir or a neobladder.

Experience with the intussuscepted nipple valve for continence in the Mainz pouch has paralleled the experience reported by Kock and Skinner with this continence mechanism in the Kock pouch. Recent results in both series report failure rates of the intussuscepted continence valve at approximately 10%. The valve mechanism is otherwise highly effective. Stone formation on staples used to stabilize the nipple valve has also been a problem. This has been reduced significantly by several modifications in technique.

The application of the Mitrofanoff procedure to the continent cutaneous reservoir has been a valuable contribution. Except in patients who have had a previous appendicectomy or who have small short appendices or inadequate blood supply, the appendix seems to make a reliable efferent limb and continence mechanism. The authors have overcome problems with stomal stenosis which are encountered with the appendical efferent limb by placing the stoma in the umbilicus. This procedure has the added advantage of giving a good cosmetic result.

Finally, the Mainz pouch also seems well suited as a neobladder. The same features that allow the pouch to function well as an augmentation or continent cutaneous reservoir also make it a satisfactory structure to serve as a neobladder. The results in 37 patients with neobladders have been excellent. All patients are dry during the daytime. Less than 10% are incontinent at night. The authors stress careful patient selection for those who will have a neobladder. Candidates are restricted to those who have solitary bladder tumors well away from the bladder neck.

The authors present helpful techniques to deal with postoperative problems. This is valuable information for the reader since all of these procedures require experience. Even with considerable experience, the surgical revision rate runs at around 10% in these procedures.

The Mainz pouch techniques apply sound principles, are versatile enough to apply to almost every circumstance, and certainly have a secure place among the other methods of urinary reconstruction.

Randall G. Rowland, Indianapolis, Indiana, USA

The Mainz Pouch Procedure (Mixed Ileum and Cecum) for Bladder Augmentation, Bladder Replacement and Continent Diversion

Introduction

In 1983 we started to use the ileocecal segment for *bladder augmentation*. The concept was to augment the bladder after subtotal resection with a low-pressure high-capacity reservoir that consisted of small *and* large bowel, the latter enabling antirefluxive ureteral implantation. In the following the operative technique was optimized.

In our first publication[1] on the Mainz pouch technique, in 1985, *bladder substitution* was mentioned only as a 'possible option'. We are still restrictive with the indications for the procedure, because a large number of our patients with bladder cancer have multifocal tumors or carcinoma *in situ*. When spontaneous voiding cannot be expected (female patients after exenteration, patients with thoracic spina bifida, patients bound to a wheelchair), we believe that catheterization through an umbilical stoma is superior to transurethral catheterization.

Our results in children with bladder exstrophy after bladder neck reconstruction and bladder replacement by an ileocecal segment were most disappointing. Urodynamic investigations have revealed that an unstable detrusor of the closed bladder is probably responsible for night incontinence,[2] and investigations in isolated muscle cells of the exstrophic bladder led us to believe that the receptors and response to neurotransmitters differ from those of a normal bladder.[3]

The construction of a safe continence mechanism represented a landmark in the development of *urinary diversion with continent stoma*, initiated by Kock[3] in 1969. All the alloplastic sphincter prostheses used in our patients had to be removed because of infection. Fixation of the ileal invaginated nipple was replaced by staples, and the umbilical stoma proved to be better than the stoma located in the lower abdominal quadrant. Today, the appendix stoma connected to the umbilical funnel is our method of choice.

Apart from the continence mechanism, a safe ureteral implantation is of utmost importance. Irradiated or wall-thickened refluxing ureters are prone to stenosis at the ureteral implantation site when a submucosal tunnel is the implantation technique. Implanting these ureters via a serous-lined extramural tunnel, as published recently by Abol-Enein and Ghoneim,[4,5] seems promising.

Our experience with the Mainz pouch technique for more than 12 years satisfies us that the initial concept is valid. The major problems (creation of a safe continence mechanism and antirefluxive ureteral implantation without a higher risk of stenosis) can be solved. Most of the late complications observed today are minor, e.g. pouch stones and stoma stenosis, which can easily be treated without anesthesia. During recent years, side-effects of urinary diversion, such as metabolic consequences and secondary malignancies, have become more and more important. Additional procedures, such as the reconstruction of the ileocecal valve,[6] have been developed, and special care (pouchoscopy, prophylactic administration of alkalinizing drugs) is taken to avoid these side-effects.

Preoperative preparation

- *Investigations*: intravenous urography gives information on the anatomy and function of the upper urinary tract, especially on the degree of ureteral dilatation. Bowel diverticulosis or polyps can be diagnosed by a water tap enema with water-soluble contrast medium

- *Bowel preparation*: oral adminstration of 4–4.7 liters of Fordtran's solution on the day before the operation; alternatively 8–10 liters of Ringer's lactate solution via a gastric tube

- *Antibiotics*: metronidazole in combination with a cephalosporine is given at the beginning of the operation

Instruments and suture material

- Basic kidney set
- Additional instruments for abdominal surgery
- Suction
- Cold light source (for preparation of the mesentery)
- Basin containing prepared iodine solution (disinfection)
- Wooden groove
- Electrocautery
- Finsterer suction
- Kidney bowel
- Two catheter tip syringes for bowel irrigation
- Sharp spoon (for roughening of the mucosa)
- TEA 55 stapler with three 4.8 magazines (ileal invagination; the first four inner staples of the magazine should be removed)

- Two ureteral stents (6–8 Fr)

- One cystostomy tube (10 Fr)

- One silicone catheter 18 Fr (ileal nipple) or 16 Fr (appendix stoma)

- Urethral anastomosis: polydioxanone 3/0, JB needle

- Stoma: polyglactin 3/0, V6 needle

- Creation of the pouch plate and pouch closure: polyglyconate 4/0, GS needle; polydioxanone 4/0, JB needle

- Ureteral implantation: chromic catgut 5/0 (anchor) and 6/0

- Stay sutures: plain catgut 4/0 (mucosa), silk 4/0 (serosa)

Operative technique step by step

- The patient is supine with the pelvis slightly elevated on a folded sheet

Bladder augmentation and replacement (Figures 1–7)
- Isolation of 10–15 cm of cecum and ascending colon, as well as two terminal ileal segments of equal length

- Restoration of bowel continuity

- Detubularization of the isolated intestinal segment

- Anastomosis of the two terminal ileal loops starting at the inferior aspect

- Anastomosis of the loop to the ascending colon

- Retroperitoneal pull-through of the left ureter to the right side

- Implantation of the ureters are at the open end of the large bowel using a submucosal tunnel of 2–3 cm length

- Stenting of the ureters by means of 6 Fr catheters

- Alternatively the ureters can be brought into the pouch through a wide incision (buttonhole) in the posterior wall of the pouch

- Anastomosis of the pouch plate to the bladder remnant

- Closure of the pouch by interrupted running sutures after placement of a transurethral catheter (20 Fr) and a cystostomy tube (10 Fr)

- Creation of the pouch plate in the same manner for bladder replacement

- Buttonhole incision at the inferior aspect of the cecal pole

- Evertion of the bowel mucosa by single stitches with chromic catgut

- Insertion of the transurethral catheter (20 Fr)

- Insertion of five sutures through the borders of the buttonhole, the everted mucosa and the urethral stump; tying of the sutures

- Ureteral implantation (open-ended or buttonhole technique) is performed adapting the site of implantation and ureteral length to the position of the pouch in the pelvis

Urinary diversion with continent stoma (Figure 8–18)

The invaginated and intussuscepted ileal nipple as continence mechanism
- An additional 8–12 cm of ileum are isolated to create the ileal intussuscepted valve

- Cecum, ascending colon and distant ileal segments are split open at their antimesenteric aspect, leaving only the segment designated for the ileal invagination and the ileocaecal valve intact

- The posterior wall of the pouch is established

- To enable invagination, the serosa of the respecting mesentery is incised and the mesenteric vessels are freed from fatty tissue

- The ileum is invaginated over a length of 5 cm and the invagination stabilized by two rows of staples placed at the 3 and 9 o'clock positions

- The mucosa of the nipple thus created is roughened to improve the following fixation into the ileocecal valve

- The ileal nipple is pulled through the ileocecal valve and fixed contralaterally to the insertion of the ileal mesentery by staples from the interior of the pouch

- The nipple is additionally fixed by two-layer interrupted 4/0 polyglyconate sutures to the ring of the ileocecal valve

- The ureters are implanted, and two 6 Fr catheters inserted

- A 10 Fr cystostomy and an 18 Fr catheter are inserted, and the pouch is closed

- For stoma formation the umbilicus is separated from the external rectus fascia and opened at the deepest point

- The fascia and the peritoneum are incised and the incision is subsequently enlarged

- The aboral end of the nipple is then pulled through

- Five to seven single sutures (3/0 Vicryl, Ethicon, Edinburgh, UK) are placed, grasping the skin of the umbilicus from the interior, the fascia and finally the border or the aboral end of the nipple

- Normally the efferent loop is too long and must be resected to a length of 2 cm

- The pouch catheter is led out through the umbilicus and the previously placed sutures are tightened

- The pouch is fixed to the abdominal wall with several interrupted sutures

The appendix as continence mechanism (Figures 19–25)
- The ileocecal and ascending colon segments are isolated with two ileal loops of identical length

- The terminal loop is incised at the antimesenteric aspect and a small bowel plate is created

- To assure that the lumen of the appendix is not obliterated, it is intubated using dilators

- The colon is split antimesenterically, leaving the caudal 4–5 cm of the cecal pole intact

- The seromuscular layer of the intact cecal pole is split along the teniae coli down to the mucosa

- By dissecting the seromuscular tissue from the mucosa a broad submucosal bed for the appendix is created

- Windows are carefully excised from the appendicular mesentery, taking care not to damage anatomic variations of the appendicular artery

- The appendix is layed back, and the seromuscular layer of the colon is closed over the embedded appendix by interrupted 4/0 polydioxanone sutures

- The creation of the stoma resembles the cutaneous implantation of the ileal nipple stoma; fewer sutures are necessary to fix the appendix to the abdominal wall and the umbilicus

- The pouch is drained via a 16 or 18 Fr transappendicular catheter and a 10 Fr pouchostomy

- A gastric tube or gastrostomy and a rectal tube are placed. For parenteral nutrition a central venous catheter has to be inserted

Surgical tricks

- With a tunnel length of 4 cm, a short mobile portion of the appendix remains for anastomosis to the umbilicus

- By incising the distal end of the appendix and the umbilical funnel in the shape of a V, the incidence of stoma stenosis can be reduced

Postoperative care

- Parenteral nutrition is maintained until bowel contractions appear, then stepwise reduced

- Antibiotics (metronidazole and cephalosporine) are given for 5 days, then metronidazole is stopped and the cephalosporine continued for another 2 days. Thereafter nitrofurantoin is administered orally as long as the pouch catheter stays in

- The rectal tube is left in place for 3 days, the gastric tube for 5–6 days

- The ureteral stents are removed starting from day 10, when intravenous urography is performed

- The pouch catheter stays for 3 weeks after bladder augmentation and for 4 weeks after urinary diversion with continent stoma. After removal, the patient is voiding spontaneously or taught to perform self-catheterization. If residual urine is less than 50 ml, the cystostomy tube is removed

References

1. Thüroff JW, Alken P, Riedmiller H, Engelmann U, Jacobi GH, Hohenfellner R. The Mainz pouch (mixed augmentation ileum and cecum) for bladder augmentation and continent urinary diversion. *World J Urol* **3** (1985) 179.
2. Hollowell JG, Hill PD, Duffy PG, Ransley PG. Bladder function and dysfunction in exstrophy and epispadias. *Lancet* **338** (1991) 926.
3. Kock NG. Intra-abdominal 'reservoir' in patients with permanent ileostomy: preliminary observations on a procedure resulting in fecal 'continence' in five ileostomy patients. *Arch Surg* 99 (1969) 223.
4. Abol-Enein H, Ghoneim MA. Optimization of uretero-intestinal anastomosis in urinary diversion: an experimental study in dogs. III. A new antireflux technique for uretero-ileal anastomosis: a serous-lined extramural tunnel. *Urol Res* **21** (1993) 135.
5. Abol-Enein H, Ghoneim MA. A novel uretero-ileal reimplantation technique: the serous lined extramural tunnel. A preliminary report. *J Urol* 151 (1994) 1193.
6. Fisch M, Wammack R, Spies F *et al*. Ileocecal valve reconstruction during continent urinary diversion. *J Urol* **151** (1994) 861.
7. Wammack R, Fisch M, Müller SC, Nawrath H, Hohenfellner R. Pharmacology, electrophysiology and immuno-histochemistry of the exstrophic bladder. (1994) (Abstract).

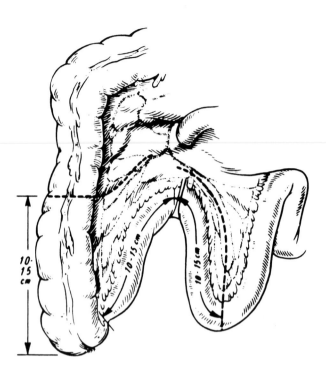

Figure 1. *The segment to be isolated for creation of a Mainz pouch bladder augmentation or replacement: 12 cm of cecum and two ileal loops of the same length.*

(a)

(b)

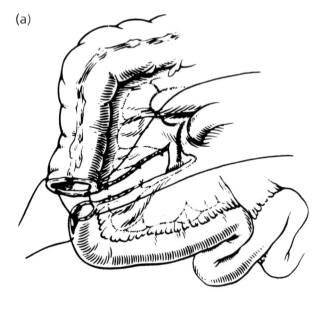

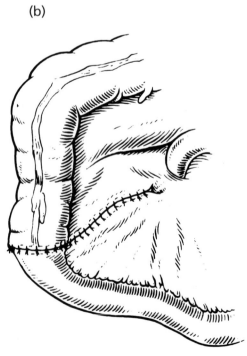

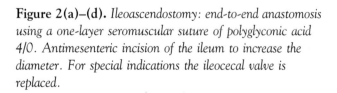

Figure 2(a)–(d). *Ileoascendostomy: end-to-end anastomosis using a one-layer seromuscular suture of polyglyconic acid 4/0. Antimesenteric incision of the ileum to increase the diameter. For special indications the ileocecal valve is replaced.*

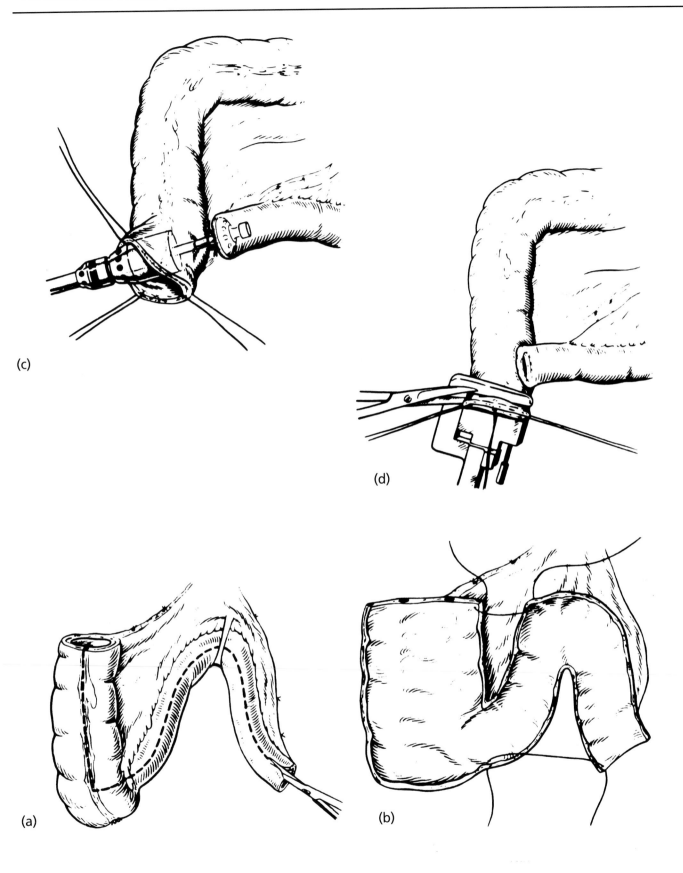

Figure 3. (a) Antimesenteric opening of the isolated segment. (b) Creation of pouch plate by side-to-side anastomosis (running suture of polyglyconate 4/0 with a straight needle).

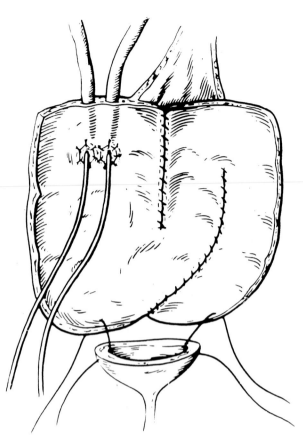

Figure 4. *Anastomosis of the pouch to the bladder remnant after subtotal cystectomy starting at the posterior aspect.*

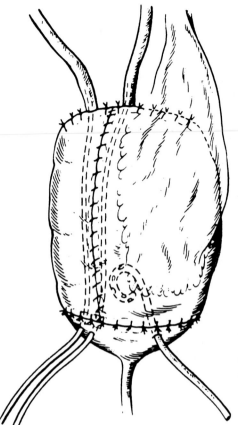

Figure 5. *Completed bladder augmentation.*

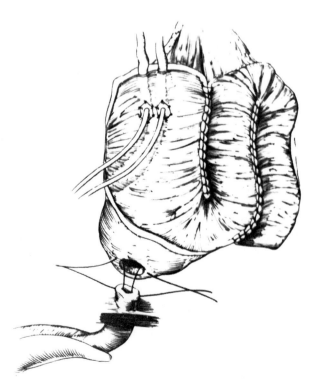

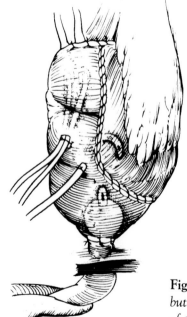

Figure 6. *Bladder replacement: buttonhole incision and anastomosis of the cecal pole to the membranous urethra.*

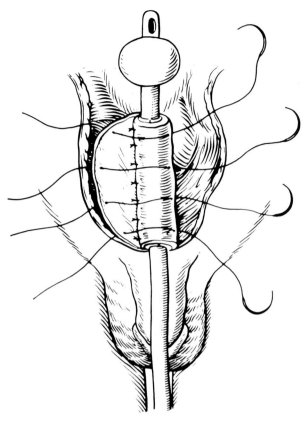

(a)

Figure 7. (a) Reconstruction of the bladder neck by closing the bladder mucosa over a catheter, subsequently duplication of the detrusor. (b) The bladder capacity is increased by augmentation with a Mainz pouch.

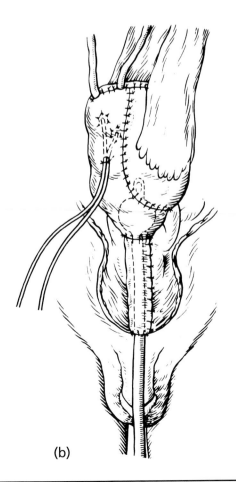

(b)

Continent Diversion

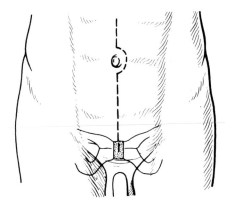

Figure 8. *Median laparotomy with left-sided circumferential incision of the skin around the umbilicus.*

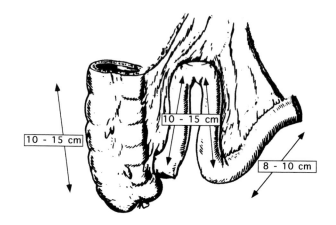

Figure 9. *Intestinal segments to be isolated for the Mainz pouch continent urinary diversion. For creation of the continence mechanism an additional segment of 8–10 cm suffices.*

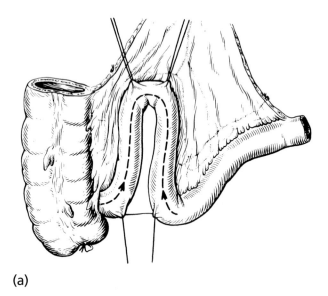

(a)

(b)

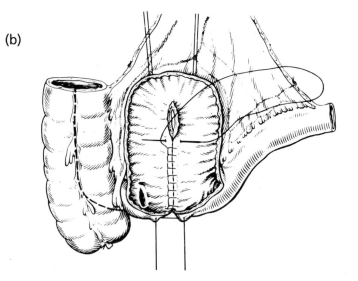

Figure 10. *(a) Antimesenteric opening of the bowel in the direction of the arrows. (b) Side-to-side anastomosis of the terminal and next proximal ileal loop; in the next step the ascending colon is split, sparing the ileocecal valve. Cecoileal anastomosis.*

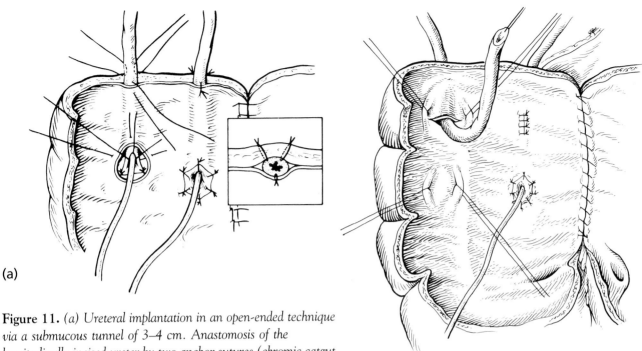

(a)

(b)

Figure 11. *(a) Ureteral implantation in an open-ended technique via a submucous tunnel of 3–4 cm. Anastomosis of the longitudinally incised ureter by two anchor sutures (chromic catgut 5/0) at the 5 and 7 o'clock positions and mucomucous sutures (chromic catgut 6/0). (b) Alternatively, ureteral implantation can be performed using the buttonhole technique. Preparation of the submucous tunnel and anastomosis are as for the open-ended technique.*

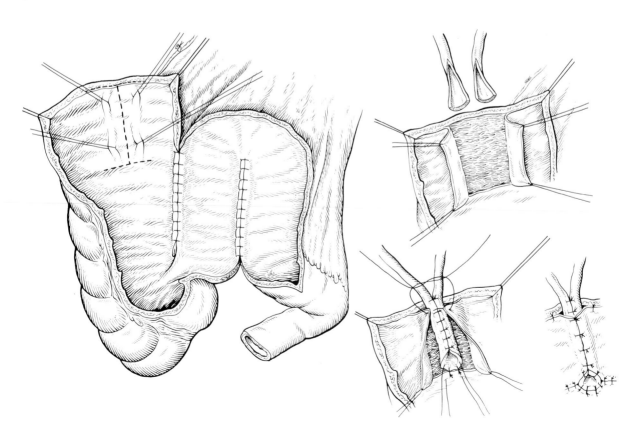

Figure 12. *Dilated ureters are implanted through a serous-lined extramural tunnel.*

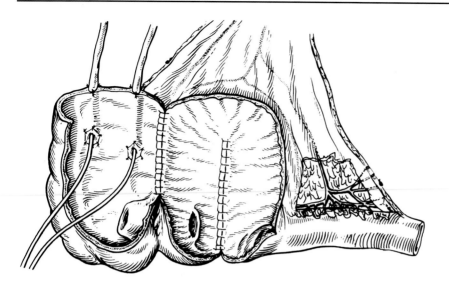

Figure 13. *Nipple construction: removal of fatty tissue and serosa leaving the vessels untouched.*

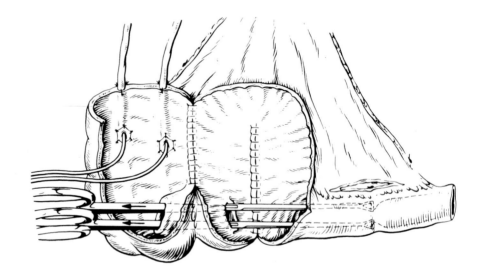

Figure 14. *Invagination of the ileum by means of two Allis clamps.*

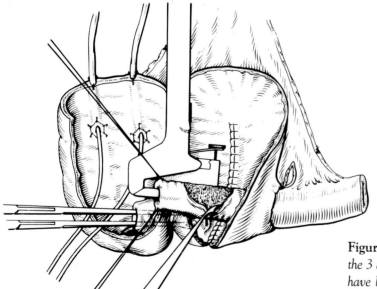

Figure 15. *Fixation of the invagination by two rows of staples at the 3 and 9 o'clock positions. The first four staples of the magazine have been removed to avoid stones at the top of the nipple. The mucosa is roughened.*

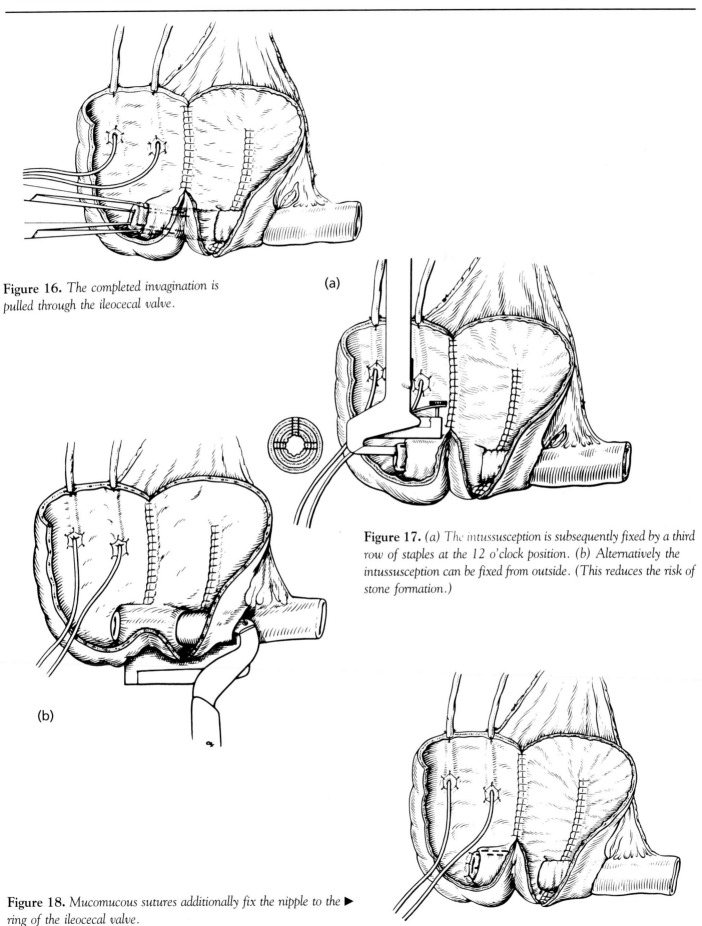

Figure 16. *The completed invagination is pulled through the ileocecal valve.*

(a)

Figure 17. *(a) The intussusception is subsequently fixed by a third row of staples at the 12 o'clock position. (b) Alternatively the intussusception can be fixed from outside. (This reduces the risk of stone formation.)*

(b)

Figure 18. *Mucomucous sutures additionally fix the nipple to the ▶ ring of the ileocecal valve.*

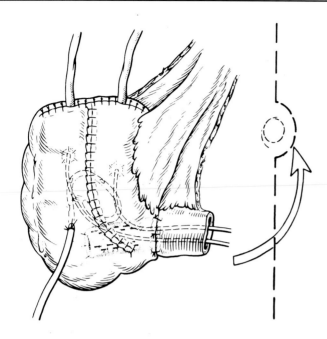

Figure 19. (a) After closure of the pouch, the efferent segment is fixed to the pouch wall by circular single sutures. Ureteral stents are led out through the efferent segment or, like the cystostomy tube, through an incision in the pouch wall. Cranial rotation of the pouch for anastomosis to the umbilicus.

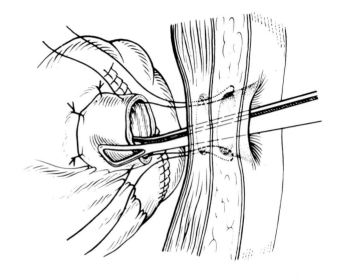

Figure 19. (b) Separation of the umbilical funnel from the abdominal fascia; crosslike incision of the fascia and peritoneum. Sutures grasp the skin, fascia and efferent segment.

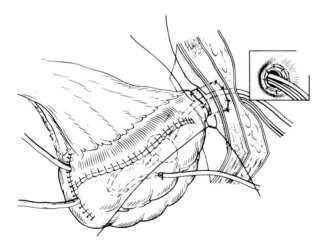

Figure 19. (c) Fixation of the pouch to the peritoneum and abdominal fascia around the efferent segment.

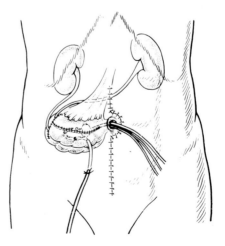

Figure 19. (d) Final position of the pouch.

Appendix - stoma

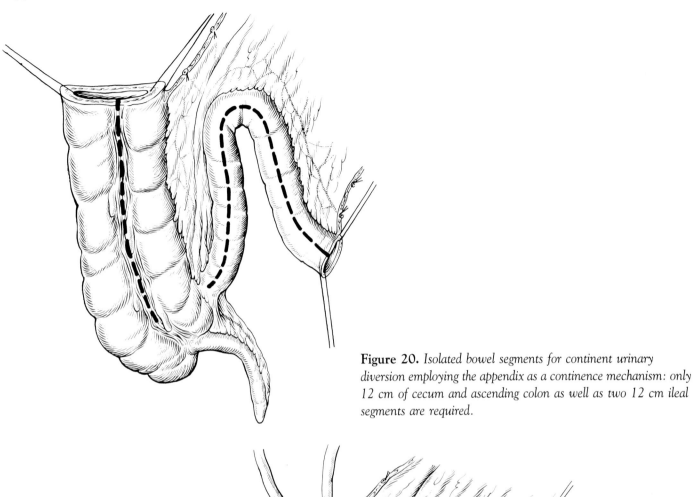

Figure 20. *Isolated bowel segments for continent urinary diversion employing the appendix as a continence mechanism: only 12 cm of cecum and ascending colon as well as two 12 cm ileal segments are required.*

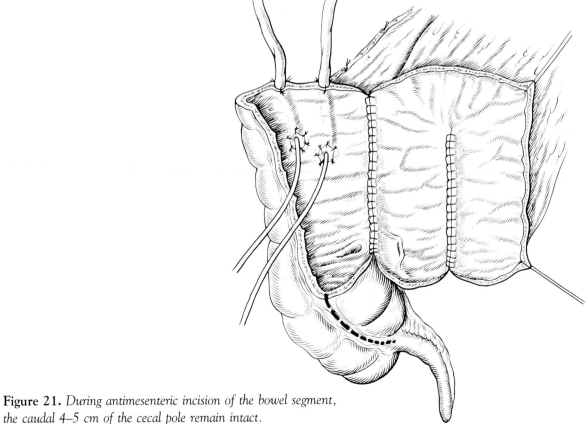

Figure 21. *During antimesenteric incision of the bowel segment, the caudal 4–5 cm of the cecal pole remain intact.*

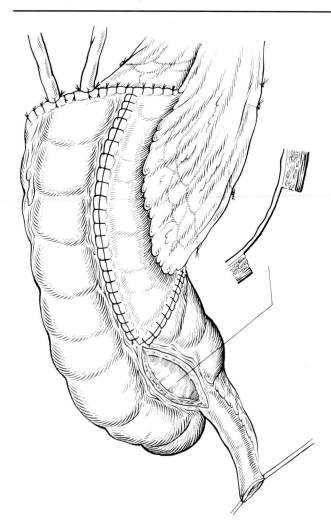

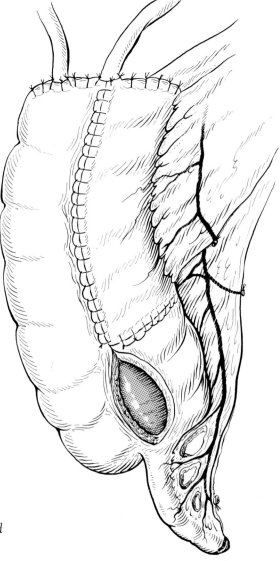

Figure 22. *After closure of the pouch, creation of a submucous tunnel 4 cm in length by incision of the seromuscular layer leaving the mucosa untouched.*

Figure 23. *Excision of mesenteric windows, avoiding the blood supply.*

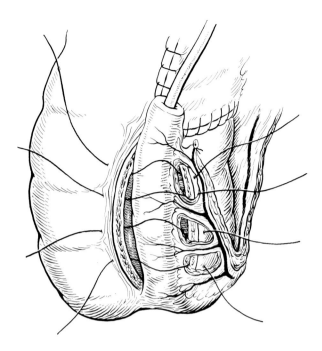

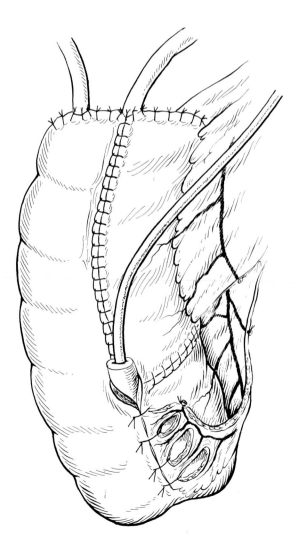

Figure 24. *Insertion of a 16 Fr catheter through the opened appendix in the pouch. The appendix is placed in the prepared bed.*

Figure 25. *Closure of the seromuscular layer over the appendix. Stoma formation to the umbilicus.*

Troubleshooting: Stoma stenosis

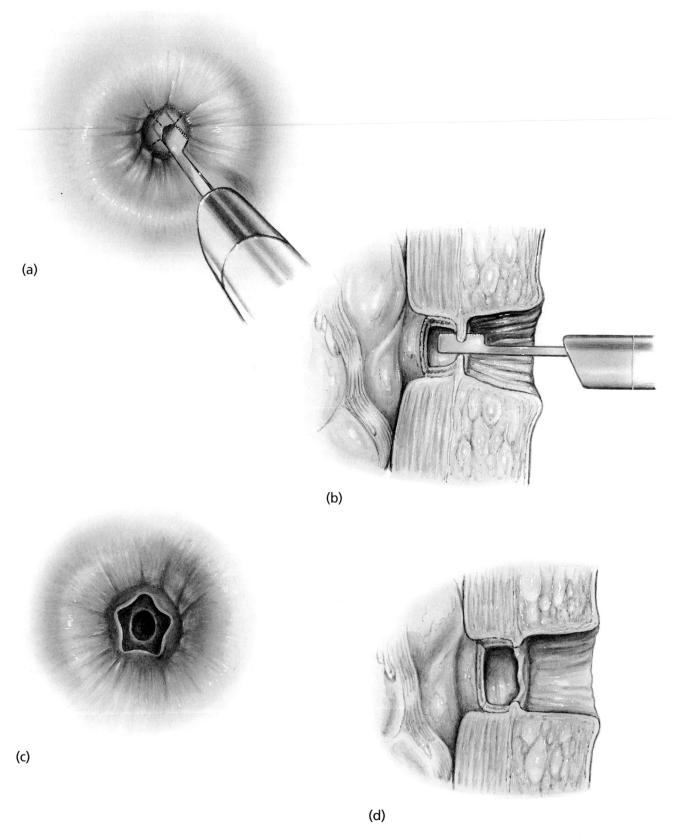

(a)

(b)

(c)

(d)

Figure 26. *Stoma stenosis at the level of the fascia: starlike incision using a Sachse knife. View inside the efferent segment after treatment.*

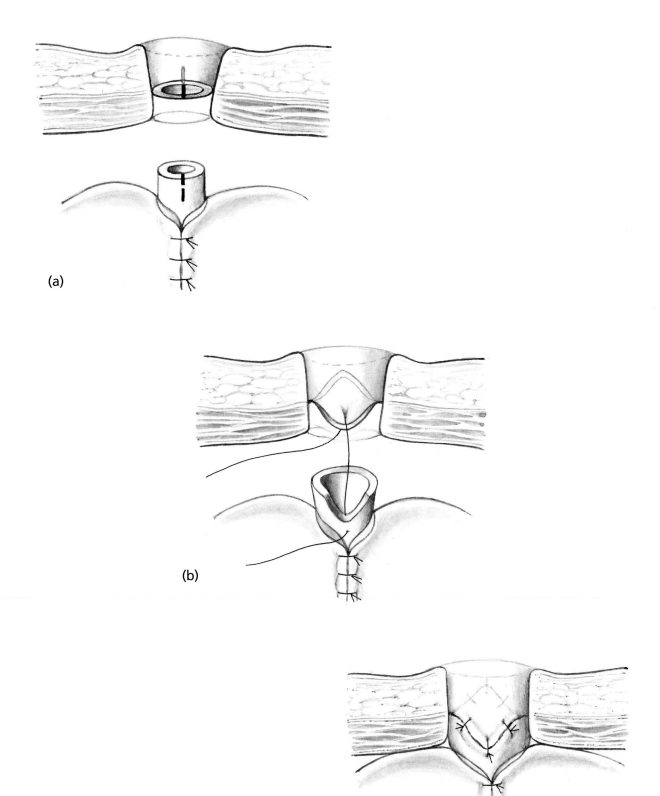

Figure 27. *To avoid stoma stenosis, the distal end of the appendix and the umbilical funnel is contralaterally incised and anastomosed in the shape of a V.*

Correction of nipple-gliding

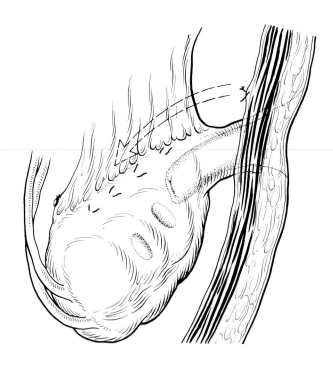

Figure 28. *Operative correction of nipple gliding. Preoperative situation: the invaginated nipple is outside the ileocecal valve. Exposure of the pouch through a right flank incision.*

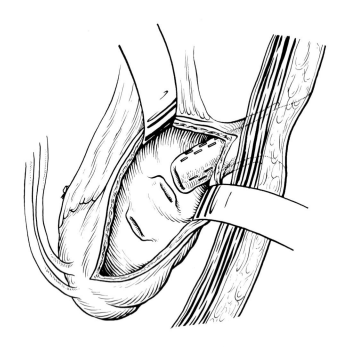

Figure 29. *An incision in the lateral wall of the pouch parallel to the ileocecal valve and the path of the dislocated nipple.*

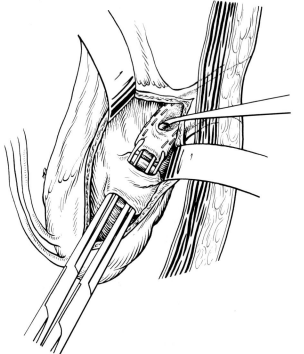

Figure 30. *The mucosa is roughened before the nipple is pulled back through the ileocecal valve.*

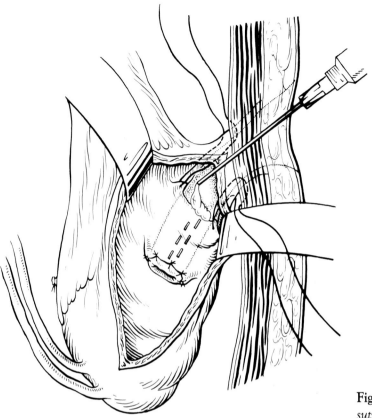

Figure 31. The tip of the mucosa of the nipple has been cut and sutured circumferentially. The space between the ileal mucosa and the inside of the ilececal valve is fixed with fibrin adhesive to improve fixation.

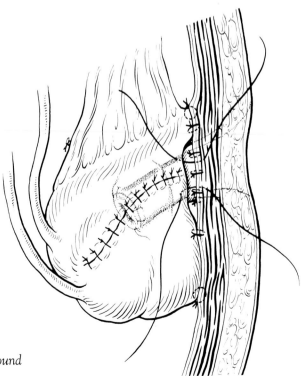

Figure 32. The pouch is fixed to the internal rectus fascia around the ileal nipple.

Ureteral reimplantation

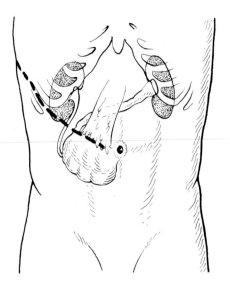

(a)

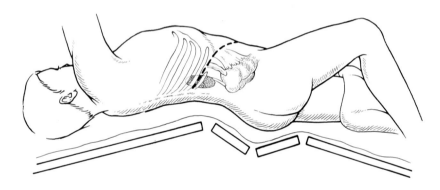

(b)

Figure 33. *Ureteral neoimplantation. (a) Right flank incision for revision of ureteral stenosis at the implantation site. (b) The patient lies in a half-left-sided position.*

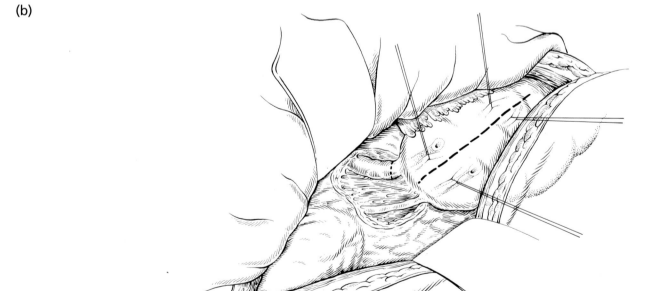

Figure 34. *Four stay sutures are placed and the pouch is opened parallel to the course of the ureters (dotted line).*

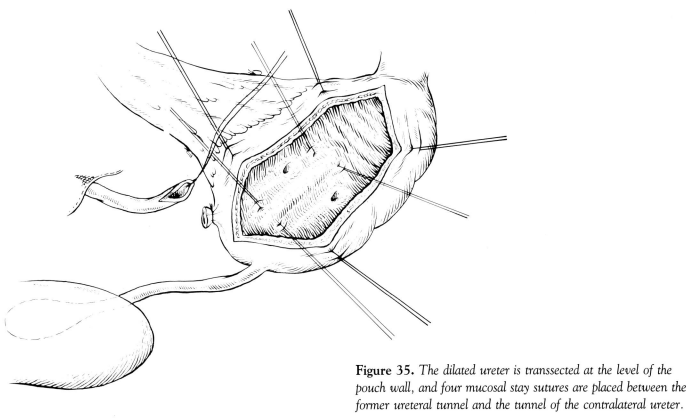

Figure 35. *The dilated ureter is transsected at the level of the pouch wall, and four mucosal stay sutures are placed between the former ureteral tunnel and the tunnel of the contralateral ureter.*

Figure 36. *The mucosa is incised and dissected from the muscular layer to form a broad bed for ureteral implantation. The ureter is brought in through a buttonhole incision at the posterior aspect of the pouch.*

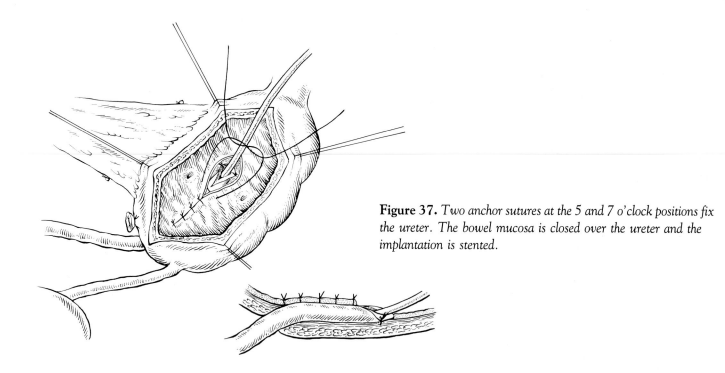

Figure 37. *Two anchor sutures at the 5 and 7 o'clock positions fix the ureter. The bowel mucosa is closed over the ureter and the implantation is stented.*

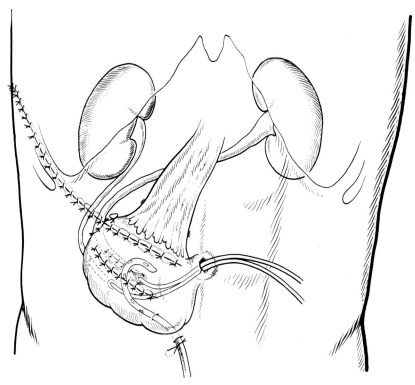

Figure 38. *Aspect after closure of the pouch.*

Follow-up

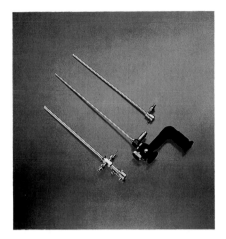

Figure 39. *Contact microcystoscope according to Hamou (Storz, Tuttlingen, Germany) for pouchoscopy.*

Figure 40. *(a) Cystoscopy allows identification of the ureters. (b) Magnification up to 150 × for evaluation of mucosal cells in suspect areas.*

(a)

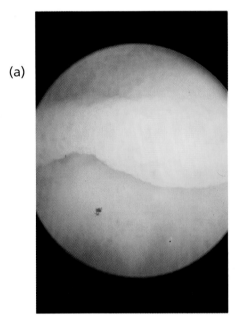

(b)

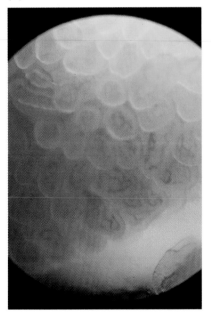

Use of Stapling Devices in Urology

U. Grein, F. Schreiter[a]
Department of Urology,
Witten University,
Schwelm, Germany
[a]*Department of Urology,*
Allgemeines Krakenhaus,
Heubers, Harburg, Germany

Introduction

Since the introduction of stapling devices into clinical practice by Hültl[1] at the beginning of this century, indications for their use have extensively broadened. The advantages of staplers (such as shorter operating times, reproducible and secure suture lines, easy use and shorter exposure of open bacteria-laden organs) have led to their wide use in abdominal surgery. In urologic practice staplers gained attention when continent diversions such as the Kock pouch, Mainz pouch[2,3] and bladder substitution replaced continent diversions at the ideal forms of urinary diversion. Bowel resection in these cases is time consuming, and staplers allow a secure and easy-to-perform anastomosis. The use of staplers in creation of a continent stoma is always necessary. Previously, the reported incontinence and catheterization problems were due to sliding of the ileal intussusception of the continence nipple.[4,5] Only the introduction of staplers could diminish these complication rates, leading to a stable nipple continence mechanism.

Prerequisites for the successful use of staplers are the same as those for general surgery: sufficient practice and correct use of the instruments, standardized operative techniques, tension-free anastomosis, preservation of the vascularization of the anastomotic site, creation of flat anastomotic margins and accurate patient preparation.

Indications

Stapling devices are often used in the closure of fascia or cutis. In addition they are used today in the creation of an ileal conduit, ileal pouch, Mainz pouch,[6] or bladder substitution with either small or large bowel. In renal surgery, indications are limited to secure vessel closure, e.g. in nephrectomy. Hemiadrenalectomy for adrenal adenomas presented big problems in hemostasis of the remaining fragile tissue, which was solved by the use of staplers.[7]

Instruments

The stapling devices used now have a high technical standard. They are characterized by easy use and permit the use of sterilizable reusable components. These instruments can be divided into six groups:

- TA staplers (US Surgical, Norwalk, Connecticut, USA). These instruments allow closure of enterotomies or cystostomies by two parallel staple suture lines. Possible uses include bladder closure, functional bowel end-to-end anastomosis, securing the antireflux and continence nipple, and vessel closure

- GIA staplers (US Surgical). These divide the bowel wall entrapped by the instrument with simultaneous closure of the bowel lumen through two staple suture lines. Possible uses include functional end-to-end anastomosis and isolation of small or large bowel segments. Their advantages include speed and avoidance of loss of bowel content in the abdominal cavity. However, there is a danger of mesenteric interposition with after-bleeding, and the anastomosis may be too tight of the instrument is not placed appropriately into the bowel lumen

- LDS staplers. These permit division and ligation of vessels. Possible uses include mesenteric preparation by isolation of bowel segments, inner and outer vasectomy, and appendicectomy. However, there is a risk of mesenteric after-bleeding due to the unsecure ligation by fat interposition

- EEA staplers (US Surgical). These may be used for circular end-to-end anastomosis in open luminal techniques, as for example in ileoascendostomy (Mainz pouch)

- Staplers for fascia and skin closure

- Vessel clips

Preoperative preparation

After 3 days of oral fluid intake, bowel cleansing is performed the day before the operation by antegrade lavage through a nasogastric tube. Perioperative antibiotic prophylaxis is given for 3 days.

Operative technique (Figures 1–19)

Numerous forms of continent urinary diversion require bowel continuity to be interrupted with the formation of either a reservoir or nipples (small bowel intussusceptions with either an antireflux technique or a catheterizable continent stoma). Resection and re-establishment of bowel continuity are optimized by the use of stapling devices.

Bowel resection
- Depending on the urinary diversion planned, a section of terminal ileum from 15 cm (ileal conduit) to 70 cm (ileal pouch) in length is mobilized at a 25 cm distance from the ileocecal valve

- Skeletization can be performed with the LDS stapler with accurate preservation of the vascularization of the bowel segment

- The bowel is divided and closed with the use of the GIA-50 stapler. Bowel content cannot therefore get lost in the abdominal cavity

- The so-called functional end-to-end anastomosis is a side-to-side anastomosis and is performed using the GIA-50 stapler.[8] The branches of the instrument are introduced in the antimesenteric triangularly opened bowel extremities. The mesentery is pulled laterally. On closing the instrument, the anastomosis and stoma are created at the same time. The result is an anastomosis wide enough for at least two fingers

- Closure of the incision used for introduction of the instrument is performed with the TA-55 stapler

- Stability of the anastomosis is established by a seromuscular Z-stitch on the dome

- After isolation of an ileocecal segment (Mainz pouch), and end-to-side ileotransversostomy may be created using the EEA stapler in an open technique

Nipple creation by pouches and bladder substitutions[3]

- A 15 cm bowel segment is used for creation of the nipple. The segment is freed from the mesentery for 5–6 cm

- A fat suction device can be used to remove fat from the vessels with accurate preservation of the bowel wall vascularization[2]

- Intussusception of bowel is achieved by the use of Allis clamps

- The nipple is stabilized by four opposite double suture lines with the use of the TA-55 stapler. The first suture line is placed antimesenterically; two further suture lines are placed on the mesenteric root; the last is placed on the posterior wall of the nipple. The last three staples are removed from the device to avoid the formation of stones by contamination of urine on the staple overlying the nipple margin

- To protect against nipple sliding, collagen may be interposed between the walls of the interposed bowel segments. Collagen leads to further stabilization of the nipple

- In the creation of a Mainz pouch, the nipple is formed in a similar manner by ileal intussusception, but the stapled invaginated segment is pulled through the ileocecal valve

Postoperative care

- Parenteral nutrition for 5–7 days to protect the bowel anastomosis

- On day 3 or 4, medical stimulation of bowel peristalsis

- Removal of the nasogastric tube at re-establishment of bowel function

- Removal of the uteteral splints (8 Fr) at days 8–10

- Control of the anastomosis of the neobladder by biplanar cystography

Complications

- Anastomotic failure after the use of stapling devices is reported as sepsis with an incidence as high as 1.5–5.5%. This rate is comparable to that of anastomotic failure after manual suture

- Endoscopy of the neobladder is mandatory to detect stones, which can form in the presence of infected urine in contact with the metal clips. Stones are routinely removed endoscopically. The development of absorbable metal clips could solve this problem

- Nipple sliding is no longer a problem since the introduction of stapling devices

References

1. Hültl H. II Kongress d. Ungarischen Gesellschaft für Chirurgie Budapest, May 1908. *Pester Med-Chir Presse* **45** (1908) 108–10, 121–2.
2. Ghoneim MH, Kock NG, Lycke G, Shebab El-Din AB. An appliance-free sphincter-controlled bladder substitution: the urethral Kock pouch. *J Urol* **138** (1987) 1150–4.
3. Schreiter F, Böttger W. Suprapubische Harnableitung heute, Ileumkonduit, Kock-Pouch, S-Blase. In: Akovbiantz A, Denck H, Denck K-J (eds) *Der Pouch der Chirurgie und Urologie – Chirurgische Gastroenterologie mit interdisziplinären Gesprächen*. TM-Verlag.
4. Kock NG, Nilson AE, Norlen L *et al.* Urinary diversion via a continent ileum reservoir: clinical experience. *Scand J Urol Nephrol Suppl* **49** (1978) 23–31.
5. Schreiter F, Noll F. Kock-pouch and S-bladder: two different ways of lower urinary tract reconstruction. *J Urol* **142** (1989) 1197–200.
6. Hohenfellner R, Alken P, Jacobi GH, Riedmiller H, Thüroff JW. Mainz-pouch mit ileozökaler Intussuszeption und umbilikalen Stoma. *Akt Urol* **18** (1987) I–IV.
7. Kearney GP, Doyle CJ, Belldegrun A. Use of surgical stapler in adrenal surgery. *Urology* **28** (1986) 320–1.

8. Steichen RM. The use of staplers in anatomical side to side and functional end to end anastomosis. *Surgery* **64** (1984) 948–52.

9. Goodwin WE, Winter CC, Baker WF. Cup-patch technique of ileocystoplasty for bladder enlargement or partial substitution. *Surg Gynecol Obstet* **108** (1959) 108–12.

10. Myers RP, Rife CC, Barret MD. Experience with the bowel stapler for ileal conduit urinary diversion. *Br J Urol* **54** (1982) 491–3.

11. Skinner DG, Lieskovsky G, Boyd SD. Continuing experience with the continent ileal reservoir (Kock-pouch) as an alternative to cutaneous urinary diversion: an update after 250 cases. *J Urol* **137** (1987) 1140–4.

Vasectomy

Figure 1. *Vasectomy. With the LDS instrument the vas is simultaneously resected and the ends closed with staples.*

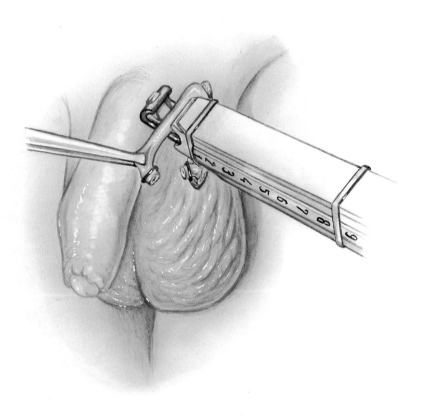

Appendectomy

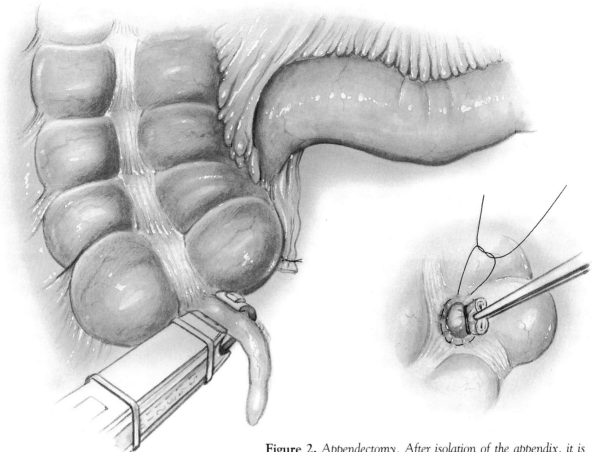

Figure 2. Appendectomy. After isolation of the appendix, it is divided at the base with the LDS instrument.

Bladder closure

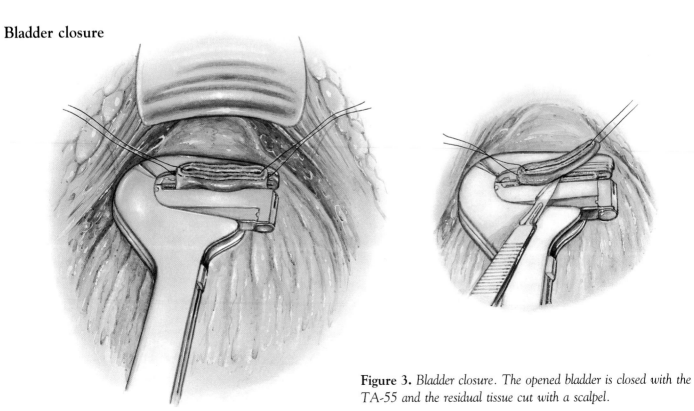

Figure 3. Bladder closure. The opened bladder is closed with the TA-55 and the residual tissue cut with a scalpel.

Nephrectomy

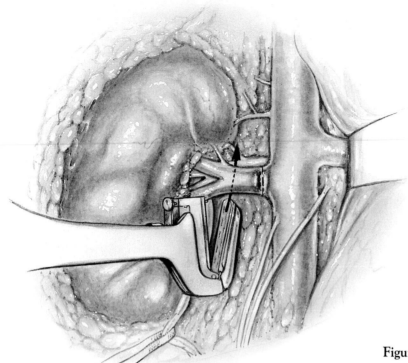

Figure 4. *Nephrectomy. A safe closure of the pedicle is assured with the TA-30.*

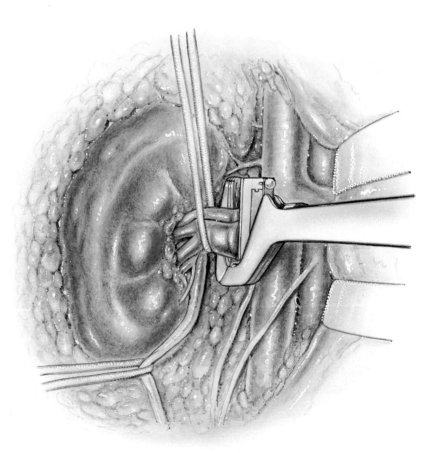

Figure 5. *Vein and artery may also be closed simultaneously.*

Small bowel resection and end-to-end anastomosis

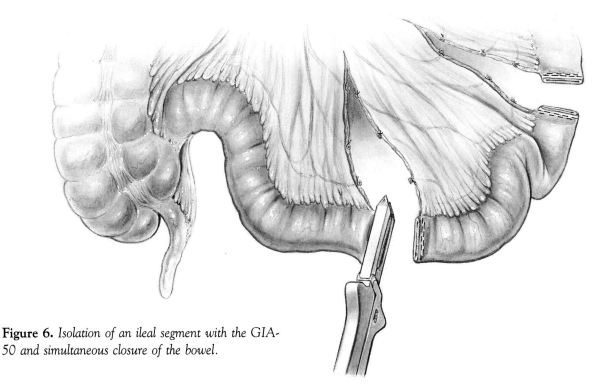

Figure 6. *Isolation of an ileal segment with the GIA-50 and simultaneous closure of the bowel.*

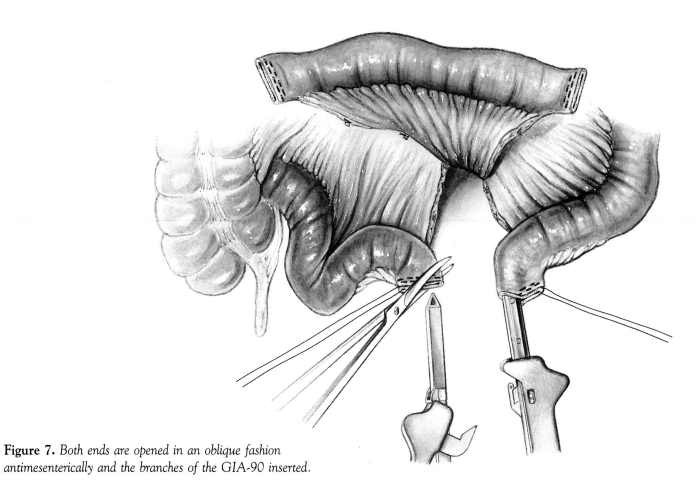

Figure 7. *Both ends are opened in an oblique fashion antimesenterically and the branches of the GIA-90 inserted.*

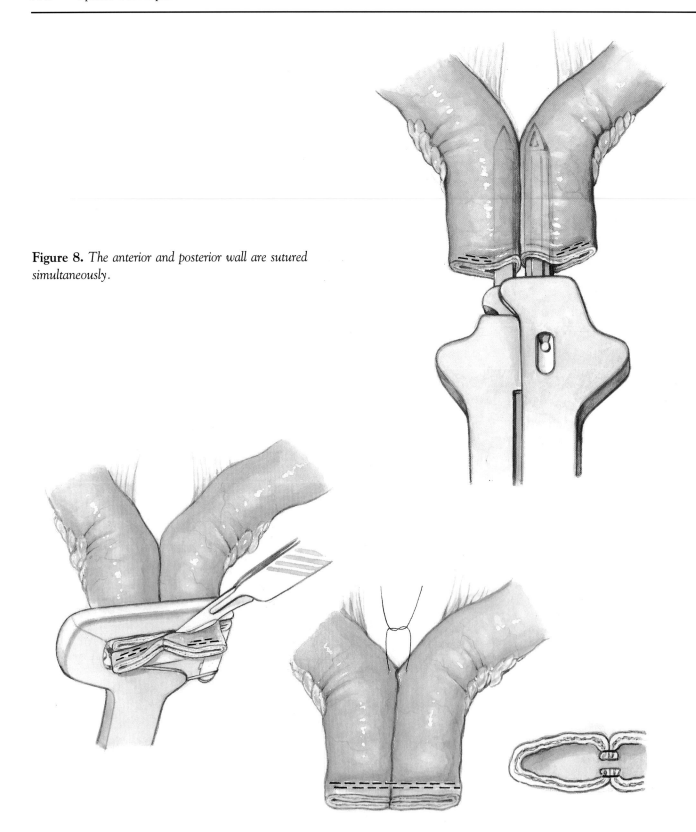

Figure 8. *The anterior and posterior wall are sutured simultaneously.*

Figure 9. *The distal openings are closed with the TA-55 and the anastomosis is secured with a Z-suture.*

Ileoascendostomy

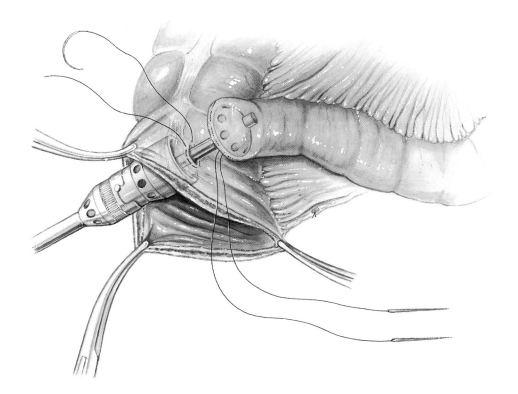

Figure 10. *After insertion of the ileocecal segment, bowel continuity is reestablished with the EEA-instrument.*

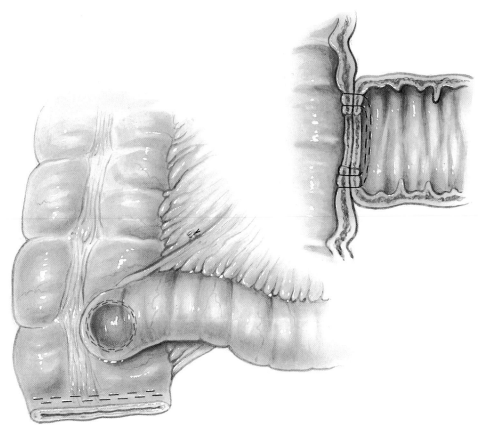

Figure 11. *For the closure of the colon the TA-55 is used.*

Nipple formation in the Kock pouch

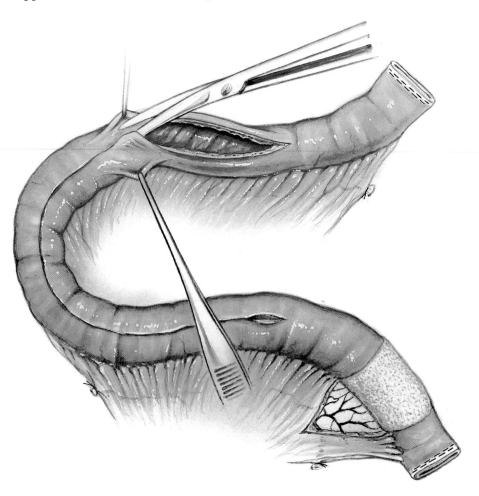

Figure 12. *The median part of the segment used for the nipple and window in the mesentery is dissected and a collagen-patch wrapped around the bowel.*

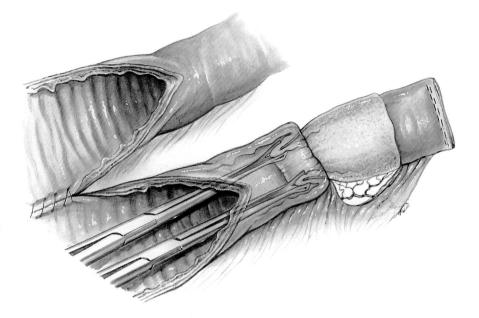

Figure 13. *Invagination with Allis clamps, while the collagen-patch assures nipple stabilization.*

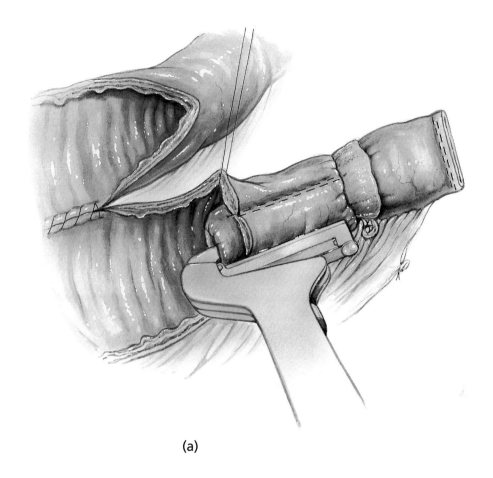

(a)

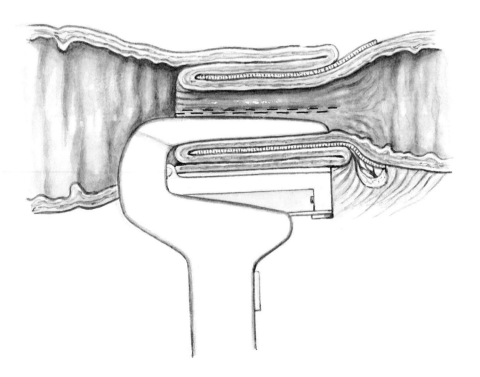

Figure 14. *Definite nipple fixation with four staple lines with the TA-55. To avoid stone formation at the nipple edge the last three staples in the magazine angle are removed.*

(b)

Nipple formation in ileal conduit

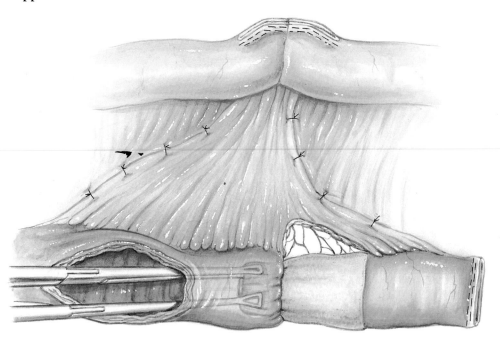

Figure 15. *Nipple formation in anology to the Kock pouch.*

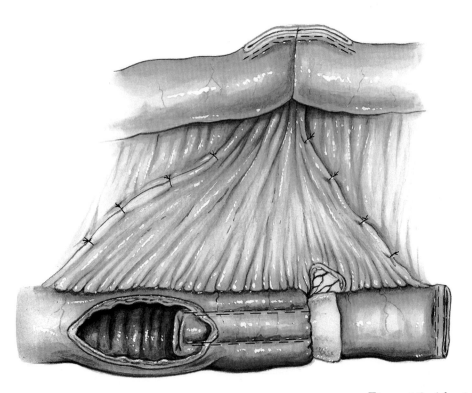

Figure 16. *After invagination, fixation of the nipple with four staple lines and the TA-55.*

Nipple formation in the Mainz Pouch I

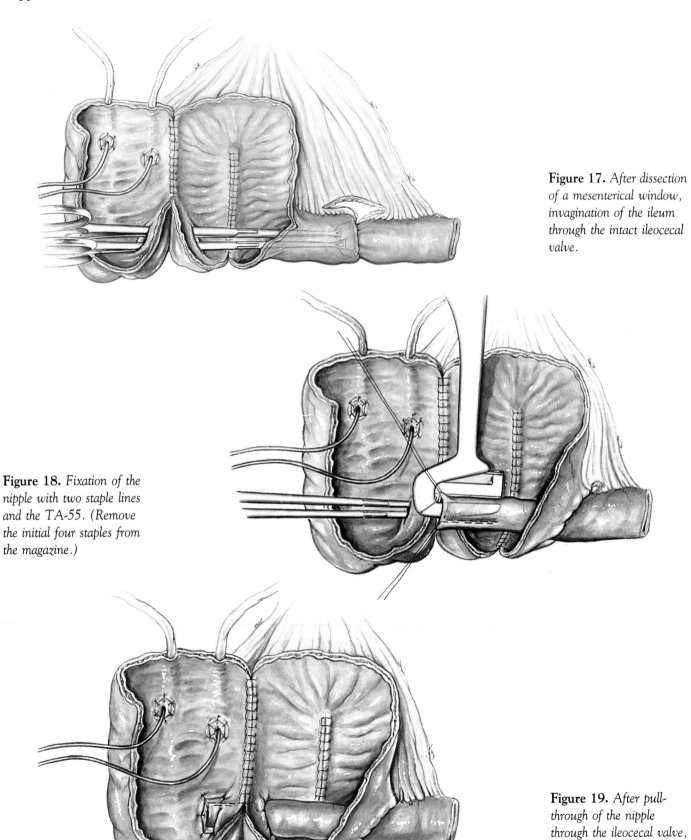

Figure 17. *After dissection of a mesenterical window, invagination of the ileum through the intact ileocecal valve.*

Figure 18. *Fixation of the nipple with two staple lines and the TA-55. (Remove the initial four staples from the magazine.)*

Figure 19. *After pull-through of the nipple through the ileocecal valve, additional fixation.*

Reconstruction of the Ileocecal Valve

M. Fisch, F. Spies, R. Hohenfellner
Department of Urology,
University of Mainz School of Medicine,
Mainz, Germany

Introduction

During reconstruction of an ileocecal reservoir, such as the Mainz or Indiana pouch, the ileocecal valve is lost. Subsequently, the intestinal transit time is shortened and ileocolic reflux occurs with bacterial colonization of the ileum.[1–3] Malabsorption, severe frequency of stools and diarrhea may result. We have functionally reconstructed the ileocecal valve by embedding the ileum into the ascending colon via the submucous tunnel, thereby avoiding the consequences of loss of the valve.

Indications

Risk factors for postoperative frequency and diarrhea after loss of the ileocecal valve are:

- Extensive bowel resection (in the history or planned)
- Neurogenic disorders, e.g. myelomeningocele
- Irradiation of the pelvis or abdomen
- Pre-existing diarrhea

Preoperative preparation

- Bowel preparation as for urinary diversion; no additional procedures are required

Instruments and suture material

- Standard set for abdominal surgery
- Sigel retractor
- Basin containing prepared iodine solution (disinfection)
- Microfeather for incision of the teniae coli
- Polyglyconic acid 4/0 for closure of the ascending colon, closure of the seromuscularis over the anastomosed ileum, and lateral adaptation stitches
- Polyglyconic acid 5/0 for anastomosis of the ileum to the mucosal incision in the colon
- Silk 4/0 stay sutures (bowel)

Surgical technique step by step (Figures 1–10)

- Isolation of the ileocecal segment

- Closure of the ascending colon by single-stitch seromuscular polyglyconic acid 4/0 sutures
- Longitudinal incision of the teniae coli for 6–7 cm starting 1 cm above the closed end
- Dissection of the muscular layer from the mucosa to create a broad trough for the ileum (sharp dissection by scissors or blunt dissection using a peanut)
- Incision of the ileum antimesenterically to obtain a large entrance without obstruction
- Defatting of the ileal mesentery and removal of the serosa
- Incision of the colonic mucosa at the cranial end over a length of 2 cm
- Ileocecal anastomosis grasping all layers of the ileum and the mucosa of the colon (5/0 polyglycolic acid sutures)
- Closure of the seromuscular layer of the colon over the anastomosed ileal loop, thereby creating a submucosal tunnel 4 cm long
- Lateral adaptation stitches to bring the ileum smoothly into the cecum and avoid mucosal diverticula or kinking with obstruction
- Additional adaptation stitches in the area of the mesentery

Surgical tricks

- At the cranial aspect, the dissection of the seromuscular layer from the mucosa of the colon should be extended laterally to the insertion of the mesentery. In this way a broad trough for the ileal loop is created and submucous embedding is facilitated
- During closure of the seromuscular layer over the ileal loop, the ileal wall should be grasped with every second stitch to prevent the loop from sliding out of the tunnel
- A tunnel length of 4 cm suffices for reflux prevention

Postoperative care

Care depends on the nature of the operation. No additional precautions are required related to the reconstruction of the ileocecal valve.

References

1. Cosnes J, Gendre JP, LeQuintrec Y. Role of the ileocecal valve and site of intestinal resection in malabsorption after

extensive small bowel resection. *Digestion* **18** (1978) 329–35.

2. Rendleman DF, Anthony JE, Davis C *et al.* Reflux pressure studies on the ileocecal valve of dogs and humans. *Surgery* **44** (1958) 640–64.

3. Richardson JD, Griffen WO Jr. Ileocecal valve substitutes as bacteriologic barriers. *Am J Surg* **123** (1972) 149–53.

4. Lie HR, Lagergren J, Rasmussen F *et al.* Bowel and bladder control of children with myelomeningocele: a Nordic study. *Dev Med Child Neurol* **33** (1991) 1053–61.

5. Singleton AO Jr, Redmond C II, McMurray E. Ileocecal resection and small bowel transit and absorption. *Ann Surg* **159** (1964) 690–3.

6. Vinograd I, Merguerian P, Udassin R, Mogle P, Nissan S. An experimental model of a submucosally tunneled valve for the replacement of the ileocecal valve. *J Pediatr Surg* (1984) 726–9.

Figure 1. *The ileocecal segment used for creation of a Mainz pouch. The ileocecal valve is lost.*

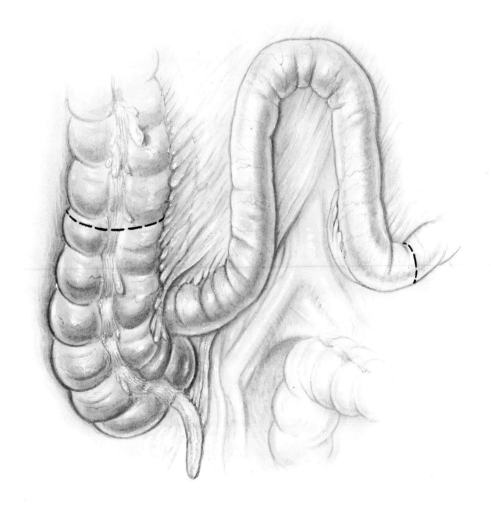

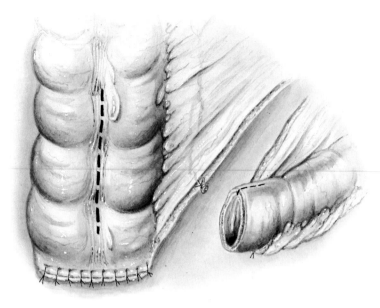

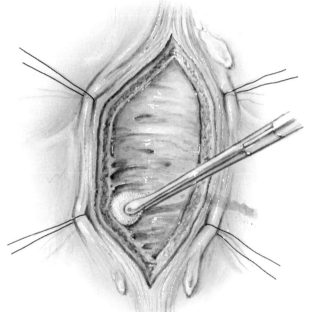

Figure 2. *The ascending colon is closed terminally and the teniae libera incised for 6–7 cm (dotted line).*

Figure 3. *Insertion of four stay sutures, and blunt dissection of the seromuscular layer from the mucosa.*

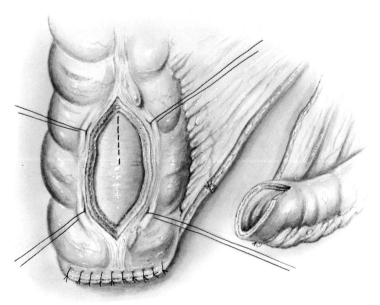

Figure 4. *Both the colonic mucosa and the ileum are incised over 2 cm at the cranial end to prepare for anastomosis.*

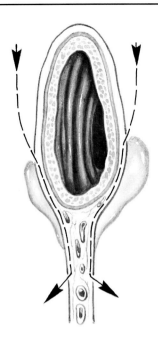

Figure 5. (a) *The arrows show the direction of dissection for defatting of the ileal mesentery to avoid the vessels.*

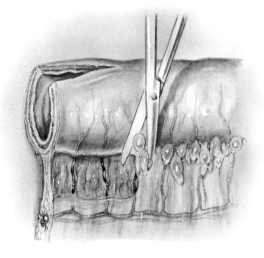

Figure 5. (b) *The mesentery is defatted.*

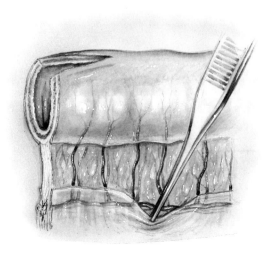

Figure 5. (c) *The serosa of the mesentery is removed.*

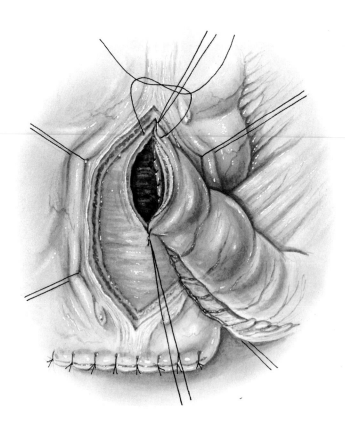

Figure 6. *Ileocecal anastomosis using either two running sutures or single stitches or polyglyconic acid 5/0. Two stay sutures facilitate anastomosis.*

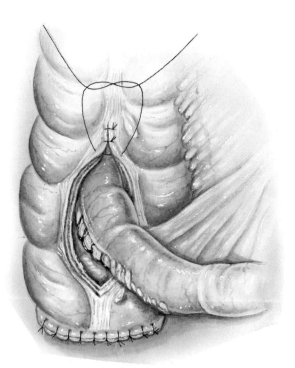

Figure 7. *Closure of the seromuscular layer (polyglyconic acid 4/0), creating a submucosal tunnel 4 cm long.*

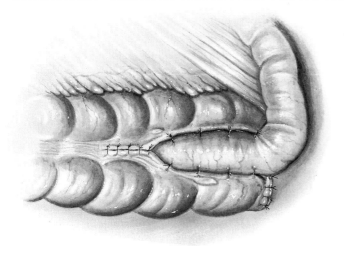

Figure 8. *Lateral adaptation stitches avoid kinking or diverticula. There are additional adaptation stitches in the area of the mesentery.*

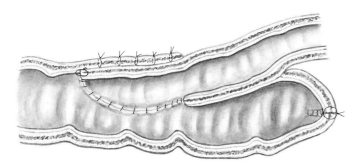

Figure 9. *Lateral view of the ileum inserted smoothly into the ascending colon.*

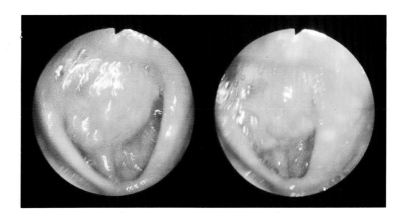

Figure 10. *Endoscopic view of the valve. The arrow marks the entrance into the ileum.*

Sigmoid Neobladder

R. Chao, P.H. Lange
Department of Urology,
University of Washington School of Medicine,
Seattle, Washington, USA

Comment

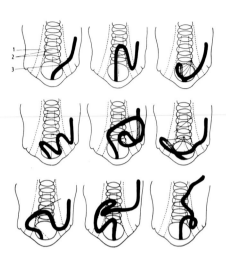

Figure 1. *Forms and different positions of the sigmoid colon.*

Initial enthusiasm for the various techniques of bladder substitution with bowel segments after radical cystoprostatectomy introduced in the middle of the 1950s, left open the question of which was the best model. As experience with these techniques grew, the results often proved disappointing, and comparison of the results obtained by different authors using the same technique was confusing. Then, in 1988, Hinman described the volume and pressure of tubularized and detubularized bowel segments,[1] creating an objective basis for judging the results of operative techniques.

Although the success of the Camey I procedure is unquestionable, despite the unacceptable rate of night incontinence,[2] Camey's modification of the tubularized Camey I to the detubularized Camey II procedure showed that a correct theory has a good influence on practical results.[3] However, a theoretical basis for many of the recognized problems is still lacking. A good example is the dependence of incontinence after bladder substitution on age: nearly half of patients older than 60 years of age are incontinent 6 months after the operation, whereas in younger patients the incontinence rate

is no more than 30%.[4] On long-term follow-up, increasing amounts of residual urine can become a problem.[4] Diarrhea (which can have similar effects to those of urine incontinence), stone formation, changes of acid–base balance and poorly defined disturbances of absorption do not facilitate selection of a special operative technique from among the increasing number of operative techniques and innovations.

However, the technique of bladder substitution using detubularized sigmoid colon presented in this chapter is an attractive method. The experienced urologic surgeon knows that disturbances in absorption are not a problem after resection of the sigmoid colon for diverticulitis or carcinoma. For bladder substitution the sigmoid colon offers adequate length,[5] suitable anatomic position and unproblematic anastomosis to the urethra, as well as the possibility of an antireflux ureteral implantation into the large bowel.

This chapter gives a clear definition of continence. Although the results are disappointing (a night incontinence rate of >30%) they are comparable to those obtained using other techniques. The authors make no special claims for the technique, but recommend it as one among many others that the urologist should master.

References

1. Hinman F Jr. Selection of intestinal segments for bladder substitution: physical characteristics. *J Urol* **139** (1988) 519–23.
2. Camey M, Botto H. The ileal neobladder: development and longterm experience: Camey I and II. *Scand J Urol Nephrol Suppl* **142** (1992) 98–100.
3. Camey M. Bladder replacement by ileocystoplasty following radical cystectomy. *World J Urol* **3** (1985) 161–6.
4. Steven K, Colding-Jørgensen M. Dynamic characteristics of intact and detubularized bowel segments for continent urinary reconstruction. *Scand J Urol Nephrol Suppl* **142** (1992) 37–41.
5. Töndury G. *Angewandte und topographische Anatomie.* Stuttgart: Georg Thieme (1970) 195.

P. Alken, Mannheim, Germany

Sigmoid Neobladder

Introduction

Bladder substitution represents an alternative to incontinent diversions after cystectomy.[1–5] The ideal neobladder should have good compliance, large capacity and reflux protection. In selected patients we achieved good results by using a detubularized sigmoid neobladder.[6,7]

Indications

- Infiltrating bladder carcinoma in men who have to undergo radical cystectomy

Contraindications

- Irritable colon
- Previous radiotherapy on the pelvis
- Polyps, tumors or severe diverticulosis of the sigmoid colon
- Tumor invasion of the prostatic urethra
- Liver or distant lymph node metastases infiltrating the surrounding tissue

Preoperative evaluation

- Bowel cleansing on the day before the operation using electrolyte solution
- Neomycin and erythromycin orally at 1, 2 and 10 p.m.
- A second-generation cephalosporin intravenously just before the operation

Operative technique step by step (Figures 1–8)

- Midline laparotomy with the patient in the lithotomy position
- Radical cystoprostatectomy with extensive lymph node dissection and preservation of the sigmoid collateral vascularization
- Anastomosis of the left colic artery and superior rectal artery (from the inferior mesenteric artery) to the medial and inferior rectal arteries (from the internal iliac artery), checking the patency of the inferior mesenteric artery by manual examination
- Preparation of the sigmoid colon, avoiding deep incisions over possible collateral circles

- Frozen sections of the urethral resection margins to exclude the presence of carcinoma *in situ* or dysplasia
- Isolation of a 30–40 cm sigmoid segment with preservation of its mesenteric vascularization
- Tension-free anastomosis with single polyglactin 3/0 stitches (e.g. Vicryl (Ethicon, Edinburgh, UK)) of the sigmoid colon (best achieved after mobilization of the left colonic flexure)
- U-configuration of the isolated sigmoid segment and longitudinal incision over the tenia medialis. The mobile sigmoid segment with few appendices epiploicae allows problem-free anastomosis with the urethral stump later. The most caudal point is chosen for urethral anastomosis
- Two-layer continuous and single-stitch closure of the posterior wall of the neobladder (Vicryl 3/0)
- Ureteral implantation before detubularization. Initially we used Leadbetter's technique,[8] but we now prefer the ureteral implantation technique of Goodwin *et al.*[9] The ureter is therefore implanted in a 3–5 cm mucosal tunnel on the posterior colonic wall. If the mucosal tunnel formation is difficult, mucosal flaps are positioned over the ureters. An alternative is given by the LeDuc technique.[10,11] Ureteral implantation is performed before urethral anastomosis and sufficient length of the ureters is therefore to be guaranteed to avoid ureteral tension during urethro-neobladder anastomosis
- Ureters are stented with 8 Fr stents, fastened tight to the mucosa with a chronic catgut stitch (5/0) and separately brought out through the neobladder wall
- Positioning of a 24 Fr Malecot catheter
- Closure of the anterior wall of the neobladder in two layers
- Filling of the pouch with saline solution to check possible leaks, which are sutured with 3/0 Vicryl
- The hole for urethral anastomosis is widened on the guide of a 30 Fr catheter
- The urethral stump is best visualized under perineal pressure and is then sutured with six stitches (2/0 Vicryl) on the guide of a 20 Fr Foley catheter to the sigmoid pouch
- All drains, including two Penrose drains placed bilaterally in the small pelvis, are brought out separately through the abdominal wall

Postoperative care

- Removal of the ureteral stents on day 10 after cystography results are normal
- Removal of the transurethral catheter at 3 weeks

- Closure and then removal of the suprapubic cystostomy only after confirmation of low postvoiding residual urinary volume

- Intravenous urography at 6 weeks

- Serum electrolytes, urinary cytology, urine culture and voiding cystourethrography at 3, 6 and 12 months

- Thereafter, urinary cytology and serum electrolytes every 6 months, with cystoscopy, intravenous urography and voiding cystourethrography every year

Results

In all, 35 patients have so far undergone this procedure. Follow-up data for longer than 1 year are available for 31 patients. One patient with a preoperative creatinine level of 2 mg/dl showed postoperatively progressive renal failure and had to receive dialysis. One patient with a left-sided ureteral obstruction underwent reimplantation surgery after balloon dilatation failed to produce improvements.

After a mean follow-up of 26.5 months, all patients are continent during the day and two-thirds during the night. In these cases we define incontinence as involuntary loss of urine or nocturia more than twice. Urodynamically measured bladder capacity was 450 cm^2 at 3 months, 580 cm^2 at 6 months and 600 cm^2 at 1 year. Pressures were minimal on maximal bladder filling. Postvoiding residual urinary volume is in all patients within normal limits.[12]

Comment by the authors

We created a neobladder with ileum, ileum and ascending colon, and stomach in over 100 patients. A reasonable alternative in selected patients with a large fat-poor sigmoid segment is the sigmoid neobladder. The sigmoid colon is dilatable and its use causes few metabolic impairments. Diarrhea, often observed in patients with isolated ileum and ascending colon, can therefore be avoided. Additionally, ureteral implantation is technically easy to perform.

Lateralization of the bowel anastomosis avoids keeping it in touch with the suture line of the pouch. The risk of intestinal pouch fistulas and bowel obstruction is thus lowered. The capacity of the sigmoid neobladder is initially sufficient and improves with time, but is less than that offered by the ileum and colon or ileum alone. Even if urgency and frequency are eventually worse than a neobladder built from other bowel segments, all our patients are to date satisfied with the results.

Comment by the editors

The left colic artery reaches the left colonic flexure or anastomoses with the marginal artery right before reaching it. The marginal artery of Drummond is composed of a series of vessel arcades that run parallel to the mesenteric margin of the large bowel at a distance of 1–8 cm. This artery may anastomose with the superior rectal artery.

References

1. Hautmann RE, Egghart G, Frohneberg D, Miller K. The ileal neobladder. *J Urol* **139** (1988) 39–42.
2. Kock NG, Ghoneim MA, Lycke KG, Mahran MR. Replacement of the bladder by the ureteral Kock pouch: functional results, urodynamics and radiological features. *J Urol* **141** (1989) 1111–16.
3. Light JK, Engelmann UJ. Le bag: total replacement of the bladder using an ileocolonic pouch. *J Urol* **136** (1986) 27–31.
4. Reddy PK, Lange PH, Fraley EE. Bladder replacement after cystoprostatectomy: efforts to achieve total continence. *J Urol* **138** (1987) 495–9.
5. Thüroff JW, Alken P, Riedmiller H, Engelmann U, Jacobi GH, Hohenfellner R. The Mainz pouch (mixed augmentation ileum and cecum) for bladder augmentation and continent diversion. *J Urol* **136** (1986) 17–26.
6. Reddy PK. Detubularized sigmoid reservoir for bladder replacement after cystoprostatectomy: preliminary report of a new configuration. *Urology* **29** (1987) 625–8.
7. Reddy PK, Lange PH. Bladder replacement with sigmoid colon after radical cystoprostatectomy. *Urology* **29** (1987) 368–71.
8. Leadbetter WF. Consideration of problems incident to performance of a ureteroenterostomy: report of a technique. *J Urol* **65** (1951) 818–30.
9. Goodwin WE, Harris AP, Kauffmann JJ, Beal JM. Open transcolonic ureterointestinal anastomosis: a new approach. *Surg Gynecol Obstet* **97** (1953) 295–300.
10. Bejany DE, Suarez GM, Penalver M, Politano VA. Nontunneled ureterocolonic anastomosis: an alternate to the tunneled reimplantation. *J Urol* **142** (1989) 961–3.
11. Camey M, LeDuc A. L'enterocystoplastie après cystoprostatectomie totale pour cancer de la vessie. *Ann Urol* **13** (1979) 114–32.
12. Reddy PK, Lange PH, Fraley EE. Total bladder replacement using detubularized sigmoid colon: technique and results. *J Urol* **145** (1991 51–5.
13. Lange PH, Reddy PK. Technical nuances and surgical results of radical retropubic prostatectomy in 150 patients. *J Urol* **138** (1987) 348–52.
14. Lange PH. "Surgeon's Corner". *Contemp Urol* March (1990) S. 12.

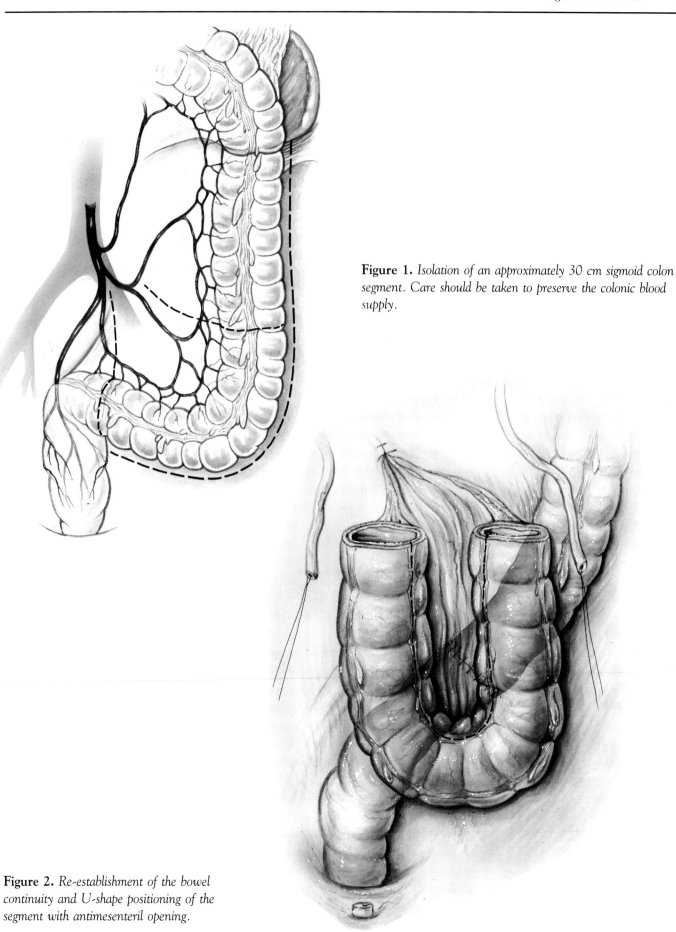

Figure 1. *Isolation of an approximately 30 cm sigmoid colon segment. Care should be taken to preserve the colonic blood supply.*

Figure 2. *Re-establishment of the bowel continuity and U-shape positioning of the segment with antimesenteril opening.*

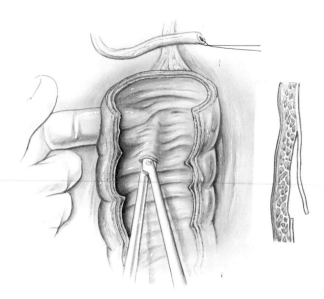

Figure 3. *Dissection of a submucosal tunnel.*

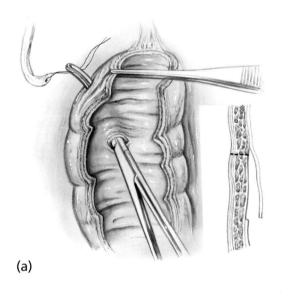

(a)

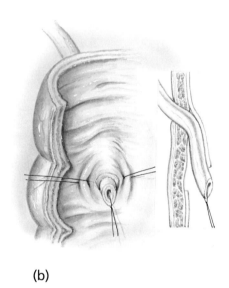

(b)

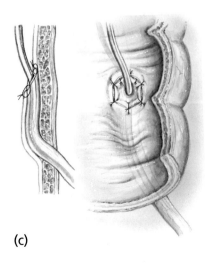

(c)

Figure 4. *Submucosal antirefluxive implantation of the ureters.*

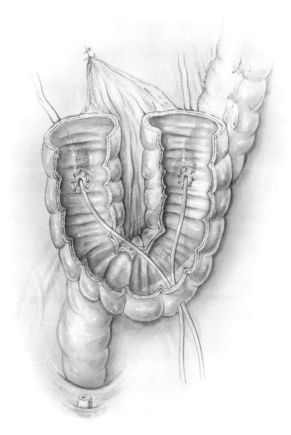

Figure 5. *Stenting of both ureters.*

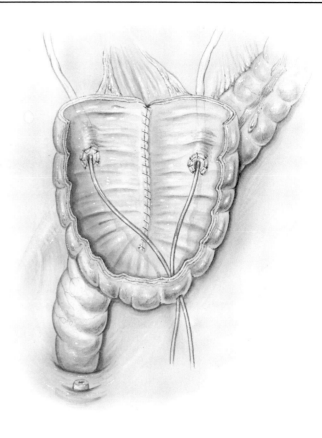

Figure 6. *2-layer closure of the posterior wall of the neobladder.*

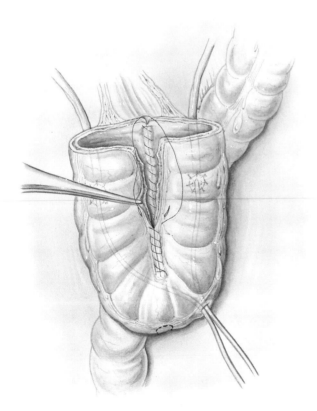

Figure 7. *2-layer closure of the anterior wall.*

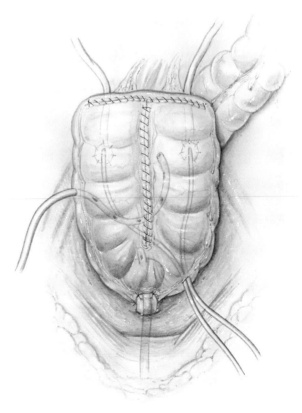

Figure 8. *Complete closure and drainage with a 24 Fr catheter. Urethral anastomosis at the lowest point with 6 sutures.*

Exposure for Abdominal and Pelvic Procedures: Peritoneum and Bowel Mobilization

F. Steinbach[a], M. Stöckle[b],
R. Stein, R. Hohenfellner
Department of Urology,
University of Mainz School of Medicine,
Mainz, Germany
[a]*University of Magdeburg, Germany*
[b]*University of Kiel, Germany*

Indications

Extensive mobilization of peritoneum and bowel with exposure of retroperitoneum is the first step of most urologic procedures, i.e.:

- Radical cystectomy with pelvic lymphadenectomy

- Reconstructive procedures with the use of bowel segments

- Ablative and reconstructive procedures in the retroperitoneal space

- Exposure of the renal pedicle in renal trauma

Instruments

- Ring retractor

- Berendt retractors and ring retractor for retroperi-toneal lymph node dissection

- 4/0 and 3/0 polyglyconate (e.g. Maxon, Davis and Geck, Gosport, UK) for closure of peritoneal incisions

- 1/0 polyglyconate for closure of the anterior parietal peritoneum

- 1/0 polyglyconate (e.g. Dexon, Davis and Geck) for suture of the muscular layer

- 1/0 polyglycolic acid for fascial closure

- Prophylactic dehiscence sutures (Ethicon, Edinburgh, UK)

Operative technique

- Overstretched dorsal position with 10–20° extension of the trunk, to increase the distance between the xiphoid process and the symphysis

- Thrombosis prophylaxis

- Marking of the stoma position on the body surface if a urinary diversion is planned

- Positioning of a rectal tube (22 Fr in adults), nasogastric tube (14 Fr) and transurethral catheter (18 Fr) under anesthesia

- Midline transperitoneal incision from the xiphoid process to the pubic symphysis

    If a prepubic urethrectomy is planned, the incision can be prolonged over the symphysis to the base of the penis. The advantages of this extensive exposure are an excellent view of the operative field, the opportunity to change the operative strategy if necessary, and a lower rate of paralytic bowel obstruction.

- If a continent umbilical stoma is planned, incision in a semicircular fashion at a distance of 4–5 cm left from the umbilicus.

- Excision of scar tissue from previous operations

- Incision of the subcutaneous tissue

- Opening of the fascia along the linea alba (easy to identify from the crossing bundles of the rectus muscles)

- Incision of the peritoneum in the cranial wound angle at the level of the liver

- Elevation of the peritoneal folds with two forceps to protect the bowel, and careful incision with scissors or a scalpel

- Check for bowel adhesions

- Complete opening of the peritoneum on the guide of the second and third fingers of the left hand

- Inspection and palpation of the whole abdominal cavity, the pelvis and retroperitoneal lymph nodes

- If radical cystectomy is planned, mobilization of the bladder bilaterally from the lateral pelvic walls before opening of the peritoneum: in this way, extensive infiltration of the pelvic wall with subsequent unresectable tumor can soon be discovered

- Ligation and section of the falciform ligament of the liver and the medial umbilical ligament

- Incision of the peritoneal folds lateral to the bladder

- Positioning of an autostatic retractor, taking care to avoid lesions of the bowel and femoral nerves

- Check that the nasogastric tube is in the correct position

- Accurate dissection of peritoneal adhesions with preservation of the omentum

- Positioning of the omentum on the thorax

- Exposure of the retroperitoneal space

- Mobilization of the cecum and ascending colon after paracolic incision of the posterior peritoneum along the avascular plane of Toldt up to Winslow's foramen (care should be taken to avoid inferior vena caval lesions): this renders eventual craniomedial mobilization of duodenum and pancreas (Kocher's manouevre) and exposure of the right renal pedicle possible

- Positioning of the small bowel in the right abdominal region

- Extension of the posterior peritoneal incision around the cecal pole, medially along the mesenteric root over the large retroperitoneal vessels up to the duodenojejunal flexure with section of Tritz's ligament

- Ligature of the inferior mesenteric vein lateral to Treitz's ligament to permit eventual mobilization of the mesentery of the descending colon

- Craniomedial mobilization of the ascending colon, small bowel mesentery, duodenum and pancreas from the retroperitoneal structures

- Positioning of Gerota's fascia on the patient's abdomen

- Mobilization of the right colic flexure

Use of ascending or transverse colon in a continent urinary diversion

- Paracolic incision along Toldt's line, and section of the hepatocolic ligament

- Preparation of the omentum in the avascular plane from the transverse colon, as incision of duodenorenal and gastro-colic ligaments near the teniae coli permit extensive mobilization of the hepatic flexure (care should be taken to avoid lesions to the right gastroepiploic artery)

- Mobilization of the descending and sigmoid colon: sufficient mobilization of the descending colon is guaranteed by adhesiolysis of adhesions between the sigmoid colon and lateral inner abdominal wall or by a paracolic incision along the avascular plane of Toldt

- Mobilization of the splenic flexure by division of the phrenicocolic ligament

- Peritoneal incision in pelvic lymphadenectomy and radical cystectomy

- Identification of the deferent ducts at the level of the inner inguinal ring, and division and ligation of the stumps using the proximal stump as a guide (the peritoneal incision falls bilaterally along the course of the ducts down to the fold of the pouch of Douglas)

- Incision on the anterior surface of the rectum near the peritoneal fusion to permit correct opening of Denonvilliers' fascia[3]

- Caudocranial incision of the peritoneum over the major pelvic vessels from the external iliac artery and vein up to the aortic bifurcation

- Bilateral identification of the ureters at the level of the crossing with the common iliac artery and vein

- On the right side, extension of the incision up to the peritoneal incision at the level of the cecum

- On the left side, extension to meet the incision along the sigmoid colon

- Wound closure

- Careful hemostasis and positioning of Robinson or Jackson–Pratt drains, taking care not to damage the inferior epigastric artery and vein

- Closure of the peritoneal incision with continuous suture (3/0 polyglyconate) to avoid intestinal obstruction: the stitches must be placed near each other

- Closure of the anterior parietal peritoneal incision with 1/0 polyglyconate continuous suture

- Dehiscence prophylaxis with Ethicon wire stitches, taking care not to include the peritoneum

- Closure of rectal muscles in the caudal wound angle

- Tight suture of the fascial layer with single stitches (1/0 polyglyconate)

- In obese patients, placement of subcutaneous drain (mandatory to avoid wound seroma)

- Subcutaneous suture (3/0 polyglycolic acid)

- Skin closure using staplers

References

1. Soeder M, Steinbach F, Hohenfellner R. Grundlagen der Stomaversorgung, *Akt Urol* **23** (1992) 1–8.
2. Von Poppeln H, Baert L. Präpubische Urethrektomie. *Akt Urol* **22** (1991) 1–10.
3. Skinner EC, Lieskovsky G, Skinner DG. Technik der radikalen Zystektomie. *Akt Urol* **22** (1991) 1–14.

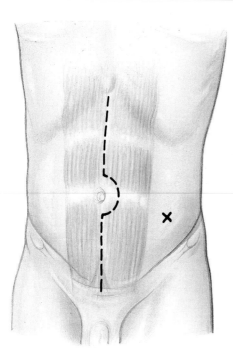

Figure 1. *Median laparotomy with wide sparing of the umbilicus for a planned continent umbilical stoma, additional preoperative marking of a possible stoma.*

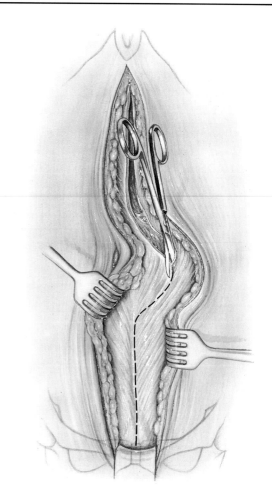

Figure 2. *Fascial incision (linea alba) with a wide margin around the umbilicus.*

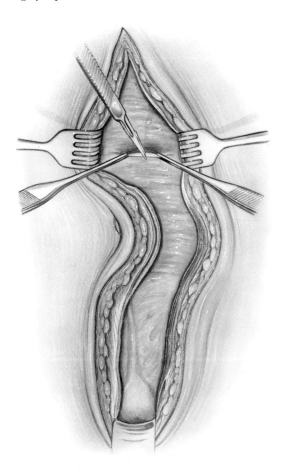

Figure 3. *Opening of the elevated peritoneum cranial to the umbilicus.*

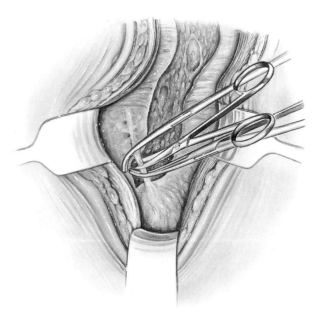

Figure 4. *Division of the median umbilical ligament between Overholt clamps.*

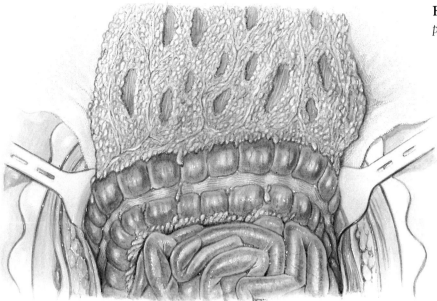

Figure 5. *Insertion of the ring retractor and positioning of the large omentum on the thorax.*

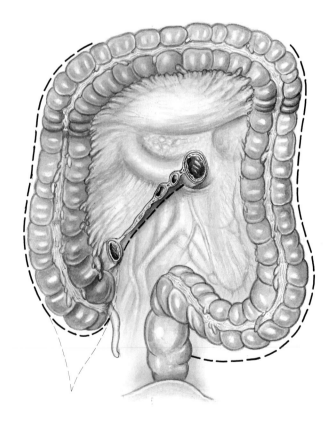

Figure 6. *Schematic drawing of possible peritoneal incisions.*

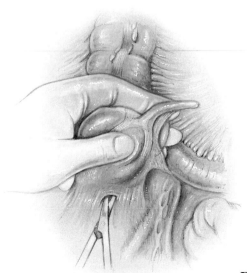

Figure 7. *Beginning of the mobilization at the cecal pole.*

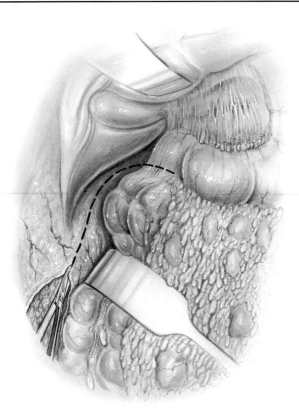

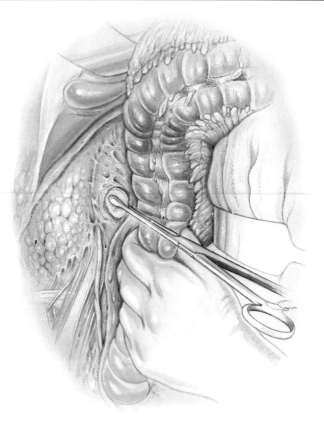

Figure 8. *Incision along the avascular line of Toldt up to Winslow's foramen. Mobilisation of the right colonic flexure and division of the hepatocolic ligament and parts of the gastrocolic ligament after separation of the omentum from the transverse colon.*

Figure 9. *Blunt medial dissection of the ascending colon and also the duodenum (Kocher) with exposure of the right retroperineal space.*

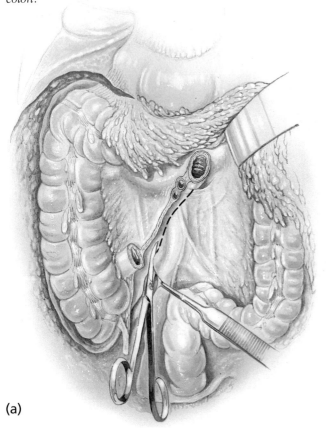

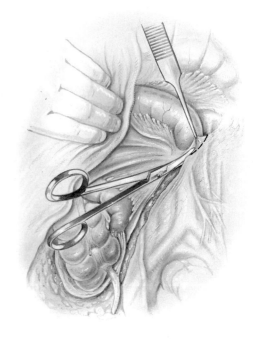

(b)

(a)

Figure 10(a) and (b). *Incision of the peritoneum along the mesenteric root of the small bowel with division of Tritz ligament. Inferior mesenteric artery and vein can be divided without problems, which however in most instances is not necessary.*

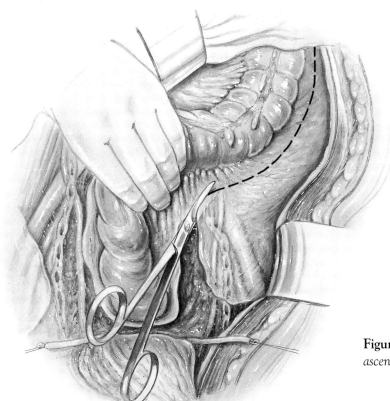

Figure 11. *Left peritoneal incision along the sigmoid and ascending colon.*

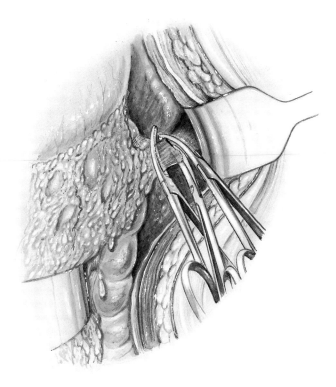

Figure 12. *Division of the phrenocolic ligament and mobilization of the left flexure.*

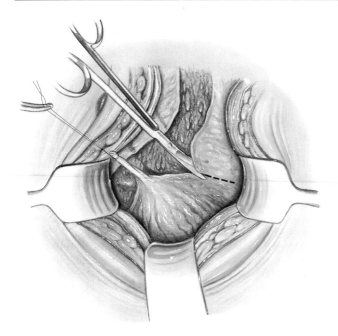

Figure 13. V-shaped division of the peritoneum to both sides of the bladder.

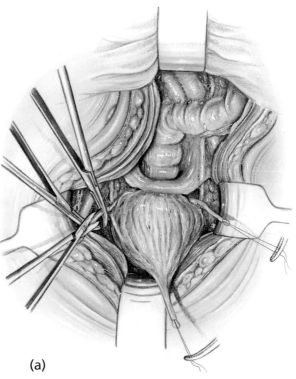

(a)

Figure 14. In radical surgeries incision of the peritoneum above the divided vas deferens with tracture on both vasa def. and the median umbilical chord for better exposure.

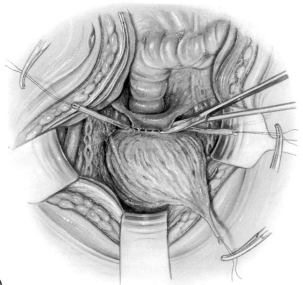

(b)

Submucosal Seromuscular Tube: A New Continence Mechanism for Mainz Pouch Continent Cutaneous Urinary Diversion

A. Lampel, M. Hohenfellner, D. Schultz-Lampel,
D. Wienold, J.W. Thüroff
Department of Urology,
Klinikum Barmen, University of Witten/Herdecke,
Wuppertal, Germany

Introduction

The *in situ* tunneled appendix stoma as a continence mechanism for Mainz pouch I continent cutaneous urinary diversion provides an easy surgical technique with a low complication rate, easy catheterization and continence without leakage.[1-4] Using the same flap-valve principle (a small-caliber conduit, which in its submucosal tunnel position is compressed against the muscular wall of the reservoir with increased filling) we have developed a new continence mechanism for patients in whom the appendix is either not available or not usable.

Advantages

- Technically easy surgery

- No additional small bowel resection for an intussusception nipple

- Universal applicability to large bowel segments (e.g. transverse colon pouch, sigmoid colon pouch)

- Suitability as a salvage procedure when the primary continence mechanism has failed

- No or only minimal secretion from the stoma because of the serosal lining

- Individual tailoring of the lumen of the seromuscular tube (the 2.5–3 cm width of the flap results in a 16–18 Fr lumen)

- No risk of stone formation by avoiding staples

Disadvantages

- The procedure takes more time than formation of an appendix stoma; approximately as long as for formation of an intussusception nipple

- Catheterization of the serosa-lined seromuscular tube requires the use of a lubricant

Indications

For use of the submucosal seromuscular tube as a continence mechanism in large bowel segment:

- Mainz pouch I ileocecal reservoir in patients after previous appendicectomy or in whom the appendix is not usable (too short, strictured or inflamed)[2,4,5]

- Salvage procedure when the primary continence mechanism has failed

- Other pouches containing large bowel segments (e.g. transverse colon pouch, sigmoid colon pouch)

Instruments and suture material

- Fine Metzenbaum scissors for dissection of the mucosa from the seromuscular layer

- Optional magnifying lenses (2.5–3 × magnification)

- Suture material: 5/0 and 4/0 polyglyconate (e.g. Maxon, Davis and Geck, Gosport, UK), 3/0 polyglycolic acid (e.g. Dexon, Davis and Geck)

Operative technique step by step (Figures 1–12)

- Marking of a 3 cm wide and 5 cm long U-shaped flap at the lower cecal pole along the teniae coli toward the confluence of the three teniae

- Insertion of four stay sutures at the corners of the flap

- Incision of the seromuscular layer, leaving the mucosa and submucosal vessels intact and maintaining the continuity of the seromuscular layer at the aboral end

- Detachment of the seromuscular layer from the underlying mucosa at the lateral and medial margins of the longitudinal incisions for 2–3 mm by blunt and sharp dissection

- Transverse incision of the mucosa for 0.5 cm at the oral end, and insertion of an 18 Fr balloon catheter into the lumen of the cecum

- Tubularization of the seromuscular flap around the catheter and closure of the open oral end of the tube by suturing it to the margin of the incised cecal mucosa using 5/0 polyglyconate interrupted sutures

- Transposition of the seromuscular tube into a submucosal

tunnel position by suturing the lateral margins of the seromuscular incisions of the cecum above it using 4/0 polyglyconate interrupted or running sutures

- Placement of three stay sutures at the outlet of the tube to pull it through the abdominal wall incision after completion of the pouch

- Detachment of the umbilical funnel from the abdominal fascia starting laterally from the margin of the abdominal incision, and excision of an 8–10 mm cuff of the umbilicus at its deepest aspect

- Crosswise incision of the peritoneum and external rectus fascia so that the index finger easily can be passed through

- Pulling the catheter and stay sutures at the outlet of the seromuscular tube through the peritoneum and abdominal fascia to the subcutaneous level

- Fixation of the pouch around the outlet of the seromuscular tube to the external rectus fascia by three or four 3/0 polyglycolic acid interrupted sutures

- Anastomosis of the skin of the umbilicus to the outlet of the seromuscular tube using 3/0 polyglycolic acid interrupted sutures with a sharp needle

- Fixation of the pouch four or five 4/0 polyglyconate interrupted sutures to the peritoneum of the anterior abdominal wall

Operative tricks

- If the continence mechanism is constructed before isolation and detubularization of the bowel segments, injury to the mucosa is less likely. Moreover, if there are unexpected findings at the cecum (such as diverticula or polyps) or if construction of the seromuscular tube fails, it still is possible to isolate a 10–12 cm proximal ileal segment for formation of an intussusception nipple as a continence mechanism

- Primary antegrade insertion of the balloon catheter through the umbilicus and the abdominal wall before completion of the continence mechanism avoids the more difficult retrograde pull-through of the balloon catheter through the umbilicus

- After completion of the seromuscular tube, changing of the balloon catheter is difficult and should be avoided within the first 3 weeks. If there is intraoperative injury to the balloon, the catheter should be left in place and fixed by sutures

- The seromuscular tube should be formed around the teniae coli. Use of the omental teniae bears a higher risk of devascularization

- To avoid injury to the mucosa when excising the seromuscular flap, fine Metzenbaum scissors are recommended rather than a scalpel

- Submucosal vessels that cross the incision lines may be preserved during preparation. The use of magnifying lenses (2.5–3× magnification) is helpful

Postoperative care

- The trans-stomal balloon catheter and an additional transmural 10 Fr pouchostomy catheter are left indwelling for 4–6 weeks

- After removal of the trans-stomal catheter, the patient is instructed in intermittent self-catheterization using a reusable 14–18 Fr Nélaton catheter to evacuate and irrigate the pouch

- The pouchostomy catheter is removed after completion of the learning phase of self-catheterization

References

1. Fisch MM, Wammack RE, Hohenfellner R. The Mainz pouch procedure (mixed augmentation, ileum and cecum). In: Webster, Kirby, King, Goldwasser (eds) *Reconstructive Urology*. Boston: Blackwell Scientific (1993) p. 470.
2. Hohenfellner R, Thüroff JW, Fisch M, Lippert C-M. Der Mainz-pouch (mixed augmentation ileum and cecum). Operative Technik, Variationen und 'troubleshooting'. *Akt Urol* **23** (1992) I–XXVI.
3. Riedmiller H, Bürger R, Müller S, Thüroff JW, Hohenfellner R. Continent appendix stoma: a modification of the Mainz pouch technique. *J Urol* **143** (1990) 1115–17.
4. Thüroff JW, Alken P, Riedmiller H, Jacobi GH, Hohenfellner R. The Mainz pouch (mixed augmentation ileum and cecum) for bladder augmentation and continent diversion. *J Urol* **136** (1986) 17–26.
5. Lampel A, Hohenfellner M, Schultz-Lampel D, Thüroff JW. *In situ* tunneled bowel flap tubes: two new techniques of a continent outlet for Mainz-pouch cutaneous diversion. *J Urol* **153** (1995) 308–15.

Figure 1. *A U-shaped incision 3 cm in width and 5 cm in length at the lower cecal pole is marked with ink. Four stay sutures are placed at the corners of the flap.*

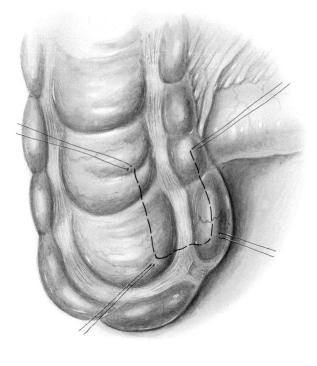

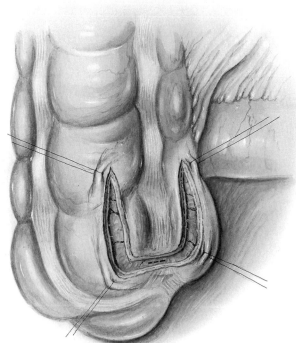

Figure 2. *The seromuscular layer is incised, leaving the mucosa and submucosal vessels intact. Detachment of the lateral and medial margins of the seromuscular incision from the underlying mucosa for 2–3 mm. Transverse incision of the mucosa at the oral end (dashed line).*

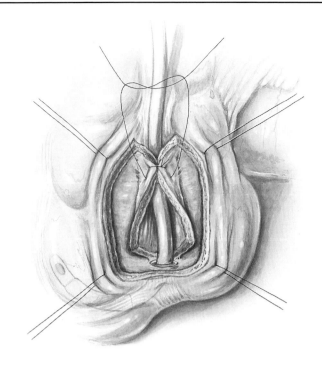

Figure 3. *Insertion of an 18 Fr balloon catheter and tubularization of the seromuscular flap over it using 5/0 polyglyconate interrupted sutures.*

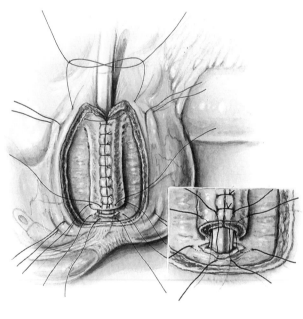

(a)

Figure 4. *Suturing of the anterior circumference of the seromuscular tube to the margin of the incised mucosa.*

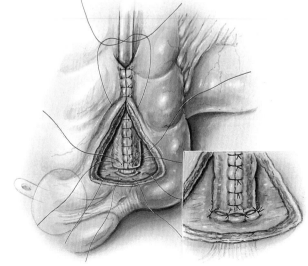

(b)

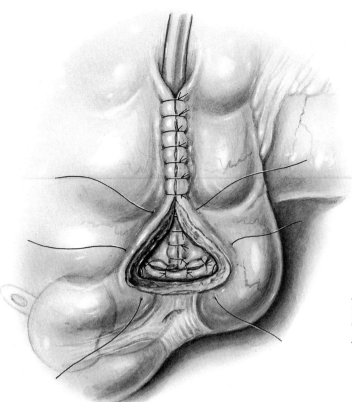

Figure 5. *Submucosal positioning of the tube by suturing the lateral seromuscular margins using 4/0 polyglyconate interrrupted sutures.*

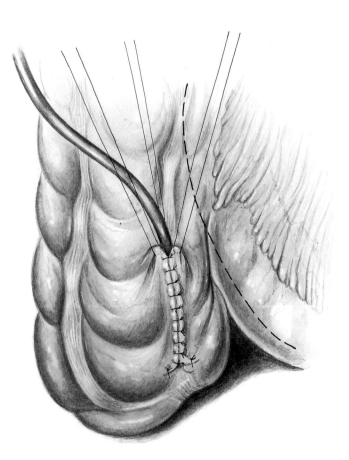

Figure 6. *Three stay sutures placed at the outlet of the seromuscular tube to pull the tube through the abdominal wall. (Dashed line: incision line for detubularization of intestinal segments and pouch formation.)*

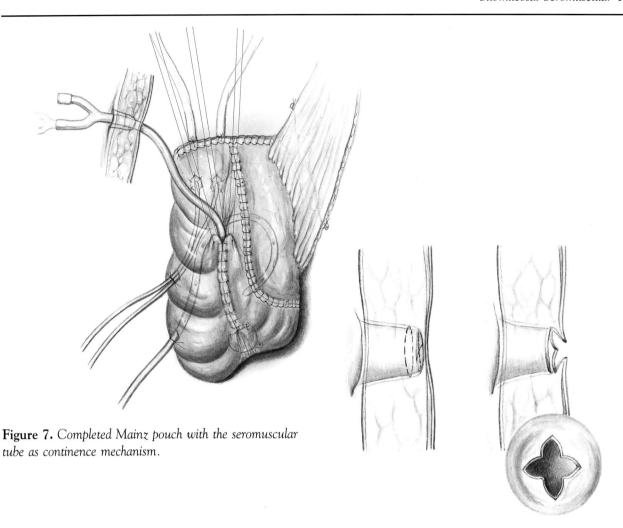

Figure 7. *Completed Mainz pouch with the seromuscular tube as continence mechanism.*

Figure 8. *Formation of the umbilical stoma. Detachment of the skin funnel of the umbilicus from the abdominal fascia and excision of an 8–10 mm cuff at its deepest aspect. Crosswise incision of peritoneum and external rectus fascia.*

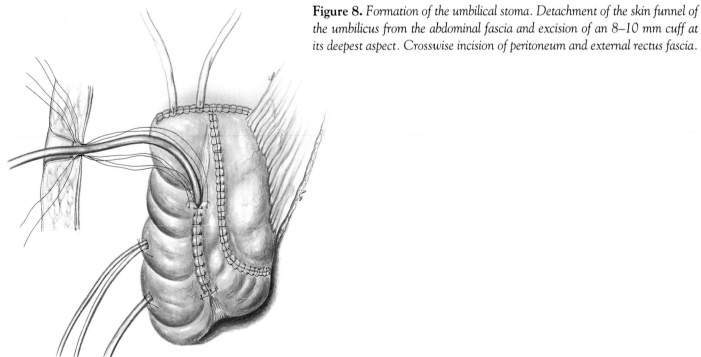

Figure 9. *Stay sutures being pulled through the abdominal wall incision to the subcutaneous level.*

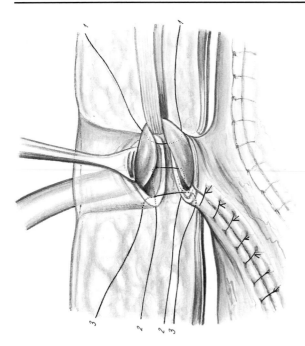

Figure 10. *Anastomosis of the outlet of the continence mechanism to the skin funnel of the umbilicus with 3/0 polyglycolic acid interrupted sutures beginning at the lateral circumference.*

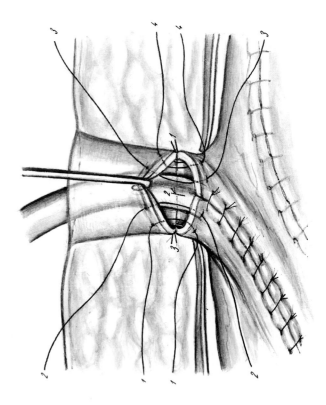

Figure 11. *Completion of the anastomosis at the medial circumference with three or four 3/0 polyglycolic acid interrupted sutures.*

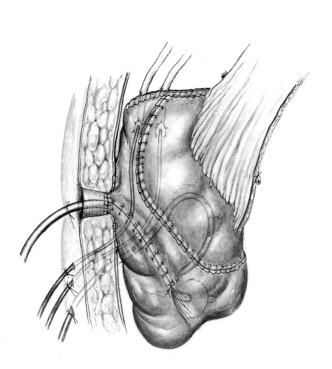

Figure 12. *Fixation of the pouch to the peritoneum of the anterior abdominal wall using 4/0 polyglyconate interrupted sutures.*

Tiflis Pouch

L. Managadze, T. Chigogidze
Institute of Urology, Tbilisi,
Republic of Georgia

Comment

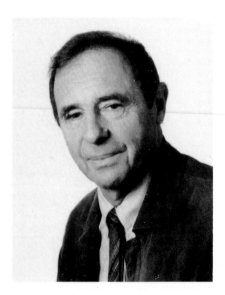

The literature[1-7] offers many different approaches to the continence problem. Generally, we have to distinguish between continence to the point of pain and continence to a specific volume with consequent overflowing. For patients more experienced in intermittent catheterization the advantages are longer intervals, greater feelings of security and an uninterrupted night's rest. Catheterization, depending on fluid intake and time of day, can be a major disadvantage of a reservoir with a leak point. Bowel invagination, ileocecal intussusception and integration of the vermiform appendix lead to "real" continence.[5]

From the beginning it was difficult to fix the nipple to the wall of the pouch. Slippage and necrosis of the nipple were frequent complications. Only when Marlex (C.R. Bard, Massachusetts, USA) and later Dexonnet were introduced was the rate of revision reduced in the now rarely applied method of Kock. Similarly long had been the trials of Mainz pouch I: after problems with narrowing of the efferent segment were recognized, this seemed to be only a "pseudo-continent" method.[3]

Rowland was able to improve the procedure by shortening and narrowing the ileal part and by fixation at the ileocecal valve.[7] In Mainz pouch I the arcades of vessels have been spared by removing mesenteric fat. By intussusception of the mucosa-free nipples (7–8 cm) into the ileocecal valve and fixation to the margin of the valve, a procedure has been developed which has a complication rate of 7–8%. The greatest disadvantage, in spite of good results, is the large scale of the technique. The main complication is a high frequency of stones in the pouch; however, these are mostly asymptomatic and treatable without surgery. The main difference from the sole ileocecal invagination is the longer nipple, which passes the complete pouch at the deepest point from the entrance of the ileocecal valve. Correspondingly, the nipple fixation at the bladder wall appeared not to be stable after traumatic loss of the urethra or damage to the bottom of the pelvis made it necessary to close the bladder neck.

Methods using the appendix have a similar long list of modifications.[4] It has been envisaged that turning the appendix through 180° and implant into the bladder or cecum would cause problems with blood circulation, with consequent incontinence. However, angiographic studies showed a double supply of blood provided by the ileocolic artery and the appendicular artery. By mesenteric slashing and *in situ* embedding very good results have been achieved.[6]

The technique introduced by Managadze considers the need for an easy and practicable method of urine drainage even if the appendix is missing. The technique published by Thüroff also deals with all these aspects. The use of interior mucosa seems not to be a disadvantage for catheterization. More results are needed to reveal the technique's advantages and disadvantages. The efferent segment is very short and rises above the pouch up to 8–10 cm. This segment can be fixed to the umbilicus without problems.

Careful attention to the operative technique is necessary.[1] If the mesentery – especially if fatty – is embedded into the teniae, problems may arise with the circulation or catheterization.

References

1. Duckett JW, Lotfi A-H. Appendicovesicostomy (and variations) in bladder reconstruction. *J Urol* **149** (1993) 567–9.
2. Gilchrist RK, Merricks JW, Hamilton MH, Rieger IT. Construction of a substitute bladder and urethra. *Surg Gynecol Obstet* **90** (1950) 752.
3. Mansson W, Colleen S, Sundin T. Continent cecal reservoir in urinary diversion. *Br J Urol* **56** (1984) 359–65.
4. Mitrofanoff P. Cystostomie continente trans-appendiculaire dans le traitement des vessieres neurologiques. *Chir Ped.* **21** (1980) 297–305.
5. Perl JL. Intussuscepted conical valve formation in jejunostomies. *Surgery* **25** (1949) 297.
6. Riedmiller H, Bürger R, Müller SC, Thüroff JW, Hohenfellner R. Continent appendix stoma: a modification of the Mainz-pouch technique. *J Urol* **143** (1990) 1115–17.
7. Rowland RG, Mitchell ME, Bihrele R, Kahnoski RJ, Piser JE. Indiana continent urinary reservoir. *J Urol* **137** (1987) 1136–9.

R. Hohenfellner, Mainz, Germany

Introduction

We have used the Mainz pouch with *in situ* submucosally embedded appendix on 41 patients. This surgical technique has been the method of choice at our hospital since 1988. In the absence of the appendix the creation of an ileocecal nipple may be useful, but there are some technical problems. Several techniques of forming a continence mechanism emphasize the problems with both continence and catheterization.[1–4] Submucosal embedding of the tapered ileum has been proposed to overcome these problems. So far, 16 of our patients without an appendix have been successfully operated on.

Preoperative preparation

- Excessive oral hydration for 2 days
- Neomycin and erythromycin for bowel sterilization
- Cleansing enemas

Operative technique step by step (Figures 1–9)

- A midline laparotomy is performed and the abdomen is opened
- To create the reservoir, 20–25 cm cecum and ascending colon and 7 cm terminal ileum are isolated
- Bowel continuity is restored by end-to-end two-layer ileocolonic anastomosis after antimesenteric spatulation of the terminal ileum
- After antimesenteric incision of the ascending colon, the caudal 4 cm of the cecal pole remain intact
- A 14 Fr silicone catheter is placed into the terminal ileum and the antimesenteric border is fixed by Allis clamps. The lumen of the ileum is narrowed with the use of a gastrointestinal stapler (GIA stapler, US Surgical, Norwalk, Connecticut, USA)
- The funnel in the distal part of the ileum is plicated with interrupted sutures using a Lambert stitch (polyglyconate, e.g. Maxon (Davis and Geck, Gosport, UK) 4/0)
- The mesenteric windows are created close to the mesenteric border of the terminal ileum
- The oblique incision in the seromuscular layer (4–5 cm) is made from the mesocolic teniae to the teniae coli with the creation of a wide submucosal bed for the ileal segment
- The seromuscular layer of the bowel is closed over the submucosally embedded tapered ileal segment with 3/0 chromic catgut sutures through mesenteric windows

- The pouch catheter is removed and the pouch recatheterized with an 18 Fr catheter. The free part of the ileum is fixed to the colon with 4/0 Maxon (Davis and Geck, Gosport, UK) sutures
- The ureters are implanted 3–4 cm into the submucosal tunnel
- The reservoir is closed using the Heineke–Mikulicz configuration (Maxon 4/0)
- The pouch is fixed to the anterior abdominal wall with 4/0 chromic catgut sutures, and the tapered ileum is fixed to the external umbilical ring

Postoperative care

- Prophylactic antibiotic therapy
- Parenteral nutrition
- The ureteral catheters are removed 10–11 days and pouch catheter 3 weeks after the surgery
- After a successful self-catheterization the pouchostomy is removed

Comments

In the absence of the appendix, Mitrofanoff used a distal ureter as a conduit. Various modifications of this method have been published, but problems with obstruction and incontinence have been observed.[5–7] We know the submucosally embedded tapered ileum to have been used in experimental studies, but as far as we know it has not been used in clinical practice.[8,9] The main advantages of the technique are:

- Easy operative technique and shorter operating time
- Short excluded intestinal segment
- Easy catheterization (14–16 Fr)

References

1. Bejany DE, Politano VA. Stapled and nonstapled tapered ileum for construction of a continent colonic urinary reservoir. *J Urol* **140** (1988) 491–4.
2. Benchecrown A, Essakalli N, Faik M, Marzouk M, Hachimi M, Abaka T. Continent urostomy with hydraulic ileum valve in 136 patients: 13 years of experience. *J Urol* **142** (1989) 46–51.
3. Rowland RG, Mitchell ME, Bihrle R, Kahnovski JR, Piser JE. Indiana continent urinary reservoir. *J Urol* **137** (1987) 1136–9.

4. Thuroff JW, Alken P, Riedmiller H, Jakobi GH, Hohen-felner R. 100 cases of Mainz-pouch: continuing experience and evolution. *J Urol* **140** (1988) 283–8.

5. Ducket JW, Snyder HM III. Continent urinary diversion: variations of Mitrofanoff principle. *J Urol* **136** (1986) 58–62.

6. Ducket JW, Snyder HM III. The Mitrofanoff principle in continent urinary reservoirs. *Semin Urol* **5** (1986) 55–60.

7. Mitrofanoff P. Cystostomie continente trans-appendiculaire dans le traitement des vessies neurologiques. *Chir Ped* **21** (1980) 297–305.

8. Eshgi M, Bronsther B, Ansong K, Hanna MK, Smith AD. Technique and trial of continent ileocystostomy. *Urology* **27** (1986) 112–17.

9. Vinograd I, Merguerian P, Udassin R, Mgle P. An experimental model of submucosally tunnelled valve for the replacement of the ileocecal valve. *J Pediatr Surg* **19** (1984) 726–31.

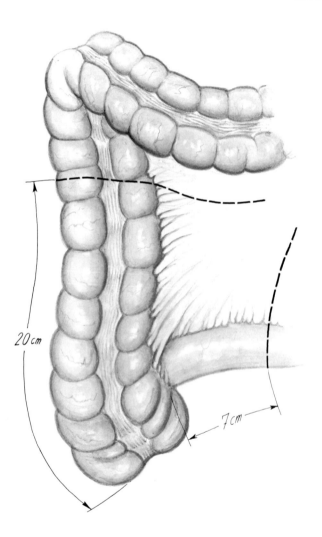

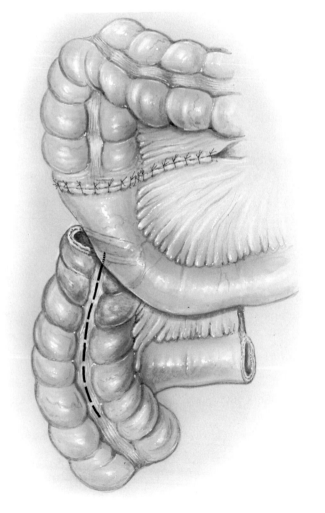

◀ **Figure 1.** *The excluded ileocecal segment (20–25 cm cecum–ascending colon, 7 cm of terminal ileum).*

Figure 2. *Two-layer ileoascendoanastomosis (first row chromic catgut 4/0, second row Maxon 4/0); antimesenteric spatulation of the ileum.*

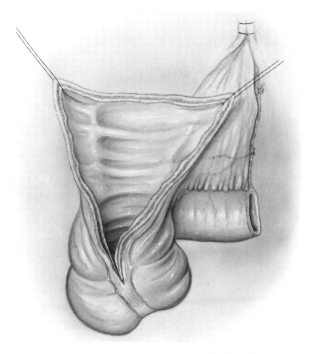

Figure 3. *Antimesenteric incision of the bowel segment. The caudal 4 cm of the cecal pole remain intact.*

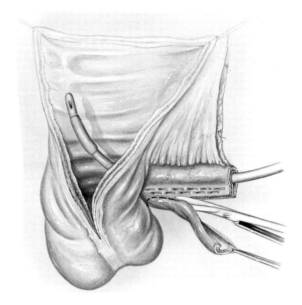

Figure 4. *Tapering of the ileum on a 14 Fr catheter by means of a GIA stapler.*

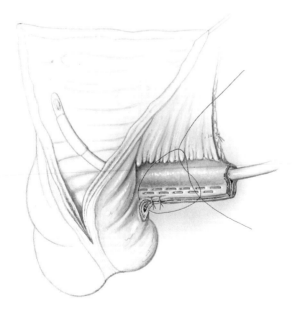

Figure 5. *The funnel of distal ileum is plicated using a Lambert stitch (Maxon 4/0).*

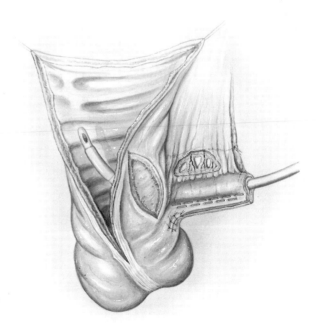

Figure 6. *An oblique incision in the seromuscular layer from the mesocolic teniae to the teniae coli. The seromuscular layer is split down to the mucosa. Mesenteric windows are created.*

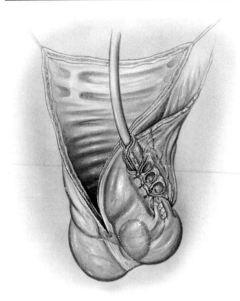

Figure 7. *Closure of the seromuscular layer over the embedded ileum (chromic catgut 4/0) through mesenteric windows.*

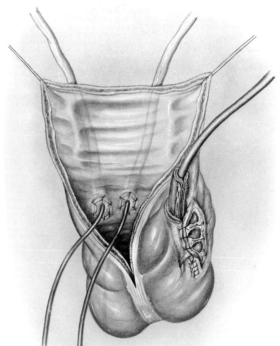

Figure 8. *Implantation of the ureters with stents.*

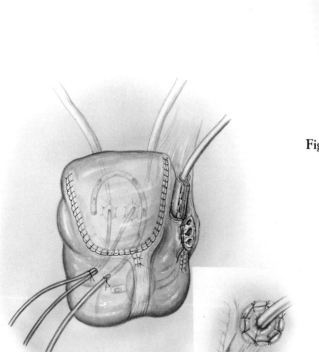

Figure 9. *The pouch is closed (Maxon 4/0) and drained. Fixation of tapered ileum to the external umbilical ring.*

Retroperitoneal Lymph Node Dissection (RPLND): A Nerve-Sparing Operative Approach

P. Albers, R.S. Foster,[a]
J.P. Donohue[a], G.E. Voges[b]
Department of Urology, Bonn University Medical Center, Bonn, Germany,
[a]Department of Urology, Indiana University Medical Center, Indianapolis,
Indiana, USA, [b]Department of Urology, University of Mainz School of
Medicine, Mainz, Germany

Comment

For many years retroperitoneal lymph node dissection (RPLND) had been the standard treatment in patients with stage I, IIA and IIB nonseminomatous germ cell tumors. In clinical stage I, RPLND is mainly a diagnostic procedure to achieve correct staging. The risk of damaging the nerve fibers responsible for antegrade ejaculation during a staging procedure is no longer acceptable. Compared with radical lymph node dissection and modified approaches, nerve-sparing techniques are able to decrease the risk of retrograde ejaculation from 100% to approximately 5%. Independent of the chosen technique (radical, modified or nerve-sparing), there is a risk of in-field relapse of 2%.[1,2]

The authors have clearly described and illustrated the surgical steps. Nerve-sparing RPLND is an elegant method of treatment, but surveillance and risk-adapted management are good alternatives to the surgical approach in clinical stage I patients. The 25–30% false-negative findings associated with first- and second-generation computed tomography do not occur with the improved image quality of third- and fourth-generation machines. The additional use of postoperative tumor marker half-life calculations may reduce staging error to less than 10%. This makes surveillance possible.

Because the histologic risk factors of tumor recurrence in nonseminomatous germ cell tumors stage I, IIA and IIB are known, a third therapeutic option has emerged.[3,4] Vascular invasion is the only risk factor that is statistically significant in multivariate analysis. Used in a treatment model, vascular invasion divides patients into two groups; low-risk patients to be treated by surveillance only, and high-risk patients to be treated by chemotherapy. Using this model, the recurrence rate is below 10%.[5] We therefore offer all three treatment options to our patients, and this approach achieves almost a 100% cure rate.[6]

RPLND has a complication rate of 10–14%, in addition to the risks associated with general anesthesia.[8] The risk of surveillance, in the absence of other risk factors, is that it will detect recurrence in an advanced stage only. The third option – risk-adapted treatment – has the lowest risks and side-effects for most patients. We have used this strategy successfully for 8 years. However, we have had no such problems in our patients. Usually, the main argument against surveillance is the psychological stress it causes patients.

During the past few years, our approach has evolved from standard treatment of all patients to individually tailored treatment. All treatment options should be offered to a patient, because all three treatment strategies are able to provide the same good results.

References

1. Weissbach L. *et al.* Stadium des Nicht-Seminoms: Vorteile und Risiken verschiedener Strategien. *Akt Urol* **20** (1989) 132–7.
2. Klepp O. *et al.* Early clinical stages of nonseminomatous testis cancer. *Scand J Urol Nephrol* **25** (1990) 179–90.
3. Sesterhenn I. *et al.* Prognosis and other clinical correlations of pathologic review in stage I and II testicular carcinoma: a report from the testicular cancer intergroup study. *J Clin Oncol* **10** (1992) 69–78.
4. Höltl W. *et al.* Testicular cancer: prognostic implications of vascular invasion. *J Urol* **137** (1987) 683–665.
5. Logothetis C. The case for relevant staging of germ cell tumors. *Cancer* **65** (1990) 709–17.
6. Gressler V. *et al.* Editorial: a third option in the management of patients with clinical stage I non-seminomatous germ cell tumor? *J Clin Oncol* **8** (1990) 4–8.
7. McLeod DG. *et al.* Staging relationships and outcome in early stage testicular cancer: a report from the testicular cancer intergroup study. *J Urol* **145** (1991) 1178–83.
8. Sandeman TF. Staging relationships and outcome in early stage testicular cancer: a report from the testicular cancer intergroup study. *J Urol* **148** (1992) 1267 (Letter).

W. Höltl, Vienna, Austria

Retroperitoneal Lymph Node Dissection

Introduction

Reasons to perform retroperitoneal lymph node dissection (RPLND) in early cancer of the testis are as follows:

- It accurately stages the patient

- There is a therapeutic benefit if small or moderate volume metastasis is resected

- If relapse occurs it is discovered early because the chest and serum are easily monitored

- The likelihood of late recurrence is lower because the retroperitoneum is cleared

- Using the nerve-sparing approach, preservation of emission and ejaculation is possible in nearly 100% of patients[1-7]

Indications

- Clinical stage I, IIA and IIB nonseminomatous testicular germ cell tumors (NSGCT)

Preoperative diagnostics

- Computed tomography of the abdomen and chest

- Tumor markers (α-fetoprotein, human chorionic gonadotropin β)

Instruments

- Self-retaining retractors

Operative technique step by step

Right-sided nerve-sparing RPLND
The borders of the template (Figure 1) are the crus of the diaphragm, the right ureter, the preaortic area (from the 12 o'clock position on the aorta down to the inferior mesenteric artery), the right psoas muscle, and bifurcation of the right internal and common iliac arteries.

Standard midline abdominal approach
- Incision of the posterior peritoneum from the cecum up to the area of Treitz's ligament (Figure 2). The inferior mesenteric artery and vein are usually not divided. Sometimes it may be necessary to divide the vein for better exposure. Retraction of the duodenum and head of the pancreas superiorly and to the right. Self-retaining retractors are used. (An alternative is full mobilization of the cecum and elevation of the small bowel onto the chest of the patient)

- The split technique is used for lymph node dissection, starting at the left renal vein and proceeding down the vena cava and aorta to the origin of the inferior mesenteric artery (Figures 3 and 4)

- The interaortocaval lymph tissue is rolled off the medial side of the vena cava, and the sympathetic fibers are identified coursing from the sympathetic chain to the preaortic plexus (Figures 5 and 6). The nerves are placed in vessel loops and the left-sided lumbar veins passing from the vena cava to the body wall are divided (Figure 7). The tissue is completely rolled off the aorta. The lumbar arteries are divided as needed. The interaortocaval lymphatic tissue is dissected sharply and bluntly from the spinal ligament preserving the sympathetic fibers (Figure 8). Lumbar arteries, veins and lymphatics are secured posteriorly with clips or cautery

- Right paracaval tissue is then removed down to the bifurcation of the common iliac artery. Finally, the right gonadal vein (which was divided at its origin from the vena cava) is dissected distally to the internal inguinal ring and removed

- Closure of the posterior peritoneum using a running absorbable suture

Left-sided nerve-sparing RPLND
The borders of the template (Figure 1) are the crus of the diaphragm, the preaortic area, the left ureter, the left psoas muscle, and the bifurcation of left internal and common iliac arteries.

Standard midline abdominal approach
- Mobilization of the left colon with division of the splenocolic attachments (or, alternatively, incision of the posterior peritoneum (as for the right-sided approach) and additional mobilization of only the lower left colon) (Figure 2)

- Visualization of the left periaortic, preaortic and upper interaortocaval zones

- Identification of the sympathetic fibers at the point where they cross the iliac artery. Placement of the nerves in vessel loops. Dissection of the left periaortic lymphatic tissue, beginning laterally and rolling tissue from the psoas. Identification of the sympathetic chain. Dissection of the efferent nerves from the lymphatic tissue

- Splitting of lymphatic tissue, starting at the left renal vein and proceeding down to the origin of the inferior mesenteric artery (Figure 9). The left periaortic lymphatic tissue is then rolled laterally and removed, carefully preserving the sympathetic fibers (Figures 10 and 11). The left lumbar arteries are usually divided

- The extreme upper interaortocaval and preaortic zone is then dissected as described for the right-sided procedure

- Finally, the left gonadal vein, which had been divided from the left renal vein, is traced distally to the cord stump and resected

- Closure of the retroperitoneal space using running absorbable sutures. No drains are necessary

Modification of the left-sided approach
- It may not always be necessary to carry out a full dissection of the interaortocaval zone. If the left periaortic nodes are unsuspicious, sampling of the preaortic area is usually sufficient

Intraoperative complications

- Ureteral laceration (requires end-to-end anastomosis using 6/0 absorbable suture)

- Laceration of the vena cava, aorta or renal vessels (suture with 5/0 absorbable suture)

Postoperative complications

- Ileus (1%)

- Lymphocele, chylous ascites (treat only if symptomatic: usually conservative management is successful;[8] if not, drainage is necessary)

References

1. Cavalli F, Monfardini S, Pizzocaro G. Report on the international workshop on staging and treatment of testicular cancer. *Eur J Cancer* **16** (1980) 1367–72.
2. Donohue JP, Foster RS, Rowland RG, Bihrle R, Jones J, Geier G. Nerve-sparing retroperitoneal lymphadenectomy with preservation of ejaculation. *J Urol* **144** (1990) 287–92.
3. Donohue JP, Thornhill JA, Foster RS, Bihrle R, Rowland RG, Einhorn LH. The role of retroperitoneal lymphadenectomy in clinical stage B testis cancer; the Indiana University experience (1965–1989). *J Urol* **153** (1995) 85–9.
4. Donohue JP, Thornhill JA, Foster RS, Rowland RG, Bihrle R. Primary retroperitoneal lymph node dissection in clinical stage A nonseminomatous germ cell testis cancer. *Br J Urol* **71** (1993) 326–35.
5. Hansen PV, Hansen SW. Gonadal function in men with testicular germ cell cancer: the influence of cisplatin-based chemotherapy. *Eur Urol* **23** (1993) 153–6.
6. Read G, Stenning SP, Cullen MH, *et al*. Medical Research Council prospective study of surveillance for stage I testicular teratoma. *J Clin Oncol* **10** (1992) 1762–8.
7. Sogani PC, Fair WR. Surveillance alone in the treatment of clinical stage I nonseminomatous germ cell tumors of the testis (NSGCT). *Semin Urol* **7** (1988) 53–6.
8. Baniel J, Foster RS, Rowland RG, Bihrle R, Donohue JP. Management of chylous ascites after retroperitoneal lymph node dissection for testicular cancer. *J Urol* **150** (1993) 1422–4.

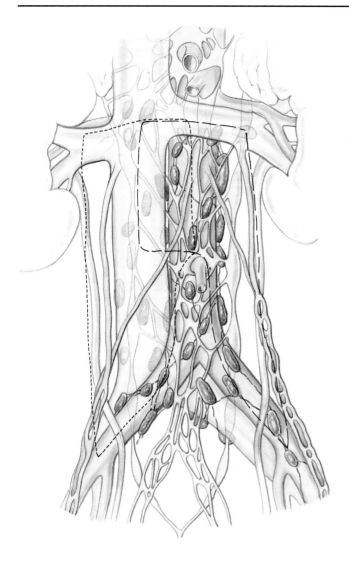

Figure 1. *Templates for right-sided and left-sided nerve-sparing retroperitoneal lymph node dissection.*

Figure 2. *(1) Right-sided approach: incision from the cecum to Treitz's ligament. (2) Left-sided approach: mobilization of the descending colon, including the splenocolic attachments. The alternative approach is the combination of the right-sided incision with a paracolic incision to remove the gonadal vessels.*

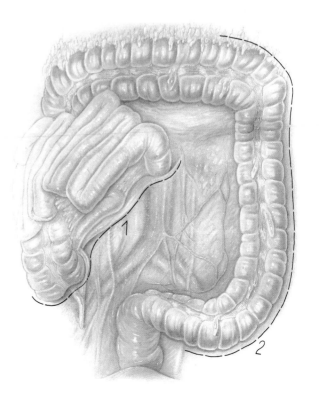

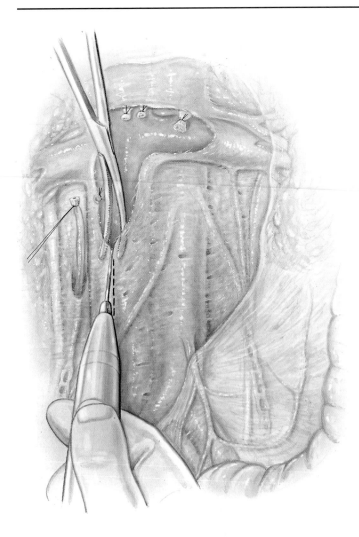

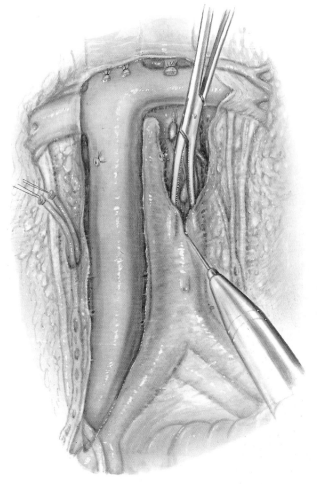

Figure 3. *Splitting of the lymphatic tissue over the left renal vein, then down the vena cava to the bifurcations of the iliac vessels. Lymphatic tissue at the upper and lower borders is carefully ligated.*

Figure 4. *Midline split over the aorta from the renal vein to the inferior mesenteric artery.*

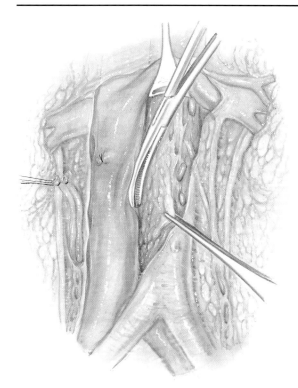

Figure 5. *Rolling the lymphatic tissue down the vena cava to the lumbar veins.*

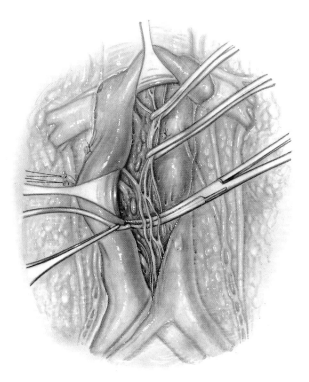

Figure 6. *Identification and dissection of the sympathetic fibers coming from the right sympathetic chain. Nerves frequently course immediately cephalad to the lumbar veins.*

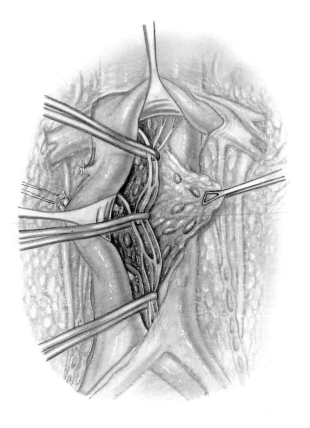

Figure 7. *Dissection of the interaortocaval lymphatic tissue after ligation of the left lumbar veins.*

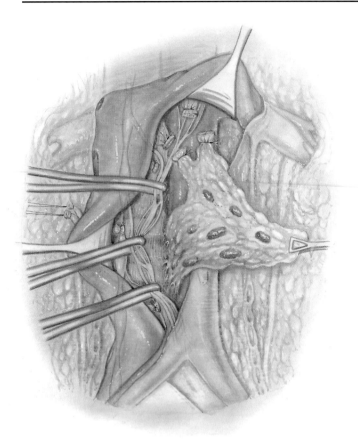

Figure 8. *Removal of the interaortocaval lymphatic tissue from the spinal ligament. Careful ligation of the upper lymphatic vessels to avoid lymphoceles. After removal of the interaortocaval portion, dissection of the paracaval lymphatic tissue and gonadal vessels completes the dissection of the right template.*

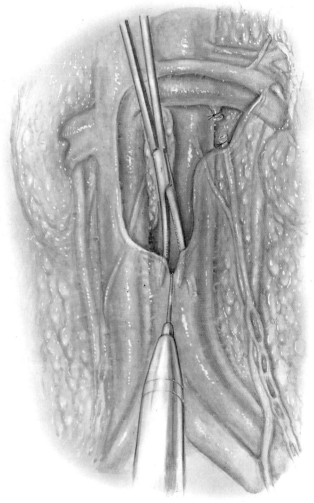

Figure 9. *Left-sided approach. The lower border of the split is the inferior mesenteric artery. The second step is dissection of the lymphatic tissue from the left ureter medially toward the aorta and identification of the left-sided sympathetic chain and fibers from the side.*

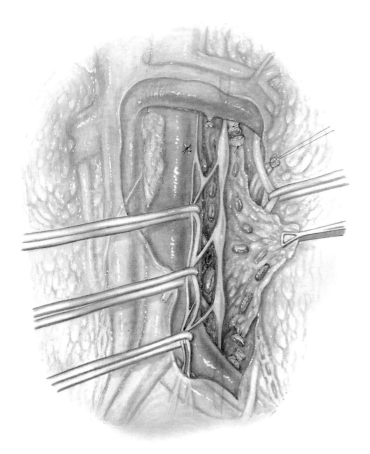

Figure 10. *Dissection of the para-aortic lymphatic tissue after identification of the left-sided nerves. Careful ligation of the upper and lower lymphatic vessels to avoid lymphoceles.*

Figure 11. *Complete removal of the para-aortic tissue after ligation of the left lumbar arteries and mobilization of the aorta. Dissection of the left template is completed by removing the left gonadal vessels and the upper interaortocaval lymph nodes.*

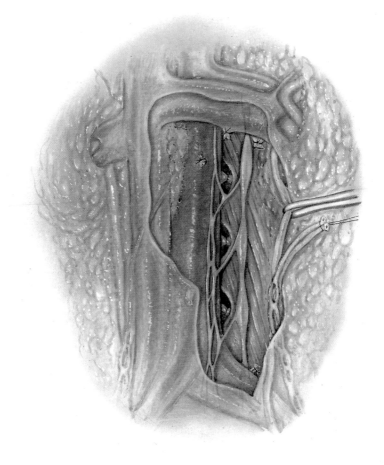

Repair of Rectourethral Fistula by the Posterior Transrectal Approach (York Mason)

B. Lytton
*Yale University School of Medicine,
New Haven, Connecticut, USA*

Introduction

Repair of rectourethral fistula presents a formidable challenge to the surgeon. These fistulas may occur as a result of congenital malformation, trauma or gunshot wounds, or as complications following operations on the prostate. Prostate operations have accounted for a recent increase in the incidence of rectourethral fistula because of the large number of radical prostatectomies that have been performed in the past few years for prostate carcinoma.

A number of different approaches have been described for the repair of rectourethral fistula:

- *Transabdominal approach.* Even with a large bladder incision, the optimal exposure of the fistula is only rarely attained

- *Transperineal approach.* The incision is placed ventral to the anus between the ischial bones, as for perineal prostatectomy.[1] The rectum is separated from the posterior surface of the prostate and bladder by dissecting between the two layers of Denonvilliers' fascia. Unfortunately, much of this fascial plane may be obliterated as a result of the fistular injury, thus making the dissection difficult.

- *Pararectal approach* according to Kraske.[2] This is technically a complex operation and may be accompanied by significant bleeding from the pararectal veins

- *Peranal approach.*[3] Indications for this procedure include small distally located fistulas, which can be exposed using a speculum after dilatation of the anal sphincter

- *Transrectal approach.* This may be either posterior (as described by York Mason) or anterior (as originally described by Gecelter). Both the anterior and the posterior approaches embody the same principles.[4,5] They provide good access to the fistula by dividing the anal sphincter, and this allows for adequate mobilization of the rectum from the prostate and bladder base. Following reconstruction of the urethral defect, a flap of rectal wall can be fashioned to cover the fistula site if necessary

The primary treatment of patients with large indurated fistula should consist of a temporary urinary and fecal diversion in the form of a suprapubic cystostomy and a sigmoid colostomy. As an alternative to colostomy, preoperative parenteral or enteral feeding with an elemental diet has been suggested in the literature.[6]

Preoperative examination

- Excretory urography will exclude ureteral obstruction or renal malformations

- Urethrocystoscopy and rectal digital examination help to determine the exact site and extent of the fistula and the integrity of the bladder. The fistula should have a clean healthy appearance and be well epithelialized before repair is attempted

- A preoperative prostate specific antigen test should be performed in patients who have had an operation for prostate cancer to detect residual disease

Patient counselling and consent

- Patients should be informed of the need for a colostomy and a suprapubic cystostomy for several weeks after the operation

- They should be warned of the possibility of urinary incontinence, especially after radical prostatectomy

Preoperative preparation

- Bowel preparation with a low-residue diet for 2 days and administration of a saline purge, or thorough antegrade mechanical cleansing of the distal rectosigmoid with enemas, if a colostomy has been established

- Bowel sterilization with metronidazole and neomycin orally administered or instilled into the rectosigmoid through the colostomy

- Systemic urinary sterilization with sulfamethoxazole (1 g) or ciprofloxacin (500 mg), twice daily, beginning 2 days before the operation

Operative technique step by step (Figures 1–8)

- Both ureters are marked by the insertion of two 5 Fr catheters to prevent iatrogenic injury. The ureteral catheters are attached to a 22 Fr Foley catheter left indwelling in the urethra

- The patient is placed prone on the operating table in the jackknife position with the head down. The buttocks are retracted by the application of adhesive tape from the buttocks to the side of the table. The skin of the anococcygeal area, perineum and anorectal canal are cleansed with an appropriate antibacterial solution such as chlorhexidine

- Incision from one side of the tip of the coccyx down to the anal margin posteriorly in the midline. Two fingers are placed in the rectum and the incision is carried down between them, through the perianal tissues in the midline to divide the rectal wall and anal sphincter. As the muscles of the external sphincter and internal sphincter ani are divided, they should be marked with silk sutures so that they can be accurately reapproximated at the completion of the procedure

- Next, the muscles of the rectum wall should be incised. Should greater access be required, the tip of the coccyx is excised; the incision can then be extended cephalad

- A small self-retaining chest retractor is inserted to hold the wound edges apart to provide optimal exposure of the fistula

- The upper part of the rectum may prolapse down and can be readily retracted over a sponge, using a wide Deaver retractor. The retractor will help to flatten out the anterior rectal wall to expose the fistula and place the opening on some tension

- The mucosal edge of the fistula is circumcised about 2–3 mm from the opening, using a sharp scalpel. The incision is deepened through the rectal wall using small sharp-pointed Metzenbaum scissors. It is probably best to work at the upper end of the incision in the midline at first to find the plane between the rectal wall and the posterior surface of the bladder. Once this has been established, the plane can be developed all around to free the entire rectal wall from the prostate and urethra

- Once the rectum has been well mobilized, the defect in the urethra or lower part of the bladder will become easily visible. The fistula may be infiltrated with a weak solution of adrenaline and saline (1/1000) to help control oozing and maintain a relatively dry field

- When the fistula is the result of a radical prostatectomy, biopsies should be taken from the edge of the fistula site to detect any residual tumor. If the biopsies are positive it is important to institute prompt postoperative treatment by hormonal manipulation with orchiectomy or luteinizing hormone releasing hormone agonists so as not to retard wound healing

- The defect of the urethra is repaired with a vertically running 0 chromic catgut suture reinforced with a few interrupted sutures of the same material. A flap of rectal wall with a wide base is developed to secure the suture

- The rectal mucosa is closed with a continuous 4/0 chromic catgut suture, and the rectal wall is reapproximated accurately with interrupted mattress sutures of 0 polyglycolic acid

- The previously marked internal and external sphincter muscles are accurately reapproximated with interrupted 0 polyglycolic mattress sutures and the skin is closed with interrupted 3/0 nylon sutures

- The ureteral catheters should be removed by the surgeon at the end of the procedure so that he or she can detect any tethering that would indicate constriction of the ureters by stitches inadvertently misplaced during the repair

Postoperative care

- The Foley catheter is left indwelling for another 4 or 5 days

- The suprapubic tube is clamped for a trial of voiding after 10 days when, if the patient is able to urinate without difficulty and has good control, the tube is removed

Complications

- Wound infections may occur, with some impairment of healing

- Difficulties with the anal sphincter cease after 3–4 weeks

- Strictures of the urethrovesical anastomosis can be successfully repaired by a small Y–V plasty

- Incontinence of urine may occur as a result of a previous injury to the membranous urethral sphincter. If no recovery of sphincter control is observed after several months, the incontinence may be corrected by the insertion of an inflatable cuff prosthesis

References

1. Goodwin WE, Turner RD, Winter CC. Rectourinary fistula: principles of management and a technique of surgical closure. *J Urol* **80** (1958) 246–54.
2. Kilpatrick FR, Thompson HR. Post-operative recto-prostatic fistula and closure by Kraske's approach. *Br J Urol* **34** (1962) 470–4.
3. Vose SN. A technique for the repair of recto-urethral fistula. *J Urol* **61** (1949) 790–4.
4. Kilpatrick FR, Mason AY. Post-operative recto-prostatic fistula. *Br J Urol* **41** (1969) 649–54.
5. Gecelter G. Transanorectal approach to the posterior urethra and bladder neck. *J Urol* **109** (1973) 1011–16.
6. Henderson DJ, Middleton RG, Dahl DS. Single stage repair of rectourinary fistula. *J Urol* **125** (1981) 592–3.

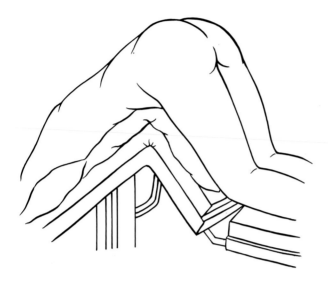

Figure 1. *Placement of the patient in the jackknife position.*

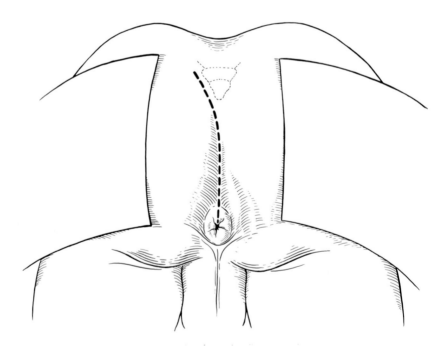

Figure 2. *Retraction of the buttocks with adhesive tape, and incision between the coccyx and anus.*

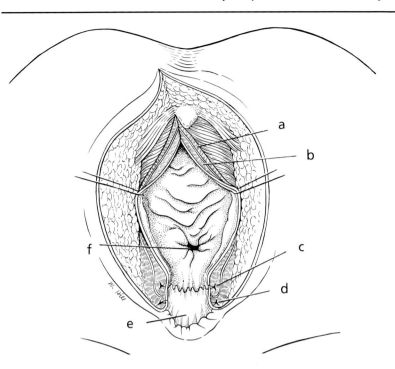

Figure 3. *Division of the posterior rectal wall, and marking of the rectum musculature and the external and internal sphincter ani musculature with holding sutures. (a) Longitudinal rectal muscle, (b) circular rectal muscle, (c) internal anal sphincter, (d) external anal sphincter, (e) anal canal and (f) rectourethral fistula.*

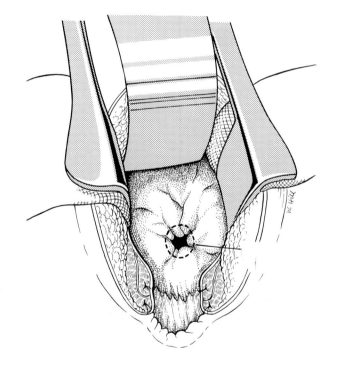

Figure 4. *Circumcision of the fistula about 2–3 mm from the mucosal edge with a sharp scalpel.*

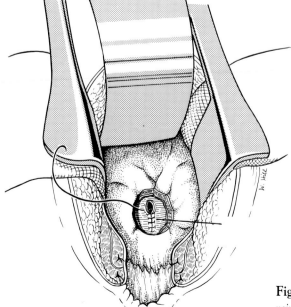

Figure 5. *Repair of the urethral defect with continuous 0 chromic catgut suture, reinforced with interrupted sutures.*

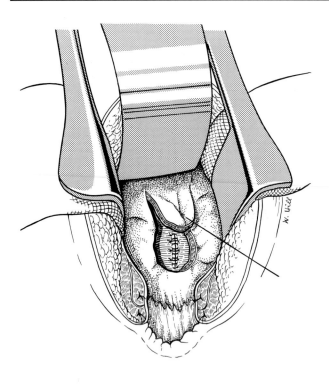

Figure 6. *Preparation of a broad rectal wall flap.*

Figure 7. *Closure of the rectal defect with the well vascularized rectal wall flap. Superimposed suture lines should be avoided.*

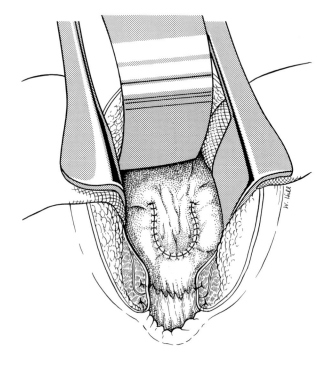

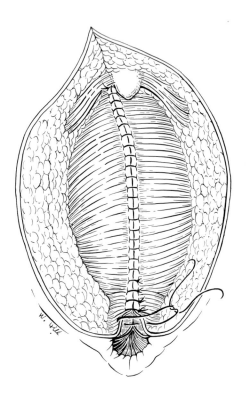

Figure 8. *Closure of the posterior rectal wall with 0 polyglycolic acid suture and careful reapproximation of the divided sphincters, also with 0 polyglycolic acid sutures.*

Continent Conversion: Incorporation of a Colonic Conduit into a Continent Diversion (Mainz Pouch I and II)

M. Fisch, R. Hohenfellner
Department of Urology,
University of Mainz School of Medicine,
Mainz, Germany

Introduction

Since Hendren coined the term 'undiversion',[1] the nomenclature of urinary diversion has changed. Incontinent *temporary* diversions (nephrostomy, pyelocutaneostomy) are differentiated from incontinent *definitive* diversions like ureterocutaneostomy, and ileal and colonic conduits. Continent diversions require anatomic sphincters as the anal sphincter (sigmoidorectal pouch) and the urethral sphincter (bladder replacement) or the creation of a continence mechanism. Because of its antirefluxive ureteral implantation, the colonic conduit offers an *intermediary* diversion with the option of incorporation into a continent form of urinary diversion (*continent conversion*).

Indications

- Elongation of the conduit with obstruction
- Stomal stenosis
- Wish for continence

Contraindications

- Impaired renal function (creatinine >1.5 mg/dl)
- Inflammatory disease of the bowel (e.g. ulcerative colitis)
- Short bowel syndrome

Instruments and suture material

- As for construction of a Mainz pouch (see p. 501)

Preoperative preparation

- As for urinary diversion using the Mainz pouch technique (see p. 502)

Operative technique step by step (Figures 1–11)

- Median laparotomy
- Circular excision of the stoma at the level of the skin, and dissection down until the conduit is freed of the subcutaneous fat and the fascia
- Pulling the conduit intra-abdominally, incision of the peritoneum lateral to the descending colon with care not to damage the conduit and its mesentery
- Reopening of the former mesenteric window (for isolation of the conduit during the first operation)

- Mobilization of the descending colon, and widening of the mesenteric window
- Pulling the conduit through the mesenteric window, thereby shifting it ventrally to the descending colon
- Antimesenteric opening of the colon, with the cranial 4–5 cm remaining intact (for ureteral implantation)
- Identification of ureteral implantation sites and insertion of ureteral stents
- Fixation of the stents at the colonic mucosa (catgut 4/0)

Incorporation of the conduit into an ileocecal pouch (Mainz pouch I)

- Isolation of a shorter bowel segment as required for the standard technique (the length is identical to that of the conduit to be incorporated)
- Creation of the pouch plate and continence mechanism using the standard technique
- When an appendix stoma is required, isolation of only one ileal loop (10–15 cm in length) in addition to the colonic segment of standard length
- Incorporation of the antimesenterically opened conduit by side-to-side anastomosis with the pouch (running polyglyconic acid suture using a straight needle)
- Closure of the pouch and formation of the stoma according to the standard technique
- Withdrawal of the ureteral stents through the pouch wall together with a 10 Fr cystostomy tube, and of the pouch catheter (16–20 Fr) through the efferent segment
- Closure of the mesenteric windows and wound closure

Incorporation of the conduit into a sigmoidorectal pouch (Mainz pouch II)

- Opening of the rectosigmoid junction and side-to-side anastomosis of the medial margins according to the standard technique
- Side-to-side anastomosis of the antimesenterically opened conduit to the thus created pouch plate by two-layer sutures: running suture polyglyconic acid 4/0 for the seromuscular layer and chromic catgut 5/0 for the mucosa
- Withdrawal of the ureteral stents peranally together with the rectal tube, and reinsertion of the rectal tube inside the pouch
- Closure of the pouch and wound closure
- Fixation of the ureteral stents and rectal tube peranally to the skin (using nonabsorbable suture material)

Postoperative care

See Chapters 6.4 and 6.8.

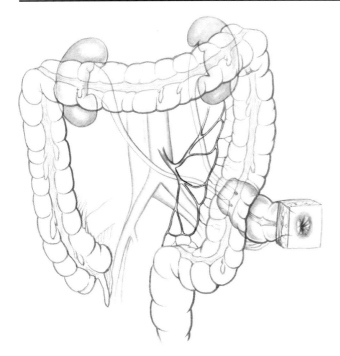

Figure 1. *The position of the stoma. The ureteral implantation lies as high as the aortic bifurcation on the psoas muscle.*

References

1. Hendren HW. Urinary undiversion. In: Glenn JF (ed.) *Urologic Surgery*, 3rd edn. Philadelphia: J.B. Lippincott (1983) 549–57.
2. Fisch M, Wammack R, Müller SC, Hohenfellner R. The Mainz pouch II (sigma rectum pouch). *J Urol* **149** (1993) 258–63.

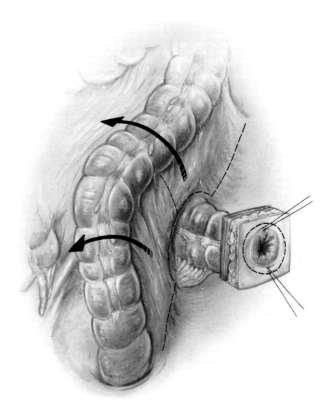

Figure 2. *Incision of the peritoneum lateral to the descending colon (dotted line). The incision is extended to the mesentery of the sigmoid colon in the area of the former mesenteric window. Circular excision of the stoma from the skin.*

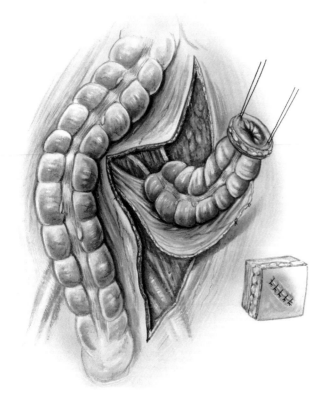

Figure 3. *Enlargement of the mesenteric window to shift the conduit ventrally. Closure of the fascia and skin in the area of the former stoma.*

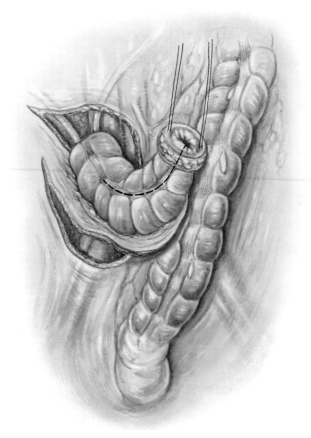

Figure 4. *The conduit is pulled through the mesenteric window and opened antimesenterically (dashed line); only the cranial 4–5 cm remain intact.*

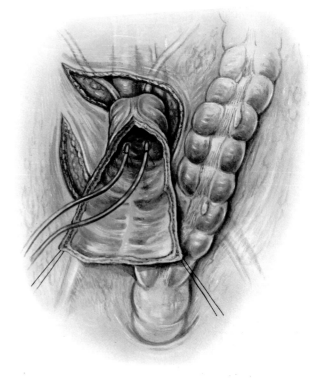

Figure 5. *Stenting of the ureteral orifices and fixation of the stents.*

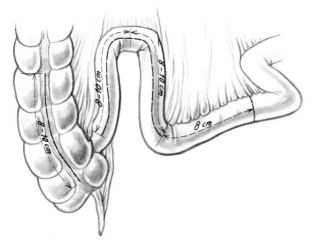

Figure 6. *The length of the ileocecal segment to be isolated for urinary diversion is reduced according to the length of the conduit.*

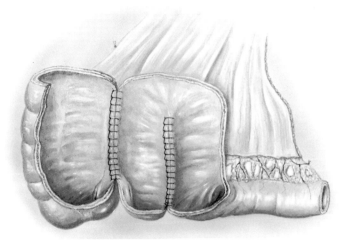

Figure 7. *Creation of the pouch plate by ileoileal and coloileal side-to-side anastomosis. The invaginated and intussuscepted ileal nipple is formed as a continence mechanism according to the standard technique.*

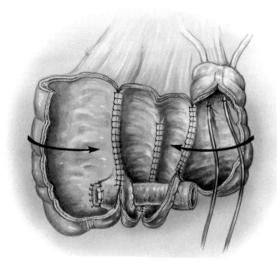

Figure 8. *Incorporation of the opened conduit into the pouch by side-to-side anastomosis with the ileal pouch margin.*

Figure 9. *When the appendix can be used to create a continence mechanism, isolation of only one ileal loop is necessary (inset), and so the ileoileal anastomosis can be abandoned. The conduit is directly anastomosed side-to-side with the ileal loop of the pouch.*

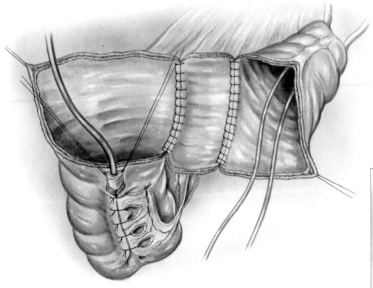

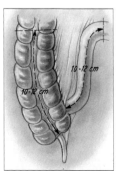

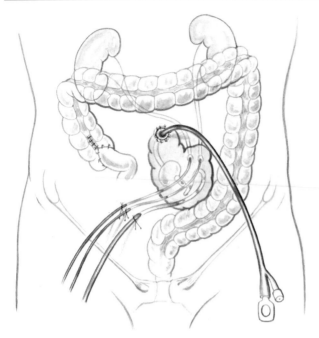

Figure 10. *Final situation. Ureteral implantation at the same position as the preoperative pouch position, in the right middle abdominal quadrant; the ileocecal valve is reconstructed.*

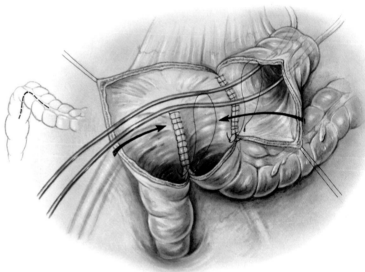

Figure 11. *Incorporation of the conduit into a sigmoidorectal pouch.*

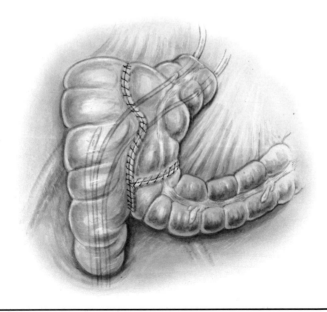

The Sigmoid Conduit

M. Fisch, R. Hohenfellner
Department of Urology,
University of Mainz School of Medicine,
Mainz, Germany

Introduction

In 1952 Übelhör first described a technique of permanent urinary diversion using a colonic segment.[1] The main advantages of the colon are the possibility of antirefluxive ureteral implantation and the reduced (minor) risk of elongation of the conduit with the growth of the body. The continent forms of urinary diversion have replaced the colonic conduit; however, it is now gaining importance as an intermediary form of diversion. Situations with uncertain outcome, such as severely dilated ureters or impaired renal function, require temporary diversion in a zero-pressure reservoir, e.g. in children with myelomeningocele. After normalization of the upper tract and stabilization of kidney function the sigmoid conduit can be incorporated into a continent reservoir (see Chapter 6.17).

Indications

- Neurogenic bladder disturbances
- Congenital malformations and severely dilated urinary tract
- Impaired renal function

Preoperative investigations

- Renal function study (MAG 3)
- Intravenous urography when creatinine <2 mg/dl (to investigate the upper urinary tract)
- Bowel enema with water-soluble contrast medium (looking for diverticula or polyposis)

Preoperative preparation

- Intestinal irrigation with Ringer's lactate solution (8–10 liters) via a gastric tube, or oral intake of 5–7 liters of Fordtran's solution. (Check the electrolyte levels!)
- Determination of the stoma position in the epigastric region: the stoma plate and bag are attached and checked with the patient in a sitting, lying and standing position. The ideal position is lateral to the rectus muscle in the line between the umbilicus and the superior anterior spine. In children, changes (in a caudal direction) of the stoma position with growth must be considered

Instruments and suture material

- Basic set for kidney surgery with additional instruments for intra-abdominal surgery

- Siegel retractor
- Basin containing prepared iodine solution (disinfection)
- Cold-light source (for preparation of the mesentery)
- Polyglyconic acid 4/0 suture for closure of the conduit, intestinal anastomosis to re-establish bowel continuity, and stoma
- Chromic catgut 5/0 and 6/0 for antirefluxive ureteral implantation
- Silk 4/0 for stay sutures (bowel)
- Catgut 4/0 for stay sutures (bowel mucosa) and fixation of the ureteral stents

Operative technique step by step (Figures 1–8)

- Patient supine and slightly overstretched with a small towel under the lumbar spine
- Insertion of a gastric tube (or gastrostomy), rectal tube and central venous catheter
- Vertical midline incision from the umbilicus to the symphysis
- Incision of the peritoneum lateral to the sigmoid colon
- Isolation of an adequate segment (12–15 cm long), respecting the blood supply; marking of the lines of the bowel incision with four stay sutures
- Incision of the peritoneum, identification and ligation of the mesenteric vessels, and incision of the bowel
- Dissection of both ureters through separate incisions in the posterior peritoneum where they cross the iliac vessels
- Division of both ureters close to the bladder wall, marking with a stay suture and ligation of the stumps
- Ureteral implantation either in an open-ended technique (see Chapter 6.2) or in an open transcolonic technique

Open transcolonic technique
- Closure of the proximal end of the conduit (seromuscular single stitches of polyglyconic acid 4/0)
- Opening of the conduit near the proximal end along the teniae coli over a length of 4 cm
- Marking the position of the implantation with stay sutures on the posterior conduit wall
- Excision of a small buttonhole of the conduit wall between the proximal stay sutures
- Dissection of a submucous tunnel of 3–4 cm length starting from the buttonhole incision
- Transfer of the ureter into the conduit in a gentle curve just below the visceral peritoneum on the mesocolon

- Ureterointestinal anastomosis by two stay sutures (chromic catgut 5/0) at the 5 and 7 o'clock positions and muco-mucosal stitches (chromic catgut 6/0)
- Insertion into the ureter of a 6 Fr stent, which is fixed to the bowel mucosa and led out through the conduit
- Implantation of the contralateral ureter in the same manner, the position of the anastomosis being about 3 cm lateral and slightly proximal to that of the first
- Closure of the anterior sigmoid incision by seromuscular single stitches using polyglyconic acid 4/0

Bowel anastomosis and stoma formation

- The continuity of the large bowel is re-established by an end-to-end anastomosis over the conduit (one-layer seromuscular single sutures with polyglyconic acid 4/0)
- For stoma formation, a button of skin and subcutaneous fat and fascia of 1.5 cm diameter is excised and the fascia incised crosswise
- The aboral end of the conduit is freed of fat and epiploic appendages
- The conduit is pulled through the fascia and the skin opening together with the ureteral stents by means of two Allis clamps
- The seromuscular layer of the conduit is fixed to the abdominal fascia by circular single stitches of polyglyconic acid 3/0
- The oral end of the conduit is anastomosed to the skin by circular single stitches (polyglyconic acid 5/0), everting the stoma

Surgical tricks

Isolation of the segment
- Transilluminating the mesentery by a cold-light source reveals the vessels and facilitates selection of the segment and preparation of the mesenteric slits. The sigmoid artery serves as a guideline: if the bowel is severed about 6 cm above and below the main stem of this vessel, the blood supply to the conduit is excellent. Usually this bowel segment is also the most mobile section of the sigmoid
- Care in the division of the mesentery is essential: mesenteric hematomas can cause serious complications, such as postoperative ureteral obstruction, so hemostasis should be meticulous during this phase of the operation
- Removal of all mesenteric fat and appendices epiploicae from the bowel where it is to be sutured facilitates reanastomosis
- Stopping the incision to divide the sigmoid at half the circumference to insert neomycin-soaked cotton swabs into the intestinal openings prevents the spilling of intestinal

contents before the incision is completed. The use of intestinal clamps should be avoided

Ureteral implantation
- A slightly bent clamp facilitates pull-through of the ureters through the buttonhole and the submucous tunnel

Formation of the stoma
- The stoma can be everted by grasping the seromuscular layer during anastomosis of the bowel to the skin

Extraperitonealization of the conduit
- The ureteral implantation site of the conduit is extraperitonealized by closure of the mesenteric window of the sigmoid colon. Extraperitonealization of the conduit is completed by attaching the reanastomosed sigmoid to the lateral abdominal wall

Postoperative care

- Antibiotics for 5 days
- Parenteral nutrition until bowel contractions appear, then gradually reduced
- Removal of the gastric tube starting from day 3 (after clamping)
- Removal of the rectal tube starting from day 3
- Removal of the central venous catheter when parenteral nutrition is stopped and the patient is eating
- Removal of the ureteral stents, first loosening them (from day 9), then removing them (from day 10), one stent at a time

Bibliography

1. Übelhör R. Die Darmblase. *Langenbecks Arch Klin Chir* **271** (1952) 202.
2. Hohenfellner R, Wulff HD. Zur Harnableitung mittels ausgeschalteter Dickdarmsegmente. *Akt Urol* **1** (1970) 18–27.
3. Skinner DG, Gottesmann JE, Ritchie JP. The isolated sigmoid segment: its value in temporary urinary diversion and reconstruction. *J Urol* **113** (1975) 614.
4. Hendren WH. Exstrophy of the bladder: an alternative method of management. *J Urol* **115** (1975) 195.
5. Kock NG, Nilson AE, Nilsson CO, Norlen LJ, Philipson BM. Urinary diversion via continent ileal reservoir: clinical results in 12 patients. *J Urol* **128** (1982) 469–75.
6. Rowland RG, Mitchell ME, Bihrle R, Kahnowski RJ, Piser E. Indiana continent urinary reservoir. *J Urol* **137** (1987) 1136–9.
7. Thüroff JW, Alken P, Riedmiller H, Engelmann U, Jacobi GH, Hohenfellner R. The Mainz pouch (mixed augmentation ileum and cecum) for bladder augmentation and continent diversion. *J Urol* **136** (1986) 17–26.

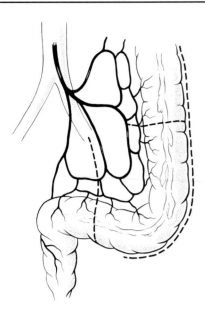

Figure 1. *Selection of a sigmoid segment to be isolated to form the conduit, respecting the course of the blood vessels.*

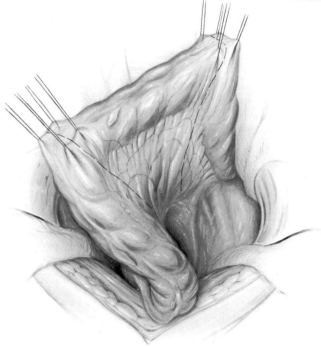

Figure 2. *The dotted line is the line of incision, the sigmoid colon is elevated with stay sutures.*

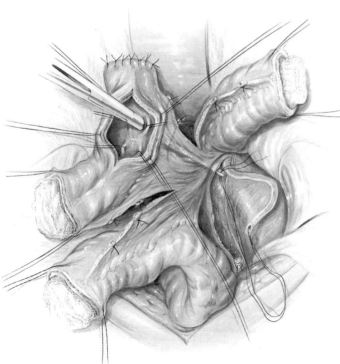

Figure 3. *The oral end of the conduit is closed. Open transcolonic ureteral implantation: the left ureter is brought into the conduit just below the peritoneal cover of the mesentery.*

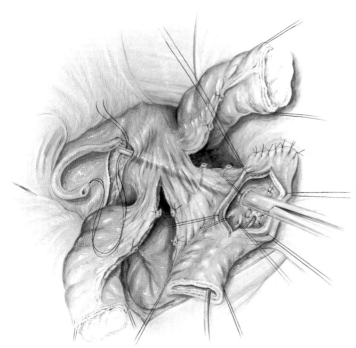

Figure 4. *The left ureter is implanted and splinted; the right ureter is brought into the conduit using an identical technique.*

Figure 5. *End-to-end anastomosis of the colon (one-layer seromuscular single sutures with polyglyconic acid 4/0).*

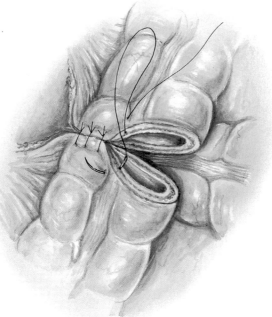

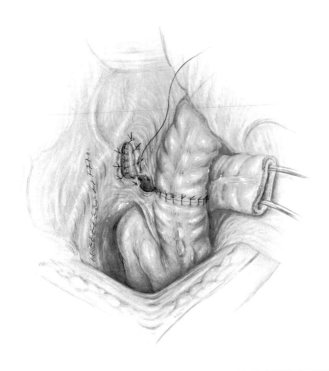

Figure 6. *Closure of the mesenteric slit.*

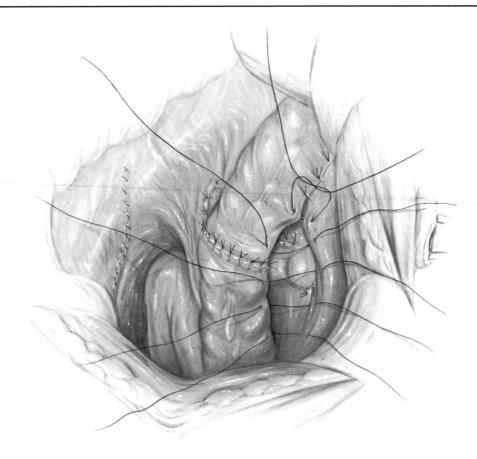

Figure 7. *Extraperitonealization of the conduit by securing the colon to the lateral abdominal wall.*

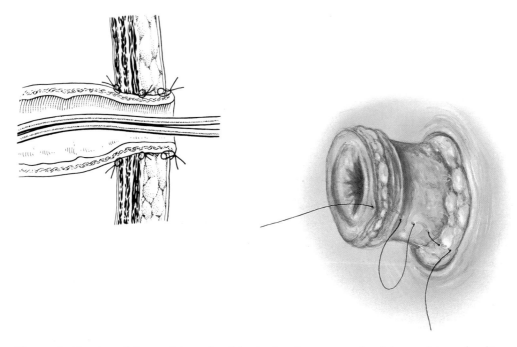

Figure 8. *Fixation of the conduit to the abdominal wall; anastomosis of the conduit to the skin.*

Operative Reconstruction of the External and Internal Genitalia in Females with Bladder Exstrophy or Incontinent Epispadias

R. Stein, M. Fisch, H. Bauer[a],
V. Friedberg[a], R. Hohenfellner
*Department of Urology,
University of Mainz School of Medicine,
Mainz, Germany, and
[a]Department of Gynecology,
University of Mainz School of Medicine,
Mainz, Germany*

Introduction

As a result of modern operative techniques and highly improved postoperative medical care, children with bladder exstrophy today have a normal life expectancy.[1] In women with bladder exstrophy or incontinent epispadias, reconstruction of the external and internal genitalia is often neglected. When the problems of urinary continence have been solved, other factors (body image, sexuality and pregnancy) become of interest to these women.

Esthetic reconstruction of the external female genitalia with adaptation of the bifid clitoris and divergent mons pubis creates good cosmetic results.[2-4] However, correction of internal genitalia during bladder neck reconstruction or urinary diversion is seldom performed. The cervix is very close to the introitus. The weak pelvic floor and poor uterine support make prolapse common. The narrow introitus prevents uterine prolapse. After episiotomy or vaginoplasty alone, without antefixation of the uterus, prolapse can occur.[1,5]

During gynecologic surgery, fixation of the uterus is very uncommon as an independent operative intervention: there are few indications for it and hysterectomy is preferred.[6] The most common operation for fixation of the uterus is shortening of the round ligament, as described by Gilliam and Doléris and modified by Simpson and others.[6] The technique described herein and developed by one of the senior authors (V.F.) permits individual adaptation to different anatomic situations caused by the varying distances between the pubic bones. It prevents ventral and lateral pockets, which can cause ileus and may result in death.[7]

Indications

- Correction of the external genitalia: esthetic operation to avoid psychological problems during childhood

- Vaginal cut-back: first minimal vaginal cut-back to allow outflow of secretion and later menstrual flow (the position of the cervix can be determined); after puberty, definitive vaginal cut-back to allow sexual intercourse

- Antefixation of the uterus: prevention or correction of uterine prolapse (e.g. after introitus plasty)

Timetable

- Reconstruction of the external genitalia and first minimal vaginal cut-back, simultaneously in primary urinary diversion, or together with bladder neck reconstruction in primary bladder closure

- Antefixation of the uterus, definitive vaginal cut-back, reconstruction of the umbilicus and correction of scars and the mons pubis (if necessary) at puberty after primary bladder closure or urinary diversion, or together with final correction after failure of primary bladder closure of urinary diversion

Operative risks

The first discussion with the parents describing the necessary operations should include not only the question of primary bladder closure and bladder neck repair *versus* urinary diversion, but also the reconstruction of the external and internal genitalia. The possibility of cohabitation and pregnancy must be mentioned explicitly.

Specific complications include:

- Shrinkage of the introitus

- Risk of uterine prolapse after first minimal vaginal cut-back (the position of the cervix can be determined and antefixation of the uterus performed at the same time as urinary diversion)

Special instruments and materials

- Bipolar electric forceps

- Scott retractor

- GORE-TEX net (PTFE, W.L. Gore, Woking, UK)

- Polyglactin sutures (e.g. Ethibond or Vicryl, Ethicon, Edinburgh, UK)

- Mersilene (Ethicon)

Anesthesia

- Insufflation anesthesia

Operative technique step by step

Reconstruction of the external genitalia and first minimal vaginal cut-back (Figures 1–10)

Independent of urinary diversion or primary bladder closure, reconstruction includes approximation of the mons pubis and the clitoris halves (taking care to preserve their sensitivity), reconstruction of the labia minora and first vaginal cut-back.

- Supine position for primary urinary diversion together with cystectomy

- Excision of the bladder plate and curved extension of the incision at both lateral sites

- After mobilization, resection of the whole bladder plate and creation of the urinary diversion (in our department the sigmoidorectal pouch is preferred[8])

- Closure of the fascia and adaptation of the rectus muscles, e.g. with polyglycolic acid 3/0 or 4/0

- If there is not enough tissue between the divergent ends of the pubic bones, crossing of the rectus muscles: division of both muscles at their insertion at the pubic bones, and fixation at the opposite side

- Tension-free closure of the skin by direct preparation, lateral mobilization of the superficial fascia and preservation of the vessels (care is needed to prevent postoperative disturbances in wound healing): careful adaptation of the superficial fascia with interrupted sutures (polyglycolic acid) guarantees tension-free closure of the skin (Mersilene) (the distal part of the wound remains open at this time)

- Change to the lithostomy position

- Circumcision of both clitoris halves and adaptation with chromic catgut 4/0, with careful preservation of the dorsal vessels and nerves

- Cranial closure of the wound with tension-free adaptation of the mons pubis

- Circumcision of the rudiments of the labia minora medially and laterally, and extension of the incision distally and laterally

- Partly sharp and partly blunt mobilization of the labia minora

- Insertion of stay sutures at both ends of the labia

- Vaginal cut-back as in Y–V plasty, a U-shaped flap of skin from the perineal region is laid into the vestibule and fixed

- Incision and mobilization of the flap

- Adjustment of the vestibule of the vagina (using two small spatulas)

- Incision of the muscle of the pelvic floor at 6 o'clock (electrocautery)

- Careful disinfection of the vagina (because of the narrow vestibule, there is a lot of secretion inside the vagina, especially in adolescents)

- Insertion of stay sutures at the top of the U-shaped skin flap (during the first minimal vaginal cut-back the incision should not be too deep: there is a risk of uterine prolapse)

- Fixation of the skin flap with single sutures (catgut 5/0)

- Tension-free adaptation of the labia minora with the distal end of the incision (adaptation of the superficial fascia with

a slightly lateral suture makes the labia minora more prominent); fixation at the same level as the vestibule

- Closure of the wound with interrupted sutures (catgut 4/0)

- Insertion and fixation of a penile glass phantom in the vagina (outflow of secretion)

- Application of a fixed dressing

Antefixation of the uterus (Figures 11–16)
- Median incision in the lower abdominal wall

- Division of the round ligaments as distally as possible, sheathing the ends with nonabsorbable suture material such as Ethibond

- Pulling of the round ligaments through the lateral fascia of the rectus muscle from the internal to the external side using an Overholt clamp

- Straightening the vagina with the help of one finger, the uterus is brought into the desired position

- Suturing together of the round ligaments over the rectus abdominis muscles and fixation at the muscle and, if possible, at the uterus (Ethibond or Vicryl)

- Fixation of the body of the uterus or, in vaginal prolapse, the anterior wall of the vagina at the ligament between two ends of the pubic rami. This is a very strong ligament that connects both ends of the pubic rami instead of the normal synostosis pubis. A prosthesis of GORE-TEX can be used as a fulcrum to avoid cutting the sutures. At the end of the operation the vaginal part of the cervix reaches the posterior vault of the vagina. The vaginal tube is now visibly larger

- In patients with primary bladder closure, antefixation at the right or left side of the closed bladder (this operation is technically more complex, especially in patients with bowel bladder augmentation)

Surgical tricks

- For reconstruction of the labia minora, the use of a Scott retractor and a small electrocauterizer is helpful

- Where there is wide diastasis of the pubic bones, the defect of the anterior abdominal wall can be covered by crossing over both rectus abdominis muscles. The round ligaments are pulled directly through the rectus abdominis muscles

- In women with urinary diversion the rectosigmoid is fixed at the long ligament of the promontory. If a sigmoidorectal pouch is created, fixation is part of the operation as it prevents rectal prolapse. After bladder neck reconstruction and fixation of the uterus the risk of rectal prolapse should always be kept in mind. To avoid this, the rectosigmoid is fixed with nonabsorbable sutures at the promontory between the two common iliac veins

Postoperative care

- The dressing is removed after 1 or 2 days

- After day 5, a hip bath with camomile lotion twice a day is beneficial; however, the closure of the abdominal wall should not be in contact with the water

- The initial tendency of the corrected vestibule to shrinkage can be prevented by inserting a special penile glass phantom for half an hour once or twice a week until the patient has regular sexual intercourse. This is not necessary in children as definitive vaginal cut-back is not performed until later

References

1. Woodhouse CRJ. Exstrophy and epispadias. In: Woodhouse CRJ (ed.) *Long-term Paediatric Urology*. Oxford: Blackwell Scientific (1991) 127–50.

2. Erich JB. Plastic repair of the female perineum in a case of exstrophy of the bladder. *Proc Staff Meet Mayo Clin* (1959) 235–7.

3. Overstreet EW, Hinman F Jr. Some gynaecologic aspects of bladder exstrophy. *West J Surg Obstet Gynaecol* **64** (1956) 131–7.

4. Ship AG, Pelzer RH. Reconstruction of the female escutcheon in exstrophy of the bladder. *Plast Reconstr Surg* **49** (1972) 643–6.

5. Dewhurst J, Toplis PJ, Shepherd JH. Ivalon sponge hysterosacropexy for genital prolapse in patients with bladder exstrophy. *Br J Obstet Gynaecol* **87** (1980) 67–9.

6. Käser O, Iklé FA. Abdominale Operationen bei Lageveränderungen des Genitales. In: Käser O, Iké FA (eds) *Operationen in der Gynäkologie*, 4th edn. Stuttgart: Thieme Verlag. Chapt. 6 pp 1–10, 1982.

7. Ruck CJ, Scholz A. Zur Antefixationsmethode nach Doléris. *Zbl Gynäk* **79** (1957) 1621–30.

8. Fisch M, Wammack R, Müller SC, Hohenfellner R. Mainz pouch II (sigma rectum pouch). *J Urol* **149** (1993) 258–64.

Reconstruction of the external genitalia, 'cut back' after primary cystectomy

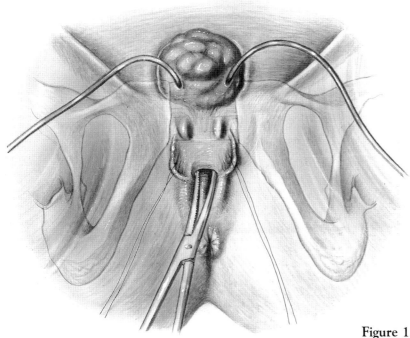

Figure 1. *Bladder exstrophy, splinted ureters, bifid clitoris and short labia minora.*

Figure 2. *Marking of the incision for cystectomy, adaptation of bifid mons pubis, reconstruction of the labia minora and first minimal vaginal cut-back.*

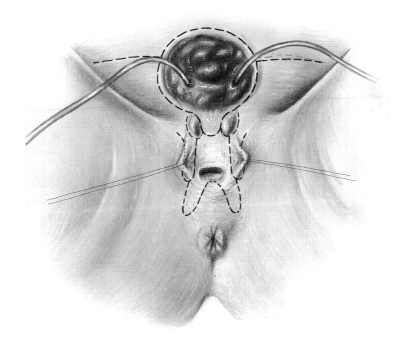

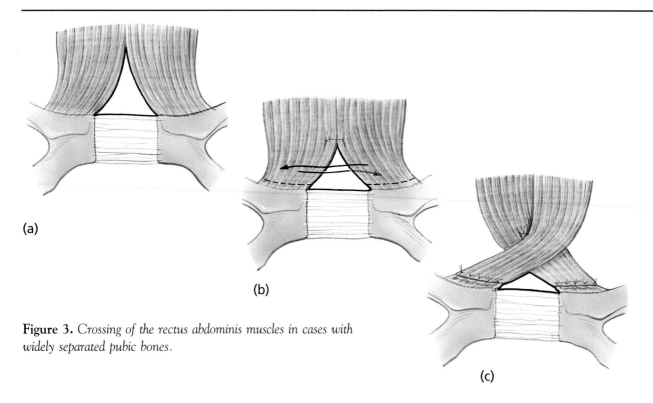

Figure 3. *Crossing of the rectus abdominis muscles in cases with widely separated pubic bones.*

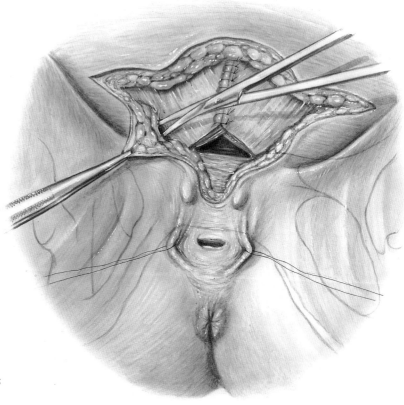

Figure 4. *After cystectomy and primary urinary diversion, adaptation of the rectus abdominis muscles and mobilization of the subcutaneous tissue to the sides.*

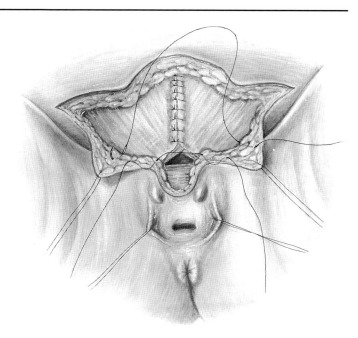

Figure 5. *Adaptation of the superficial fascia with polyglycolic acid 4/0.*

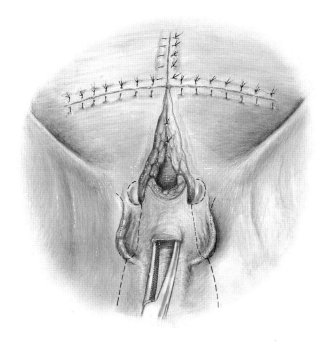

Figure 6. *Closure of the skin with interrupted sutures (Mersilene). The distal part of the wound remains open.*

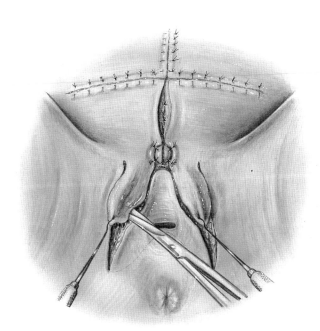

Figure 7. *Lengthening of the labia minor after adaptation of the bifid clitoris and cystectomy.*

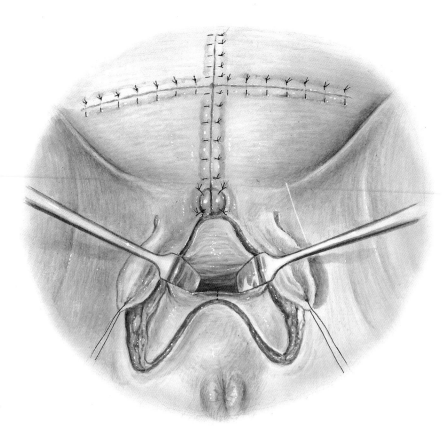

Figure 8. *For reconstruction of the vestibule, completion of the incision for creation of a U-shaped flap of perineum and demonstration of the vestibule of the vagina.*

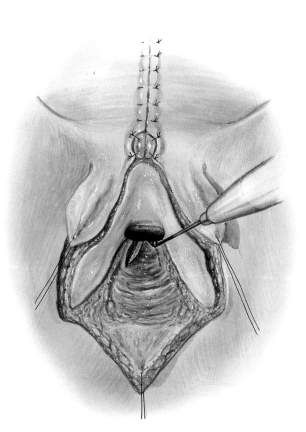

Figure 9. *Incision of the vestibule with the electrocauterizer.*

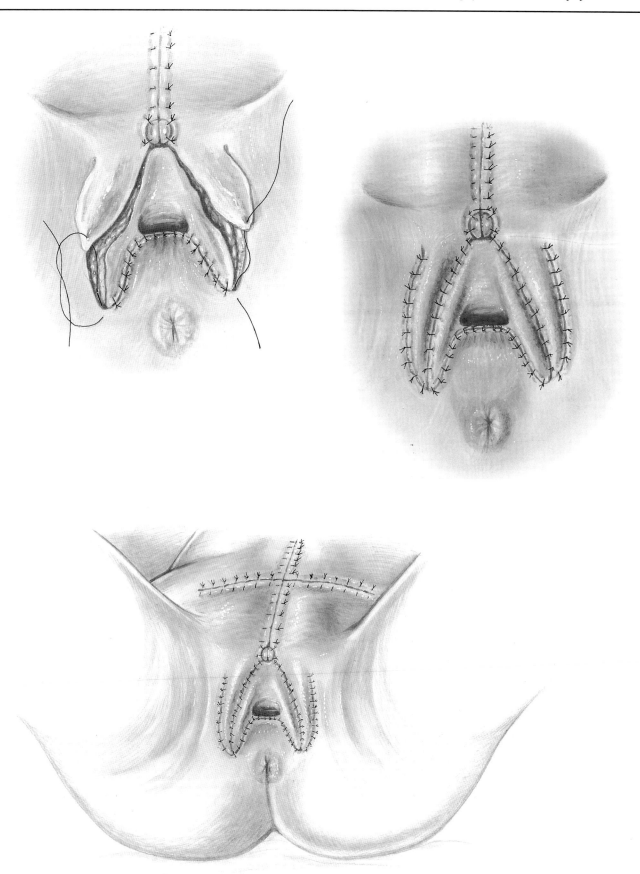

Figure 10. *Fixation of the U-shaped flap at the vestibule and closure of the wound with interrupted sutures. The distal ends of the labia minora should be fixed at the distal part of the incision.*

Antefixation of the uterus

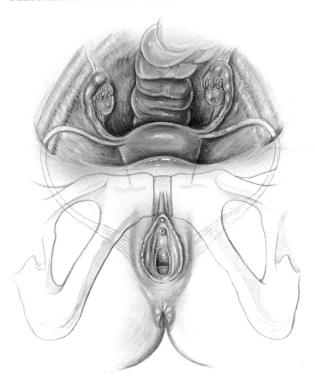

Figure 11. *Normal female internal and external genitalia.*

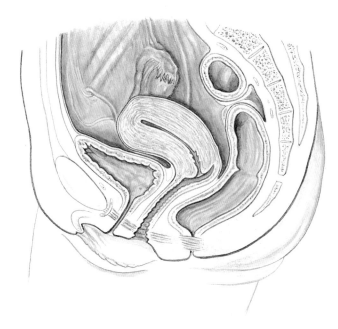

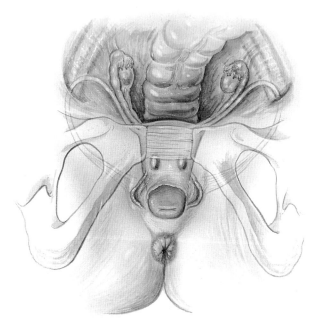

Figure 12. *Anatomy of the exstrophic female: normal internal genitalia and uterine prolapse, e.g. after reconstruction of the vestibule. The vagina and anus are displaced forwards because the anterior abdominal wall and parts of the bladder are missing. The vagina appears short and runs directly posterior. The clitoris is bifid; the labia and mons pubis are divergent.*

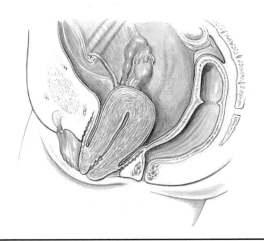

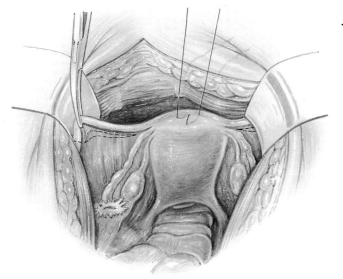

◀ **Figure 13.** *Stay suture at the corpus uteri, preparation of the round ligaments and division as distally as possible.*

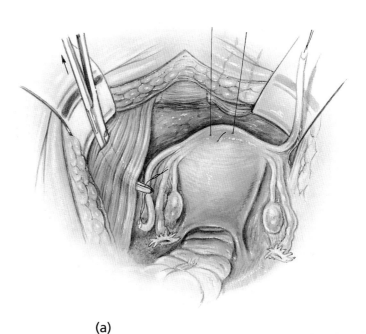

(a)

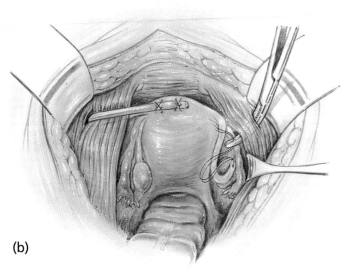

(b)

Figure 14. *The ends of the round ligaments are sheathed with nonabsorbable suture material (e.g. Ethibond). Together with the suture, the ligament is pulled through from the internal to the external side and fixed at the uterus.*

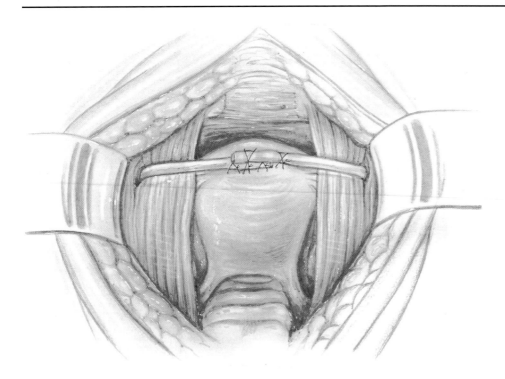

Figure 15. *If necessary, the ligaments may be crossed over the uterus.*

Figure 16. *Additionally the body of the uterus or, in vaginal prolapse, the anterior wall of the vagina is fixed at the ligament between the two ends of the pubic rami. A prosthesis of GORE-TEX can be used as a fulcrum to avoid cutting the sutures.*

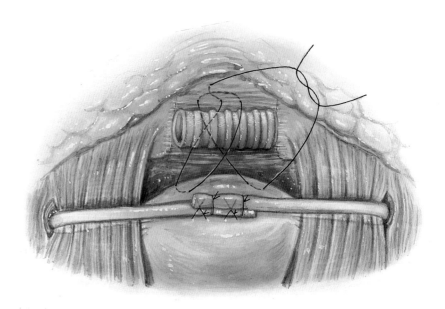

Gastrostomy

C.P. Gilfrich, F. Steinbach, M. Stöckle
Department of Urology,
University of Mainz School of Medicine,
Mainz, Germany

Introduction

Gastrostomy is one of the oldest operations in abdominal surgery, having been introduced in 1873 by Egeberg. In extensive urologic surgery requiring gastric decompression, gastrostomy is gaining influence as an alternative to the nasogastric tube. The advantages are as follows:

- It is better tolerated by the patient
- It causes significantly fewer postoperative respiratory complications (especially in old, very young or immunocompromised and those with respiratory diseases)
- It causes no coughing or vomiting because of pharyngeal irritation
- Complete gastric decompression is achieved (with the nasogastric tube, this is not always the case)

Indications

- Every operation requiring gastric decompression for 24 hours or longer
- Operations for which a nasogastric tube is indicated, for example cystectomy with bladder substitution and other operations with opening of the intestine

Contraindications

- Previous gastric surgery or suspicion of stomach cancer

Instruments

- Suprapubic catheter (e.g. 10 Fr polyurethane)

Operative technique step by step (Figures 1–3)

- Insufflate air through the nasogastric tube
- Make a caudal incision. The stomach can then be pulled down easily by slight traction on the greater omentum
- Insert a purse-string suture of diameter about 2 cm on a vertical area of the stomach that is nearly free of vessels, near to the small curvature
- Push the trocar of a suprapubic catheter (10 Fr, polyurethane) through the anterior abdominal wall on the left side of the abdominal incision, cranial to the umbilicus, in the direction of the purse-string suture
- Push the trocar through the gastric wall in the middle of the purse-string (taking care that the stomach is well filled with air). Move the catheter into the stomach
- Remove and separate the trocar
- Aspirate air through the nasogastric tube, which can then be withdrawn
- Fill the catheter balloon with 5 ml of 0.9% saline. The catheter placement can be judged by palpating the balloon. The balloon should be palpated while gently pushing it directly under the gastric wall
- Fix the stomach on the peritoneum with the free needle of the purse string. Close the purse-string suture
- Suture the catheter in place (with Vicryl 3/0, for example)

Complications

- Local peritonitis and wound healing problems, sometimes leading to fistula, can result after removal of the gastrostomy
- Perforation of the back-wall of the stomach may occur when the stomach is not filled with enough air

Postoperative care

- Gastrostomy drainage until normal bowel activity returns
- Small amounts of clear liquids orally until normal bowel activity returns
- Closure of the gastrostomy when normal bowel peristalsis resumes
- Removal of the catheter at 2 weeks (no earlier, even if it is no longer necessary)

Bibliography

1. Grant GN, Elliott DW, Frederick PL. Postoperative decompression by temporary gastrostomy or nasogastric tube. *Arch Surg* **85** (1962) 164–71.
2. Van Poppel H, Baert L. The percutaneous operative gastrostomy for gastric decompression in major urological surgery. *J Urol* **145** (1991) 100–2.

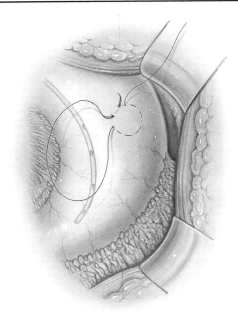

Figure 1. *A purse-string suture of diameter about 2 cm on a vertical area of the stomach that is nearly free from vessels, near to the large curvature.*

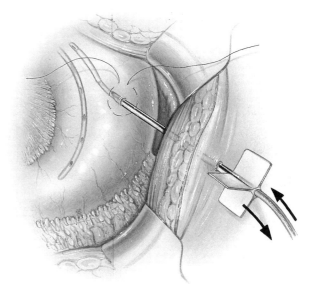

Figure 2. *The trocar is pushed through the abdominal and gastric walls in the middle of the purse-string. The catheter is moved into the stomach. The trocar is separated and removed.*

Figure 3. *Fixation of the stomach on the peritoneum with the free needle of the purse-string. Closure of the purse string. The catheter is sutured in place.*

Orthotopic Ileal Bladder Substitution with Serous Lined Extramural Ureteral Reimplantation

H. Abol-Enein, M.A. Ghoneim
Urology and Nephrology Center,
Mansoura, Egypt

Comment

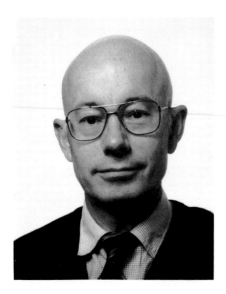

Some publications during the last years have seriously questioned the need for reflux prevention in continent urinary reconstruction.[1,2] This attitude is based on three assumptions:

- That the receptacle for urine has a low pressure
- That, in bladder substitution, the urine is sterile
- That the risk of ureterointestinal obstruction is higher with antireflux than with a refluxive technique

It is most unfortunate that the expression 'low-pressure pouch' has been so widely adopted in urologic circles. By sheer word-power, its indiscriminate use has led many to believe that, when the intestinal segment to receive and collect urine is detubularized, the increase in intraluminal pressure with filling is virtually abolished. This is not the case. The volume capacity increases and the spontaneous activity of the intestine is reduced, but considerable intraluminal pressure can be achieved[3] and this must be borne in mind.

Sterile urine is not typical of urinary tracts reconstructed with intestinal segments. Cultures are always positive in conduits, most often positive after continent cutaneous diversion, and positive in at least 50% after bladder substitution, with a very unstable flora.[4]

There are three main causes of ureterointestinal anastomotic stricture:

- Inadequate blood supply to the ureter
- Failure to use a no-touch surgical technique
- Inflammatory changes induced by urine and/or the healing process

There is no evidence that antireflux implantation techniques are associated with a higher incidence of stricture than refluxing techniques. In a prospective randomized study of conduits, we found stricture to be unrelated to mode of ureteric implantation.[5]

There are several studies suggesting that reflux damages renal function after reconstruction involving intestinal segments. In experiments in dogs, the use of a refluxing technique for implantation into conduits was associated with a higher incidence of pyelonephritis than an antireflux technique.[6] Similar results were obtained in dogs with a continent cutaneous diversion[7] and ileocystoplasty.[8,9] In our clinical study,[5] glomerular filtration rate (GFR) did not differ significantly between kidneys with and without reflux protection. However, upper tract bacteriuria and renal scarring were more common in refluxing renal units than in non-refluxing, and in kidneys with renal scarring there was a significant decrease in GFR.[10] Although these results concern patients with conduits, it is my strong belief that ureters should not be implanted into pouches with a refluxing technique until carefully conducted prospective studies clearly show that this can be done without endangering renal function.

The antireflux technique shown in this chapter uses a serous-lined extramural tunnel for the ureter.[11] As is demonstrated, the method can be used whenever detubularized intestinal segments are used for the urine receptacle. By variations in the established techniques for the Mainz pouch I and II, this type of antireflux implantation can be applied. I think there are two main advantages of the technique. One is that it is also suitable for dilated ureters. Such ureters are otherwise difficult to implant in a reflux-preventing way, and usually require an interposed ileal nipple valve. The other is that it should be easy to find the ureteric orifices at endoscopy (as they are always situated at the end of a suture line) should endoscopic manipulation of the ureter become necessary. One point needs to be emphasized and that is that the back wall of the serous-lined trough is created using nonabsorbable seromuscular sutures joining two serosal surfaces. Loss of this suture line implies that the antireflux mechanism is lost.

Whether this technique is superior to the standard antireflux implantation for nondilated ureters (i.e. the submucosal tunnel or the Le Duc technique) remains to be shown in prospective randomized trials. In Lund the Le Duc technique is the standard procedure in continent urinary reconstruction. In 157 operations during the years 1989–1993 we had stricture requiring surgery or resulting in a nonfunctioning kidney in three patients (2%). We have this year examined the 18 patients with 35 kidneys operated on in the period October 1989 to April 1991. Among these patients there was no stricture and in only one case could reflux be proved at enterocystography.

References

1. Helal M, Pow-Sang J, Sanford E, Figueroa D, Lockhart J. Direct (non-tunneled) ureterocolonic reimplantation in association with continent reservoirs. *J Urol* **150** (1993) 835–7.

2. Studer UE, Turner WH. Is reflux prevention important in urinary diversion? In: Webster GD, Goldwasser B (eds) *Urinary Diversion: Scientific Foundations and Clinical Practice.* Oxford: Isis Medical Media (1995) 282–93.

3. Colding-Jørgensen M, Steven K. The mechanics of tubular and detubularized bowel for bladder substitution. In: Webster GD, Goldwasser B (eds) *Urinary Diversion: Scientific Foundation and Clinical Practice.* Oxford: Isis Medical Media (1995) 45–52.

4. Månsson W, Colleen S, Wullt B. Microbial ecology in urinary tracts reconstructed with intestinal segments. In: Webster GD, Goldwasser B (eds) *Urinary Diversion: Scientific Foundation and Clinical Practice.* Oxford: Isis Medical Media (1995) 53–63.

5. Kristjansson A, Wallin L, Månsson W. Renal function up to 16 years after conduit (refluxing or antireflux anastomosis) or continent urinary diversion. I. Glomerular filtration rate and patency or uretero-intestinal anastomosis. *Br J Urol* (in press).

6. Richie JP, Skinner DG, Wajsman J. The effect of reflux on the development of pyelonephritis in urinary diversion: an experimental study. *J Surg Res* **16** (1974) 256–61.

7. Kock NG, Nilson AE, Norlén L, Sundin T, Trasti H. Changes in renal parenchyma and the upper urinary tracts following urinary diversion via a continent ileum reservoir: an experimental study in dogs. *Scand J Urol Nephrol* suppl. **49** (1978) 11–12.

8. Clair SR, Hixon CJ, Ritchey ML. Enterocystoplasty and reflux nephroplasty in the canine model. *J Urol* **148** (1992) 728–32.

9. Kristjansson A, Abol-Enein H, Alm P, Mokthar AA, Ghoneim MA, Månsson W. Substitution cystoplasty and reflux nephropathy in a canine model: a preliminary report. In: *Continent Urinary Reconstruction Second International Meeting.* Abstract book, Mainz (1995) 102.

10. Kristjansson A, Bajc M, Wallin L, Willner J, Månsson W. Renal function up to 16 years after conduit (refluxing or anti-reflux anastomosis) or continent urinary diversion. II. Renal scarring and location of bacteriuria. *Br J Urol* (in press).

11. Abol-Enein H, Ghoneim MA. Optimization of ureterointestinal anastomosis in urinary diversion: an experimental study in dogs. III. A new antireflux technique for uretero-ileal anastomosis: a serous-lined extramural tunnel. *Urol Res* **21** (1993) 135–9.

Wiking Månsson, Lund, Sweden

Introduction

A sound ureterointestinal reimplantation in continent urinary diversion should offer:

- Technical simplicity and clinical reproducibility

- Unidirectional unobstructed flow of urine

- The use of an extra length of bowel (staples and/or synthetic materials should be avoided)

- The feasibility of retrograde endoscopic manipulation of the upper tracts

- A technique for dilated as well as normal ureters

The intussuscepted nipple valve[1] and the long afferent intact ileal loop[2] lack most of these. The technique of Le Duc[3] is associated with a high complication rate due to irregular healing of the implanted uncovered ureters, resulting in stenosis and/or reflux.[4,5]

Indications

This technique is suitable for implantation of normal as well as the dilated ureters whenever detubularized intestinal reservoirs are indicated.

Contraindications

- Concomitant pathology in the distal ureters, necessitating high excision

Instruments

- Standard instruments for radical cystectomy and bowel surgery, including adequate self-retaining retractors and adequate illumination in the depth of the pelvis

- Suture material: 3/0 nonabsorbable silk suture, 3/0 and 4/0 polyglactin sutures and 4/0 catgut sutures

Patient preparation

- No special preparation is required except those for any abdominal surgery

- Oral fluids are allowed only until 24 hours before the operation

- Nothing by mouth for at least 6 hours before the operation

Operative technique step by step (Figures 1–6)

- Following lymphadenectomy the final stages of cystectomy must be carefully executed to preserve the integrity of the urethra and periurethral musculature

- A 40 cm segment of the distal ileum is isolated and arranged in a W configuration

- The lateral limbs of the W are joined together by a seromuscular continuous suture of 3/0 silk

- The antimesenteric border of the intestine is incised using a diathermy knife. The edges of the two medial flaps are joined by a running through-and-through suture of 3/0 polyglactin. The result is the creation of two serous-lined intestinal troughs

- The most lateral ileal flaps are joined by a continuous 3/0 polyglactin suture closing the lower aspect of the reservoir

- The most dependent point in close proximity to the urethral stump is determined and a 2 cm hole is created, or preferably the median suture line is reopened for 2 cm, and the security of the suture line is maintained by two interrupted sutures at both ends of the aperture

- 4/0 polyglactin stay sutures are inserted to hold the urethral stump around a 20 Fr silicone Foley catheter

- The urethral stump is anastomosed to the hole using the stay sutures

- The left ureter is brought medially through a suitable mesenteric window in the left mesocolon, providing a downward smooth curve without angulation

- Each ureter is laid in its corresponding trough. A mucosa-to-mucosa anastomosis between the stented and spatulated end of the ureter and the ileal flaps is performed using 4/0 polyglactin suture

- The implanted ureter is then covered by approximation and an interrupted polyglactin suture is inserted

- The ureteral stents are fixed to the pouch mucosa close to the ureteral hiatus and secured to their exits (made by stabbing through the anterior wall of the reservoir) using 4/0 gut sutures

- Closure of the pouch is then completed at the anterior aspect and the dome

- Two tube drains are placed in the pelvic cavity and brought out through separate exists in the abdominal wall. Gravity drainage only is used

Surgical tricks

- Light diathermy coagulation of the seromuscular suture lines at the base of the intestinal troughs induces adhesions, reinforcing the suture lines

- During the antimesenteric splitting of the bowel, each intestinal trough should be tailored according to the caliber of its corresponding ureter

- Eversion of the ileal mucosa at the pouch aperture using 5/0 plain catgut sutures ensures adequate adaptation of the urethroileal anastomosis

- Stay sutures of 4/0 polyglactin at the 3, 9 and 12 o'clock positions, incorporating the mucosa and periurethral muscles, prevent retraction of the urethral stump and can be used for urethroileal anastomosis

- The divided Denonvilliers' fascia is included in the posterior stay sutures at the 5 and 7 o'clock positions for later incorporation in the urethrointestinal anastomosis

Postoperative care

- Intravenous alimentation is necessary until normal bowel function resumes

- Antibiotic therapy is given for 5–7 days

- The drainage tubes are removed once drainage has ceased

- The ureteral stents are removed at 10 and 11 days

- Control sonography and intravenous urography are necessary before removal of the urethral catheter at the end of week 3

References

1. Kock NG, Nilson AE, Norlén L, Sundin T, Trasti H. Urinary diversion via a continent reservoir: clinical experience. *J Urol Nephrol* Suppl **49** (1982) 23.
2. Studer UE, Gerber E, Springer J, Zingg EJ. Bladder reconstruction with bowel after radical cystectomy. *World J Urol* **10** (1992) 11.
3. Le Duc A, Camey M, Teillac P. An original antireflux ureteroileal implantation technique: long-term follow up. *J Urol* **137** (1987) 1156.
4. Abol-Enein H, El-Baz M, Ghoneim MA. Optimization of uretero-intestinal anastomosis in urinary diversion: an experimental study in dogs. I. Evaluation of the Le Duc technique. *Urol Res* **21** (1993) 125.
5. Abol-Einen H, El-Baz M, Ghoneim MA. Optimization of uretero-intestinal anastomosis in urinary diversion: an experimental study in dogs. II. Influence of exposure to urine on the healing of the ureter and ileum. *Urol Res* **21** (1993) 131.

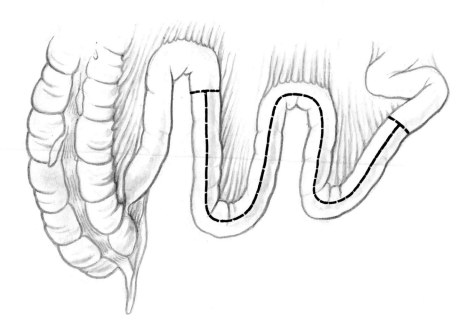

Figure 1. *A 40 cm segment from the distal ileum is isolated and arranged in a W-shaped configuration.*

Figure 2. *The antimesenteric border is incised (using a diathermy knife); the medial flaps are joined using a 3/0 polyglactin continuous suture.*

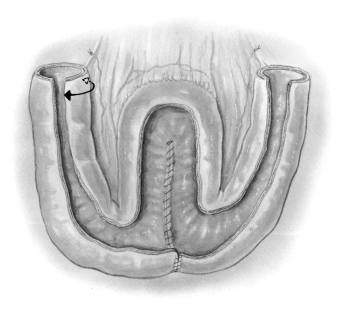

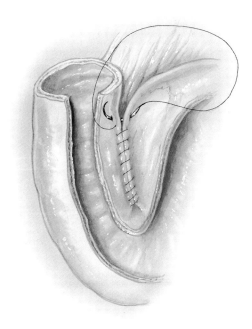

Figure 3. *The lateral ileal limbs are joined together by seromuscular continuous 3/0 silk to create two serous-lined intestinal troughs.*

Figure 4. *The spatulated ureter is anastomosed to the intestinal mucosa and the tunnel is then closed over the implanted ureter using interrupted 4/0 polyglactin sutures (the length of the tunnel should be 2 cm for a normal ureter).*

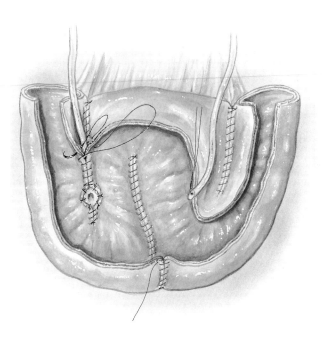

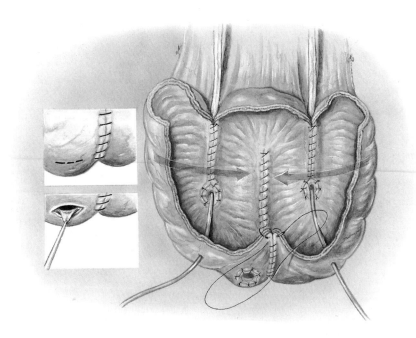

Figure 5. *A 2 cm aperture is created in a dependent position or through the suture line and its mucosa is everted using 5/0 catgut suture.*

Figure 6. *The pouch is closed after urethroileal anastomosis. The ureteral stents are brought out through separate exits in the anterior pouch wall.*

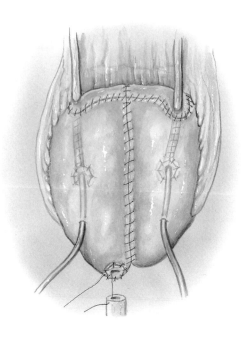

Ureteral Implantation into a Mainz Pouch I and Sigmoidorectal Pouch via a Serous Lined Extramural Tunnel

M. Fisch, H. Abol-Enein, R. Hohenfellner
Department of Urology,
University of Mainz School of Medicine,
Mainz, Germany

Introduction

The submucous tunnel offers an excellent implantation technique for normal undilated ureters with a low risk of stenosis or reflux, but it is associated with an increased complication rate when dilated or thick-walled ureters are present. For these ureters the technique recently published by Abol-Einen, with promising experimental and clinical results, represents an alternative.[1,2] The technique described first for the ileal neobladder is also applicable for the Mainz pouch I procedure. To facilitate ureteral implantation the original technique of the Mainz pouch procedure has slightly been modified.

As the procedure requires two suture lines, an additional sigmoid loop is used for creation of the sigmoidorectal pouch when an anal reservoir is planned.

Indications

Ureteral implantation during continent urinary diversion when dilated or thick-walled ureters are present:

- After irradiation
- After long-lasting dilatation
- In refluxing ureters (e.g. in neurogenic bladder disturbances)
- In tuberculosis and bilharziasis

Instruments

As for continent urinary diversion using the Mainz pouch I or the sigmoidorectal pouch procedure (see Chapters 6.4 and 6.8).

Operative technique step by step

- Midline incision
- For creation of a Mainz pouch I: median laparotomy with left-sided circumferential incision around the umbilicus

Ureteral implantation into a Mainz pouch I (Figures 1–9)
- Right paracolonic incision and mobilization of the cecal pole, ascending colon and right colonic flexure
- Dissection of the omentum from the transverse colon; opening of the omental bursa
- Identification and dissection of the right ureter, which is cut at its entrance into the bladder
- Left paracolonic incision; identification and dissection of the left ureter, cutting it as deep as possible

- Transposition of the ureter behind the mesentery to the right side (above the superior mesenteric artery) according to the standard technique
- Creation of the pouch: isolation of two colonic segments (cecum and ascending colon) of 10–15 cm length and one *ileal* loop of equal length (in contrast to the standard technique); if an ileal intussuscepted nipple is planned as a continence mechanism, an additional 8–12 cm segment of ileum is required
- Restoration of bowel continuity by simple ileocolonic anastomosis or by replacing the ileocecal valve
- Creation of the continence mechanism according to the standard technique, and insertion of a catheter into the pouch
- Flushing of the isolated bowel segment and opening it antimesenterically except in the area of the continence mechanism
- Positioning of the aboral end of the isolated segment in the shape of an upside-down V
- Anastomosis of the medial margins of the V by a serous running suture (nonabsorbable suture material) close to the mesentery, thus creating a serous-lined groove; in the edge of the V an opening is left to pull the right ureter through later
- Anastomosis of the ileal loop with the colonic part of the pouch by an identical serous running suture close to the mesentery, creating a second groove
- Incision of the mesentery above the ileocolonic anastomosis
- Pulling of the left ureter through this incision and the right ureter through the opening above the right groove
- Positioning of the ureters in the irrespective grooves
- Anastomosis of the seromuscular borders over the ureter by an all-layer running suture, whereby the ureter is incorporated into the back wall of the pouch lying in a serous-lined tunnel: the length of the tunnel should be four times the diameter of the ureter
- For definitive implantation, cutting of the ureter to its required length and spatulation
- Placing of four anchor sutures at the 11 and 1 and the 5 and 7 o'clock positions, grasping all layers of the ureter as well as all layers of the bowel wall (chromic catgut 4/0)
- Exact mucomucous stitches between the anchor sutures to complete the anastomosis (chromic catgut 5/0)
- Continuation of the serous running suture to the end of the antimesenteric incision by enlarging the distance to the mesentery, thereby grasping the seromuscular borders

- Implantation of the contralateral ureter in the same manner

- Ureteral implantation, secured by the insertion of two stents (size to depend on the thickness of the ureter)

- Fixation of the ureteral stents to the bowel mucosa (catgut 5/0)

- Insertion of a cystostomy tube through the pouch wall and closure of the pouch (running suture polyglyconic acid 4/0)

Surgical tricks
- By using two colonic and only one ileal loop, in contrast to the standard technique, the required slit in the mesentery to pull the left ureter through comes in an area of the mesentery which is free of vessels

- The closer to the mesentery the serous continuous suture grasps the bowel wall, the larger the tunnel will be; in this way, the diameter of the tunnel can be adjusted to the ureteral diameter

Implantation into a sigmoidorectal pouch (Mainz II) (Figures 10–16)
- Left paracolic incision

- Mobilization of the descending colon including the left colonic flexure in cases of a short sigmoid colon

- Identification and dissection of the left ureter

- Right paracolic incision, continued along the root of the mesentery of the small bowel

- Identification and dissection of the right ureter

- Cutting of the ureters, as deep as possible

- Transposition of the left ureter, behind mesentery, to the right side

- Marking of an S-shaped sigmoid segment by stay sutures, each limb being of 10–12 cm to give a total length of 30–36 cm

- Antimesenteric opening of the S in the area of the teniae coli

- Side-to-side adaptation of the limbs by two serous running sutures close to the mesentery (nonabsorbable suture, e.g. 4/0 silk Prolene (Ethicon, Edinburgh, UK)) creating two serous-lined grooves: on the right side, an entrance for the right ureter is left at the cranial aspect of the running suture

- Incision of the mesentery cranial to the left running suture and pull-through of the left ureter

- Placing of the ureters in their respective grooves and anastomosis of the borders of the bowel over the ureter by a running suture grasping all layers of the bowel wall

- Definitive implantation identical to the implantation into a Mainz pouch I

- Insertion of two ureteral stents, which are led out with the rectal tube after fixation to the bowel mucosa (catgut 5/0)

- Closure of the anterior pouch wall by seromuscular single sutures (polyglyconic acid 4/0)

Postoperative care

- As after the standard procedure

- The ureteral stents are removed starting from day 8

References

1. Abol-Enein H, Ghoneim MA. Optimization of uretero-intestinal anastomosis in urinary diversion: an experimental study in dogs. III. A new antireflux technique for uretero-ileal anastomosis: a serous-linked extramural tunnel. *Urol Res* **21** (1993) 135–9.
2. Abol-Enein H, Ghoneim MA. A novel uretero-ileal reimplantation technique: the serous lined extramural tunnel. A preliminary report. *J Urol* **151** (1995) 1193–7.

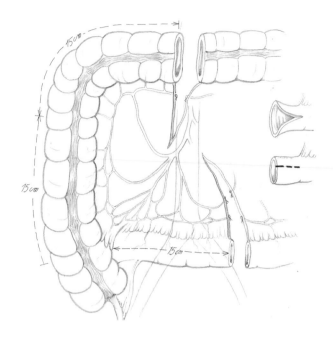

Figure 1. *Segment to be isolated: two colonic segments (cecum and ascending colon) of 10–15 cm length and only one ileal loop of equal length; fishmouth-like incision of the ileal margin for the following ileoascendostomy.*

Figure 2. *Appendix stoma according to the standard technique.*

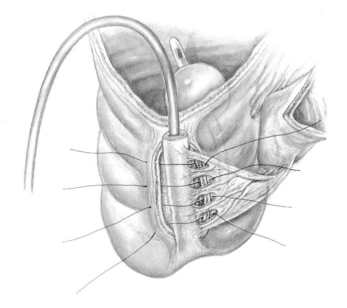

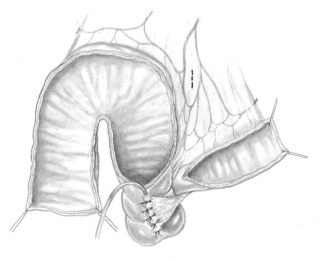

Figure 3. *Antimesenteric opening of the bowel; only the part required for creation of the continence mechanism remains intact. The aboral end of the outlined segment is laid down in an upside-down V. The incision for pull-through of the ureter lies in an area of the mesentery free of vessels.*

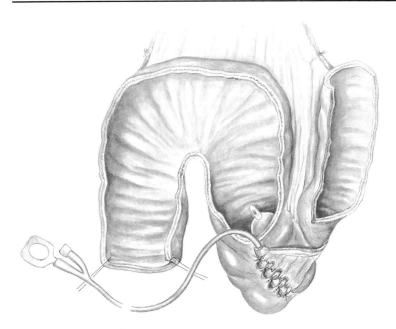

Figure 4. *The ileal loop is rotated upwards.*

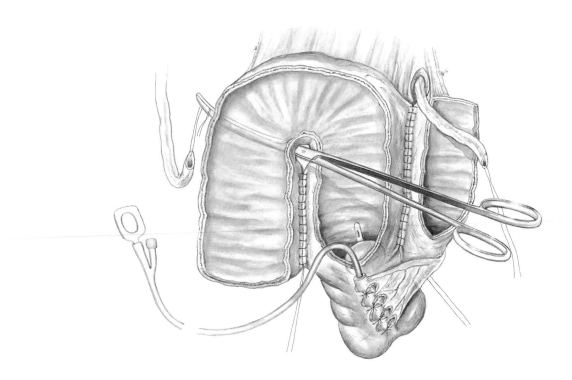

Figure 5. *Serous running suture (of nonabsorbable suture material) close to the mesentery for adaptation of the medial margins of the V, thus creating a serous lined groove. In the edge of the V, space is left for pull-through of the right ureter. Anastomosis of the ileal loop with the colonic part of the pouch by an identical serous running suture close to the mesentery, creating a second groove. The left ureter is pulled through the mesenteric slit.*

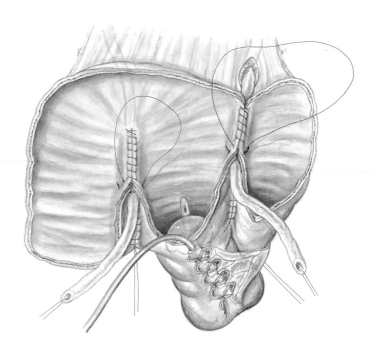

Figure 6. (a) Each ureter is laid down in its trough. The bowel borders are anastomosed over the ureter (using resorbable synthetic suture material 4/0).

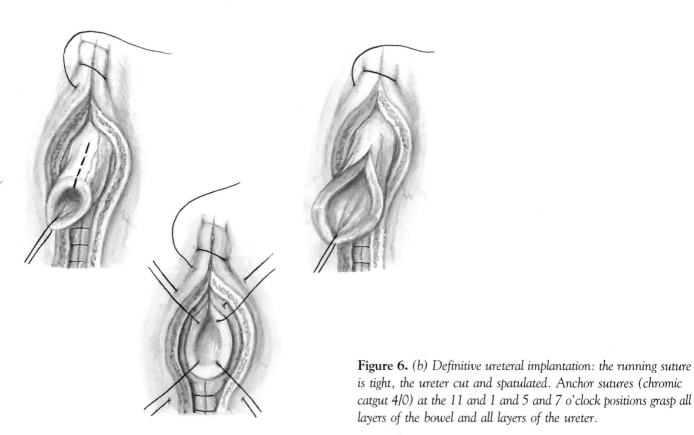

Figure 6. (b) Definitive ureteral implantation: the running suture is tight, the ureter cut and spatulated. Anchor sutures (chromic catgut 4/0) at the 11 and 1 and 5 and 7 o'clock positions grasp all layers of the bowel and all layers of the ureter.

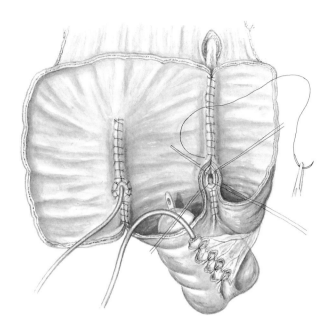

Figure 7. *Completion of ureteral anastomosis by exact mucomucous adaptation (singe stitches of chromic catgut 5/0 or 6/0). The running suture is continued to the end of the antimesenteric incision.*

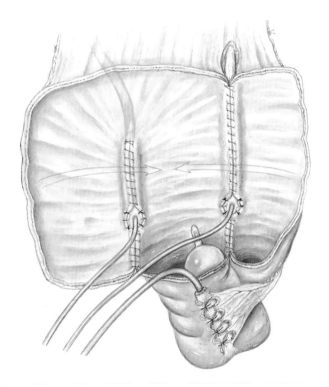

Figure 8. *Implantation of the contralateral ureter in the same manner. The implantations are stented. The pouch is closed horizontally.*

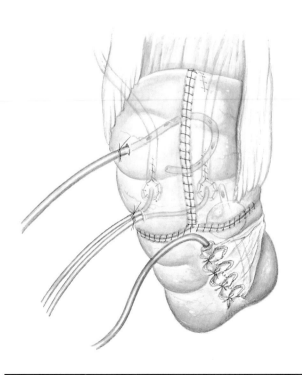

Figure 9. *Completed pouch. The pouchostomy and the ureteral stents are led out separately through the pouch wall.*

Implantation into a sigma-rectum pouch (Mainz-pouch II)

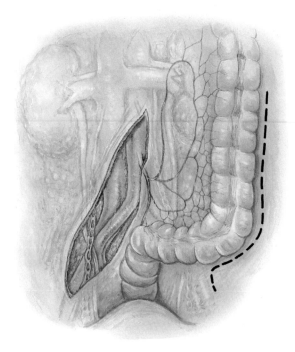

Figure 10. *Right and left paracolic incision; identification of the ureters.*

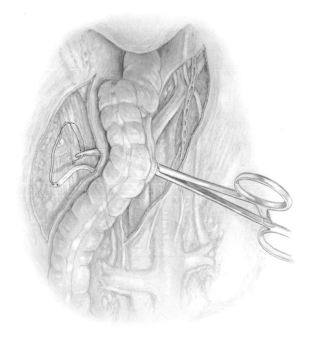

Figure 11. *The ureters are cut and the left is pulled through behind the mesentery to the right side (above the inferior mesenteric artery).*

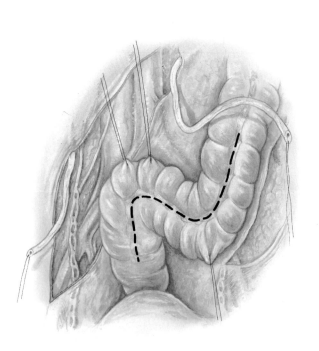

Figure 12. *An S-shaped sigmoid segment of two 10–12 cm sections, starting at the rectosigmoid junction (standard technique), plus an additional 10–12 cm section of the descending colon is marked by stay sutures.*

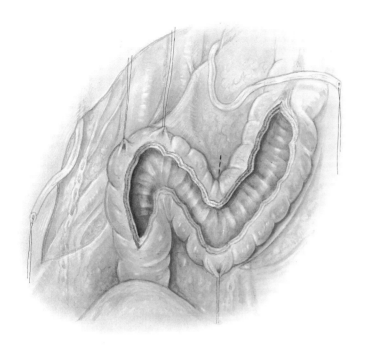

Figure 13. *Antimesenteric opening of the S-shaped segment in the area of the teniae coli. Excision of a mesenteric window to pull the left ureter through.*

Figure 14. *Side-to-side adaptation of the limbs of the S by two serous running sutures close to the mesentery (nonabsorbable suture 4/0), creating two serous-lined grooves. On the right side, an entrance for the right ureter is left at the cranial aspect of the running suture and the ureter is pulled through. The ureters are laid down in their grooves.*

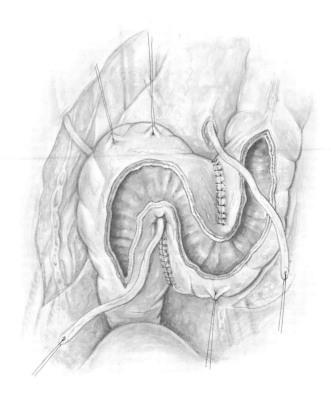

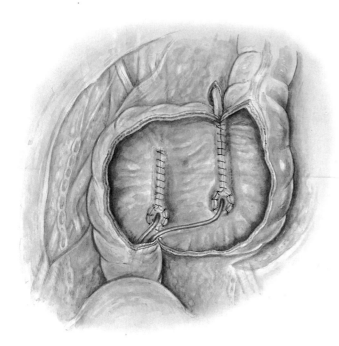

Figure 15. *Definitive ureteral implantation identical to that of the Mainz pouch I technique in its continuous suture line. The anastomosis is secured by ureteral stents.*

Figure 16. *The stents are led out transanally and the pouch is closed with a two-layer running suture or single sutures through all layers, using absorbable synthetic material.*

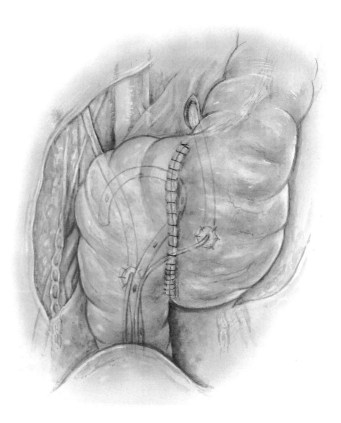

Index